Drugs Used in Psychiatry

This guide contains color reproductions of some commonly prescribed psychotherapeutic drugs. This guide mainly illustrates tablets and capsules. A † symbol preceding the name of a drug indicates that other doses are available. Check directly with the manufacturer. *(Although the photos are intended as accurate reproductions of the drug, this guide should be used only as a quick identification aid.)*

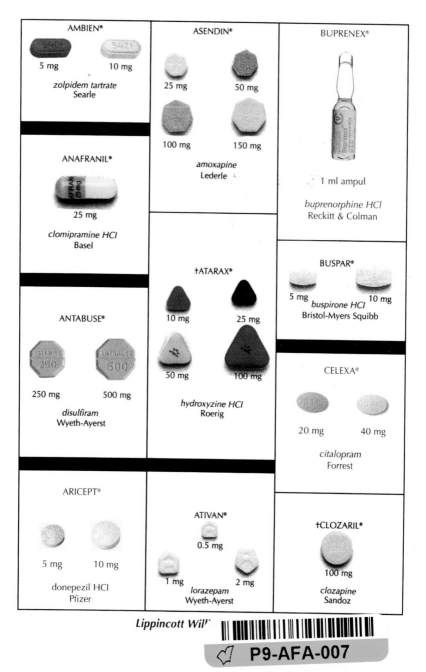

AMBIEN®		ASENDIN®		BUPRENEX®
5 mg	10 mg	25 mg	50 mg	
zolpidem tartrate Searle		100 mg	150 mg	1 ml ampul
		amoxapine Lederle		*buprenorphine HCl* Reckitt & Colman

ANAFRANIL®
25 mg
clomipramine HCl
Basel

†ATARAX®
10 mg   25 mg
50 mg   100 mg
hydroxyzine HCl
Roerig

BUSPAR®
5 mg   10 mg
buspirone HCl
Bristol-Myers Squibb

ANTABUSE®
250 mg   500 mg
disulfiram
Wyeth-Ayerst

CELEXA®
20 mg   40 mg
citalopram
Forrest

ARICEPT®
5 mg   10 mg
donepezil HCl
Pfizer

ATIVAN®
0.5 mg
1 mg   2 mg
lorazepam
Wyeth-Ayerst

†CLOZARIL®
100 mg
clozapine
Sandoz

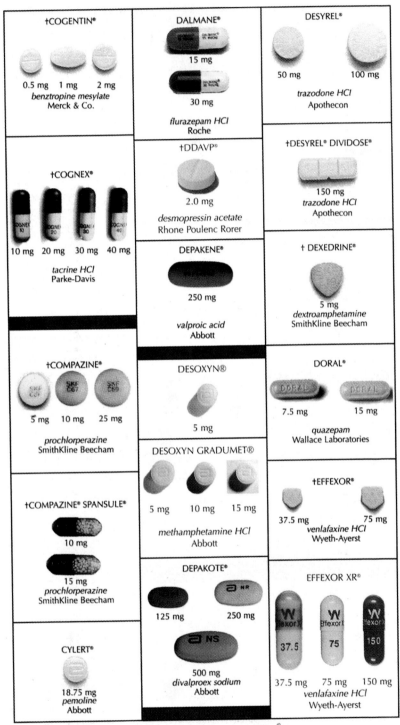

†COGENTIN®

0.5 mg   1 mg   2 mg
benztropine mesylate
Merck & Co.

†COGNEX®

10 mg   20 mg   30 mg   40 mg
tacrine HCl
Parke-Davis

†COMPAZINE®

5 mg   10 mg   25 mg
prochlorperazine
SmithKline Beecham

†COMPAZINE® SPANSULE®

10 mg

15 mg
prochlorperazine
SmithKline Beecham

CYLERT®

18.75 mg
pemoline
Abbott

DALMANE®

15 mg

30 mg

flurazepam HCl
Roche

†DDAVP®

2.0 mg

desmopressin acetate
Rhone Poulenc Rorer

DEPAKENE®

250 mg

valproic acid
Abbott

DESOXYN®

5 mg

DESOXYN GRADUMET®

5 mg   10 mg   15 mg

methamphetamine HCl
Abbott

DEPAKOTE®

125 mg   250 mg

500 mg
divalproex sodium
Abbott

DESYREL®

50 mg   100 mg

trazodone HCl
Apothecon

†DESYREL® DIVIDOSE®

150 mg
trazodone HCl
Apothecon

† DEXEDRINE®

5 mg
dextroamphetamine
SmithKline Beecham

DORAL®

7.5 mg   15 mg

quazepam
Wallace Laboratories

†EFFEXOR®

37.5 mg   75 mg
venlafaxine HCl
Wyeth-Ayerst

EFFEXOR XR®

37.5 mg   75 mg   150 mg
venlafaxine HCl
Wyeth-Ayerst

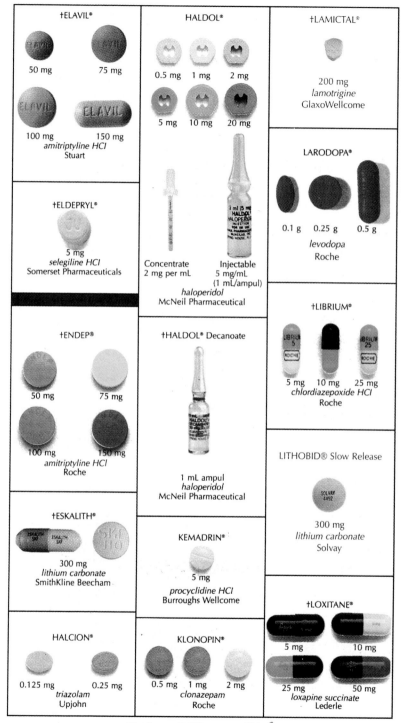

†ELAVIL®

50 mg
75 mg
100 mg
150 mg
amitriptyline HCl
Stuart

†ELDEPRYL®

5 mg
selegiline HCl
Somerset Pharmaceuticals

†ENDEP®

50 mg
75 mg
100 mg
150 mg
amitriptyline HCl
Roche

†ESKALITH®

300 mg
lithium carbonate
SmithKline Beecham

HALCION®

0.125 mg
0.25 mg
triazolam
Upjohn

HALDOL®

0.5 mg
1 mg
2 mg
5 mg
10 mg
20 mg

Concentrate
2 mg per mL

Injectable
5 mg/mL
(1 mL/ampul)
haloperidol
McNeil Pharmaceutical

†HALDOL® Decanoate

1 mL ampul
haloperidol
McNeil Pharmaceutical

KEMADRIN®

5 mg
procyclidine HCl
Burroughs Wellcome

KLONOPIN®

0.5 mg
1 mg
2 mg
clonazepam
Roche

†LAMICTAL®

200 mg
lamotrigine
GlaxoWellcome

LARODOPA®

0.1 g
0.25 g
0.5 g
levodopa
Roche

†LIBRIUM®

5 mg
10 mg
25 mg
chlordiazepoxide HCl
Roche

LITHOBID® Slow Release

300 mg
lithium carbonate
Solvay

†LOXITANE®

5 mg
10 mg
25 mg
50 mg
loxapine succinate
Lederle

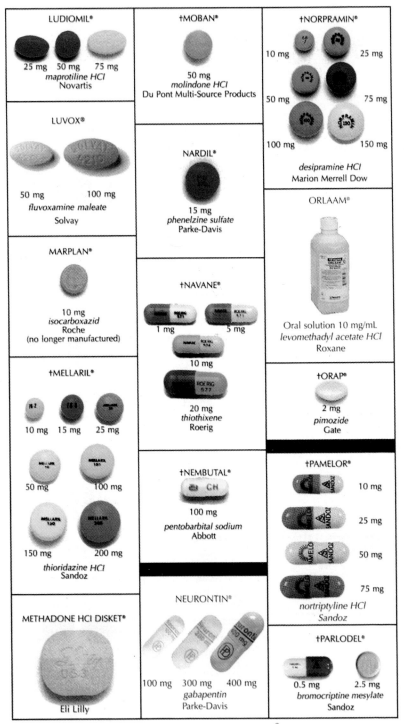

LUDIOMIL®

25 mg 50 mg 75 mg
maprotiline HCl
Novartis

LUVOX®

50 mg 100 mg
fluvoxamine maleate
Solvay

MARPLAN®

10 mg
isocarboxazid
Roche
(no longer manufactured)

†MELLARIL®

10 mg 15 mg 25 mg

50 mg 100 mg

150 mg 200 mg

thioridazine HCl
Sandoz

METHADONE HCl DISKET®

Eli Lilly

†MOBAN®

50 mg
molindone HCl
Du Pont Multi-Source Products

NARDIL®

15 mg
phenelzine sulfate
Parke-Davis

†NAVANE®

1 mg 5 mg

10 mg

20 mg
thiothixene
Roerig

†NEMBUTAL®

100 mg
pentobarbital sodium
Abbott

NEURONTIN®

100 mg 300 mg 400 mg
gabapentin
Parke-Davis

†NORPRAMIN®

10 mg 25 mg

50 mg 75 mg

100 mg 150 mg

desipramine HCl
Marion Merrell Dow

ORLAAM®

Oral solution 10 mg/mL
levomethadyl acetate HCl
Roxane

†ORAP®

2 mg
pimozide
Gate

†PAMELOR®

10 mg

25 mg

50 mg

75 mg

nortriptyline HCl
Sandoz

†PARLODEL®

0.5 mg 2.5 mg
bromocriptine mesylate
Sandoz

Lippincott Williams & Wilkins©

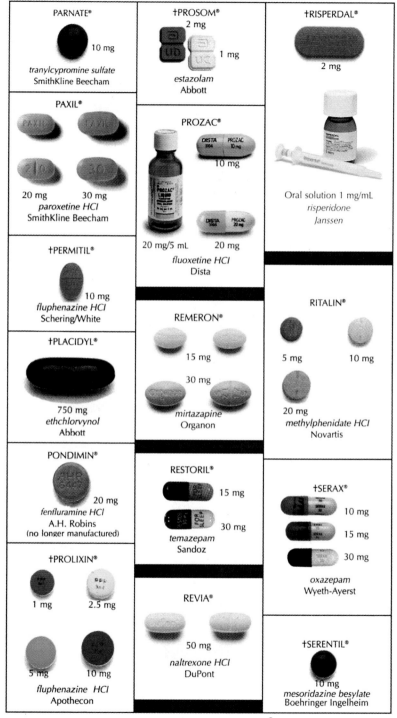

PARNATE®
10 mg
tranylcypromine sulfate
SmithKline Beecham

PAXIL®
PAXIL · PAXIL
20 mg · 30 mg
paroxetine HCl
SmithKline Beecham

†PERMITIL®
10 mg
fluphenazine HCl
Schering/White

†PLACIDYL®
750 mg
ethchlorvynol
Abbott

PONDIMIN®
20 mg
fenfluramine HCl
A.H. Robins
(no longer manufactured)

†PROLIXIN®
1 mg · 2.5 mg
5 mg · 10 mg
fluphenazine HCl
Apothecon

†PROSOM®
2 mg
1 mg
estazolam
Abbott

PROZAC®
10 mg
20 mg/5 mL · 20 mg
fluoxetine HCl
Dista

REMERON®
15 mg
30 mg
mirtazapine
Organon

RESTORIL®
15 mg
30 mg
temazepam
Sandoz

REVIA®
50 mg
naltrexone HCl
DuPont

†RISPERDAL®
2 mg
Oral solution 1 mg/mL
risperidone
Janssen

RITALIN®
5 mg · 10 mg
20 mg
methylphenidate HCl
Novartis

†SERAX®
10 mg
15 mg
30 mg
oxazepam
Wyeth-Ayerst

†SERENTIL®
10 mg
mesoridazine besylate
Boehringer Ingelheim

Lippincott Williams & Wilkins©

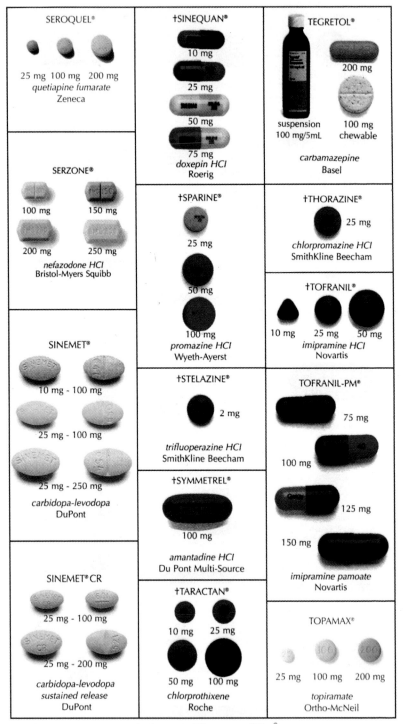

SEROQUEL®

25 mg   100 mg   200 mg
quetiapine fumarate
Zeneca

SERZONE®

100 mg   150 mg

200 mg   250 mg
nefazodone HCl
Bristol-Myers Squibb

SINEMET®

10 mg - 100 mg

25 mg - 100 mg

25 mg - 250 mg

carbidopa-levodopa
DuPont

SINEMET® CR

25 mg - 100 mg

25 mg - 200 mg

carbidopa-levodopa
sustained release
DuPont

†SINEQUAN®

10 mg

25 mg

50 mg

75 mg
doxepin HCl
Roerig

†SPARINE®

25 mg

50 mg

100 mg
promazine HCl
Wyeth-Ayerst

†STELAZINE®

2 mg

trifluoperazine HCl
SmithKline Beecham

†SYMMETREL®

100 mg

amantadine HCl
Du Pont Multi-Source

†TARACTAN®

10 mg   25 mg

50 mg   100 mg
chlorprothixene
Roche

TEGRETOL®

200 mg

suspension   100 mg
100 mg/5mL   chewable

carbamazepine
Basel

†THORAZINE®

25 mg

chlorpromazine HCl
SmithKline Beecham

†TOFRANIL®

10 mg   25 mg   50 mg
imipramine HCl
Novartis

TOFRANIL-PM®

75 mg

100 mg

125 mg

150 mg

imipramine pamoate
Novartis

TOPAMAX®

25 mg   100 mg   200 mg

topiramate
Ortho-McNeil

Lippincott Williams & Wilkins©

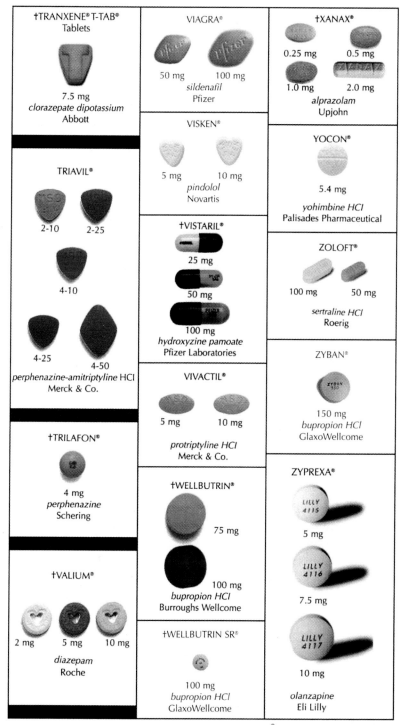

†TRANXENE® T-TAB®
Tablets

7.5 mg
clorazepate dipotassium
Abbott

TRIAVIL®

2-10   2-25

4-10

4-25   4-50
perphenazine-amitriptyline HCl
Merck & Co.

†TRILAFON®

4 mg
perphenazine
Schering

†VALIUM®

2 mg   5 mg   10 mg

diazepam
Roche

VIAGRA®

50 mg   100 mg
sildenafil
Pfizer

VISKEN®

5 mg   10 mg
pindolol
Novartis

†VISTARIL®

25 mg

50 mg

100 mg
hydroxyzine pamoate
Pfizer Laboratories

VIVACTIL®

5 mg   10 mg

protriptyline HCl
Merck & Co.

†WELLBUTRIN®

75 mg

100 mg
bupropion HCl
Burroughs Wellcome

†WELLBUTRIN SR®

100 mg
bupropion HCl
GlaxoWellcome

†XANAX®

0.25 mg   0.5 mg

1.0 mg   2.0 mg
alprazolam
Upjohn

YOCON®

5.4 mg

yohimbine HCl
Palisades Pharmaceutical

ZOLOFT®

100 mg   50 mg

sertraline HCl
Roerig

ZYBAN®

150 mg
bupropion HCl
GlaxoWellcome

ZYPREXA®

5 mg

7.5 mg

10 mg

olanzapine
Eli Lilly

Lippincott Williams & Wilkins©

KAPLAN & SADOCK'S POCKET HANDBOOK OF PSYCHIATRIC DRUG TREATMENT

Third Edition

Senior Consulting Editor

ROBERT CANCRO, M.D., MED. D.SC.
Lucius N. Littauer Professor and Chairman, Department of Psychiatry,
New York University School of Medicine,
New York, New York;
Director, Department of Psychiatry, Tisch Hospital,
New York, New York;
Director, Nathan S. Kline Institute for Psychiatric Research,
Orangeburg, New York

Contributing Editors

JAMES C. EDMONDSON, M.D., Ph.D.
Clinical Assistant Professor of Neurology,
State University of New York at Brooklyn College of Medicine;
Assistant Attending Physician, Department of Neurology,
Long Island College Hospital,
Brooklyn, New York

NORMAN SUSSMAN, M.D.
Clinical Professor of Psychiatry,
New York University School of Medicine;
Director, Psychopharmacology Research and Consultation Service,
Bellevue Hospital Center,
New York, New York

Collaborating Authors

Joseph Belanoff, M.D.
Assistant Professor of Clinical Psychiatry,
Stanford University School of Medicine,
Stanford, California

Marianne Guschwan, M.D.
Clinical Assistant Professor of Psychiatry,
New York University Medical Center,
New York, New York

Eugene Rubin, M.D.
Assistant Professor of Clinical Psychiatry,
Wayne State University School of Medicine,
Detroit, Michigan

KAPLAN & SADOCK'S POCKET HANDBOOK OF PSYCHIATRIC DRUG TREATMENT

Third Edition

BENJAMIN J. SADOCK, M.D.

Menas S. Gregory Professor of Psychiatry and Vice Chairman,
Department of Psychiatry, New York University School of Medicine;
Attending Psychiatrist, Tisch Hospital;
Attending Psychiatrist, Bellevue Hospital Center;
Consultant Psychiatrist, Lenox Hill Hospital,
New York, New York

VIRGINIA A. SADOCK, M.D.

Clinical Professor of Psychiatry, Department of Psychiatry,
New York University School of Medicine;
Attending Psychiatrist, Tisch Hospital;
Attending Psychiatrist, Bellevue Hospital Center,
New York, New York

 LIPPINCOTT WILLIAMS & WILKINS
A **Wolters Kluwer** Company
Philadelphia · Baltimore · New York · London
Buenos Aires · Hong Kong · Sydney · Tokyo

Acquisitions Editor: Charles W. Mitchell
Developmental Editor: Lisa R. Kairis
Production Editor: Melanie Bennitt
Manufacturing Manager: Benjamin Rivera
Cover Designer: Christine Jenny
Compositor: Maryland Composition
Printer: R.R. Donnelly-Crawfordsville
Project Editor (New York): Justin A. Hollingsworth

© **2001 by LIPPINCOTT WILLIAMS & WILKINS**
530 Walnut Street
Philadelphia, PA 19106 USA
LWW.com

"Kaplan Sadock Psychiatry" with the pyramid logo is a trademark of Lippincott Williams & Wilkins.

Notice. The indications and dosages of all drugs in this book have been recommended in the medical literature and conform to the practices of the general medical community. The medications described do not necessarily have specific approval by the Food and Drug Administration (FDA) for use in the diseases and dosages for which they are recommended. The package insert for each drug should be consulted for use and dosage as approved by the FDA. Because standards for usage change, it is advisable to keep abreast of revised recommendations, particularly those concerning new drugs.

Printed in the USA

First Edition 1993
Second Edition 1996

Library of Congress Cataloging-in-Publication Data

Sadock, Benjamin J.
    Kaplan & Sadock's pocket handbook of psychiatric drug treatment / Benjamin J. Sadock, Virginia A. Sadock.—3rd ed.
    p. ; cm.
    Rev. ed. of: Pocket handbook of psychiatric drug treatment / Harold I. Kaplan, Benjamin J. Sadock, 2nd ed. c1996
    Includes bibliographical references and index.
    ISBN 0-7817-2531-3
    1. Psychopharmacology—Handbooks, manuals, etc. 2. Psychotropic drugs—Handbooks, manuals, etc. I. Title: Kaplan and Sadock's pocket handbook of psychiatric drug treatment. II. Title: Pocket handbook of psychiatric drug treatment. III. Title: Psychiatric drug treatment. IV. Sadock, Virginia A. V. Kaplan, Harold I., 1927–1998, Pocket handbook of psychiatric drug treatment. VI. Title.
    [DNLM: 1. Mental Disorders—drug therapy—Handbooks. 2. Psychotropic Drugs—therapeutic use—Handbooks. WM 34 S126k 2000]
    RC483 .K35 2000
    616.89'18—dc21   00-033095

10 9 8 7 6 5 4 3 2 1

*Dedicated
to our
Parents*

About the Authors

BENJAMIN J. SADOCK, M.D.

Benjamin James Sadock, M.D., is the Menas S. Gregory Professor of Psychiatry and Vice Chairman of the Department of Psychiatry at the New York University (NYU) School of Medicine. He was graduated from Union College, received his Doctor of Medicine degree from New York Medical College, and did his internship at Albany Hospital. He completed his residency at Bellevue Psychiatric Hospital and then entered military service where he served as acting chief of neuropsychiatry at Sheppard Air Force Base, Texas. He has held faculty and teaching appointments at Southwestern Medical School and Parkland Hospital in Dallas, and at New York Medical College, St. Luke's Hospital, New York State Psychiatric Institute, and Metropolitan Hospital in New York City. He joined the faculty of the NYU School of Medicine in 1980 and served in various positions: director of medical student education in psychiatry, co-director of the Residency Training Program in Psychiatry, and director of Graduate Medical Education.

Dr. Sadock is currently director of Student Mental Health Services, psychiatric consultant to the Admissions Committee, and co-director of Continuing Education in Psychiatry at the NYU School of Medicine. He is attending psychiatrist at Bellevue Hospital and Tisch Hospital and is consultant psychiatrist at Lenox Hill Hospital. Dr. Sadock is a diplomate of the American Board of Psychiatry and Neurology and served as an assistant and associate examiner for the board for over a decade. He is a Fellow of the American Psychiatric Association, a Fellow of the American College of Physicians, a Fellow of the New York Academy of Medicine, and a member of Alpha Omega Alpha Honor Society. He is active in numerous psychiatric organizations and is president and founder of the NYU-Bellevue Psychiatric Society.

Dr. Sadock was a member of the National Committee in Continuing Education in Psychiatry of the American Psychiatric Association, served on the Ad Hoc Committee on Sex Therapy Clinics of the American Medical Association, was delegate to the Conference on Recertification of the American Board of Medical Specialists, and was a representative of the American Psychiatric Association's Task Force on the National Board of Medical Examiners and the American Board of Psychiatry and Neurology. In 1985 he received the Academic Achievement Award from New York Medical College and in 2000 he was appointed Faculty Scholar at NYU School of Medicine. He is both author and editor of over 100 publications, a book reviewer for psychiatric journals, and lectures on a broad range of topics in general psychiatry.

Dr. Sadock maintains a private practice for diagnostic consultations, psychotherapy, and pharmacotherapy. He has been married to Virginia Alcott Sadock, M.D., clinical professor of psychiatry at NYU School of Medicine, since completing his residency. Dr. Sadock enjoys opera, skiing, and traveling, and is an avid fly-fisherman.

Virginia A. Sadock, M.D.

Virginia Alcott Sadock, M.D., is a member of the faculty of the New York University (NYU) School of Medicine, where she is clinical professor of psychiatry and attending psychiatrist at Tisch Hospital and Bellevue Hospital. She is director of the Program in Human Sexuality and Sex Therapy at the NYU Medical Center, one of the largest treatment and training programs of its kind in the United States.

She is the author of over 50 articles and chapters on sexual behavior, including the effects of drugs on sexual function, and was the developmental editor of *The Sexual Experience*, published by Williams & Wilkins—one of the first major textbooks on human sexuality. She serves as referee and book reviewer for several medical journals including the *American Journal of Psychiatry* and the *Journal of the American Medical Association*.

She has had a long-standing interest in the role of women in medicine and psychiatry and was a founder of the Committee on Women in Psychiatry of the New York County District Branch of the American Psychiatric Association. She is active in academic matters, has served as an assistant and associate examiner for the American Board of Psychiatry and Neurology for over 15 years, and was also a member of the test committee in psychiatry for both the American Board of Psychiatry and the Psychiatric Knowledge and Self-Assessment Program (PKSAP) of the American Psychiatric Association. She served as chairperson of the Committee on Public Relations, New York County District Branch of the American Psychiatric Association, and also participated in the National Medical Television Network series *Women in Medicine* and the Emmy Award winning PBS television documentary *Women and Depression*. She has been vice-president of the Society of Sex Therapy and Research, a regional council member of the American Association of Sex Education Counselors and Therapists, and is president of the Alumni Association of Sex Therapists. She lectures extensively both in the United States and abroad on sexual dysfunction, relational problems, and depression and anxiety disorders.

She is a Fellow of the American Psychiatric Association, a Fellow of the New York Academy of Medicine, and a diplomate of the American Board of Psychiatry and Neurology. Dr. Sadock was graduated from Bennington College, received her M.D. from New York Medical College, and trained in psychiatry at Metropolitan Hospital. She lives in Manhattan with her husband, Dr. Benjamin Sadock, where she maintains an active psychiatric practice that includes individual psychotherapy, couples and marital therapy, sex therapy, psychiatric consultation, and pharmacotherapy. They have two children, James and Victoria, both physicians in emergency medicine. In her leisure time, Dr. Sadock enjoys theater, film, reading fiction, and travel.

Preface

This is the third edition of *Kaplan and Sadock's Pocket Handbook of Psychiatric Drug Treatment*, which covers the entire spectrum of drug therapy as used in the everyday practice of psychiatry. Every section was updated and revised. New sections were added and all of the latest drugs included.

It is written for psychiatrists, psychiatric residents, and medical students who require up-to-date information about the use of drugs in the treatment of psychiatric disorders in both adults and children.

Nonpsychiatric physicians, especially primary care specialists who prescribe psychotropic medications, will also find this book valuable. Other mental health professionals including nurses, psychologists, and social workers, can use the book to provide them with information about the psychiatric drugs prescribed for their patients or clients.

How To Use This Book

Following the Contents, the reader will find a shaded chart of drugs (Table A) and the chapter where each drug is discussed. In addition, Table B lists the various medications used to treat a particular psychiatric disorder. It is completely up to date.

Drugs are listed alphabetically and each section provides a wealth of data that includes (1) the drug's name and molecular structure; (2) preparation and dosages; (3) pharmacological actions including its pharmacokinetics and pharmacodynamics; (4) the indications for use and clinical applications; (5) use in children, elderly persons, and pregnant and nursing women; (6) side effects and adverse and allergic reactions; and (7) drug-drug interactions.

Illustrated Drug Identification Guide

A unique aspect of this and other *Kaplan & Sadock* books are the colored plates of major drugs used in psychiatry, the forms in which they are commercially available, and their dose ranges to help the physician recognize and prescribe the medications. The plates also have been useful in helping patients identify, to their physicians and therapists, medications that they are taking.

Laboratory Tests

A special section on laboratory tests is included to aid the clinician in understanding the relation of psychopharmacologic agents and their effects on laboratory values, and in monitoring baseline values necessary for effective drug treatment.

Toxicity

We include a special section in tabular form (Chapter 43) that lists the toxic and lethal doses of each drug, the signs and symptoms of overdose, and emergency management measures.

References

Each chapter ends with a reference to the seventh edition of *Kaplan and Sadock's Comprehensive Textbook of Psychiatry*, for the reader who requires further information about the particular drug. The *Pocket Handbook* cannot substitute for a major textbook of psychiatry, such as *Kaplan and Sadock's Comprehensive Textbook of Psychiatry* or its companion, *Kaplan and Sadock's Synopsis of Psychiatry*. The purpose of the *Pocket Handbook* is to serve as an easily-accessible reference for busy doctors-in-training or clinical practitioners.

Classification

We classify drugs according to their pharmacological activity and mechanism of action. We introduced this approach to replace the categories of antidepressants, antimanics, antipsychotics, anxiolytics, and mood stabilizers, which are broad terms that do not accurately reflect the clinical use of psychotropics. For example, many of the so-called antidepressant drugs are used to treat anxiety disorders; some anxiolytics are used to treat psychosis, depression, and bipolar disorders; and drugs for all categories are used to treat other clinical disorders, such as eating disorders, panic disorders, and impulse-control disorders. Finally, such drugs as clonidine (Catapres), propranolol (Inderal), and verapamil (Isoptin) can effectively treat a variety of psychiatric disorders but do not fit into any broad classification of drugs. This classification follows that used in major textbooks of pharmacology and is equally applicable to psychopharmacology.

ACKNOWLEDGMENTS

We thank our two contributing editors, James Edmondson, M.D., and Norman Sussman, M.D., for their extraordinary help. Together, these distinguished physicians insured that the material about the pharmacologic actions and clinical applications of each drug was thoroughly and completely up-to-date. Dr. Edmondson is a highly skilled clinical neurologist with expertise in drugs that affect the nervous system, which by definition includes psychotropic medication. Dr. Sussman directs the psychopharmalogic consultation service at Bellevue Hospital Center and has vast clinical experience and breadth of knowledge in this specialized and complex area of psychiatry.

We also thank our collaborating authors for their assistance. Marianne Gushwan, M.D., Clinical Assistant Professor of Psychiatry at NYU Medical Center, assisted in the area of opioids and naltrexone; Joseph Belanoff, M.D., Assistant Professor of Clinical Psychiatry at Stanford University School of Medicine, assisted in the area of lithium and tricyclic and tetracyclic drugs; and Eugene Rubin, M.D., Assistant Professor of Clinical Psychiatry at Wayne State University School of Medicine, assisted in the area of biological psychiatry.

Justin Hollingsworth served as project editor, as he has for many of our other publications and for which we are deeply appreciative. He carries out his complex tasks with skill and enthusiasm. Linda Kenevich processed the manuscripts, and we thank her for her prodigious efforts. We also thank Margaret Cuzzolino, Yande McMillan,

Henna Ahmad, M.D., and Eileen Lee, M.D., for their valuable assistance in this project.

We especially thank Victoria Sadock, M.D., and James Sadock, M.D., for their help in the area of emergency management of drug reactions and overdose.

The authors also acknowledge Jack Grebb, M.D., coauthor of the seventh edition of *Kaplan and Sadock's Synopsis of Psychiatry* and contributing editor of the seventh edition of *Kaplan and Sadock's Comprehensive Textbook of Psychiatry*, for his helpful advice.

Finally, we thank Robert Cancro, M.D., Professor and Chairman of the Department of Psychiatry at New York University Medical Center, who served as Senior Consulting Editor. He is an outstanding researcher, clinician, and educator, and we are deeply grateful for his encouragement and support over the years.

Benjamin J. Sadock, M.D.
Virginia A. Sadock, M.D.

June 26, 2000
New York University
New York, New York

Contents

Generic Name	Brand Name	Section Title	Chapter Number
Acebutolol	Sectral	β-Adrenergic Receptor Antagonists	3
Acetophenazine[a]	Tindal	Dopamine Receptor Antagonists	18
Alprazolam	Xanax	Benzodiazepines	8
Amantadine	Symmetrel	Amantadine	4
Amitriptyline	Elavil, Endep	Tricyclics and Tetracyclics	35
Amlodipine	Lotrel, Norvasc	Calcium Channel Inhibitors	11
Amobarbital	Amytal	Barbiturates and Similarly Acting Substances	7
Amoxapine	Asendin	Tricyclics and Tetracyclics	35
Amphetamine	—	Sympathomimetics and Related Drugs	32
Apomorphine[b]	Uprima	Dopamine Receptor Agonists	17
Aprobarbital	Alurate	Barbiturates and Similarly Acting Substances	7
Atenolol	Tenormin	β-Adrenergic Receptor Antagonists	3
Befloxatone[b]	—	Monoamine Oxidase Inhibitors	21
Benzphetamine	Didrex	Sympathomimetics and Related Drugs	32
Benztropine	Cogentin	Anticholinergics	5
Biperiden	Akineton	Anticholinergics	5
Bromocriptine	Parlodel	Dopamine Receptor Agonists	17
Buprenorphine	Buprenex	Opioid Receptor Agonists	24
Bupropion	Wellbutrin, Zyban	Bupropion	9
Buspirone	BuSpar	Buspirone	10
Butabarbital	Butisol	Barbiturates and Similarly Acting Substances	7
Butalbital	—	Barbiturates and Similarly Acting Substances	7
Butaperazine[b]	Repoise	Dopamine Receptor Antagonists	18
Carbamazepine	Tegretol	Carbamazepine	12
Carbidopa	Lodosyn	Dopamine Receptor Agonists	17
Carphenazine[b]	Proketazine	Dopamine Receptor Antagonists	18
Chloral hydrate	—	Chloral Hydrate	13
Chlorpromazine	Thorazine	Dopamine Receptor Antagonists	18
Chlorprothixene[a]	Taractan	Dopamine Receptor Antagonists	18
Citalopram	Celexa	Selective Serotonin Reuptake Inhibitors	28
Clomipramine	Anafranil	Tricyclics and Tetracyclics	35
Clonazepam	Klonopin	Benzodiazepines	8
Clonidine	Catapres	α_2-Adrenergic Receptor Agonists	2
Clozapine	Clozaril	Serotonin-Dopamine Antagonists	29
Cyproheptadine	Periactin	Antihistamines	6
Dantrolene	Dantrium	Dantrolene	15
Desipramine	Norpramin, Pertofane	Tricyclics and Tetracyclics	35
Dextroamphetamine	Dexedrine	Sympathomimetics and Related Drugs	32
Diazepam	Valium	Benzodiazepines	8
Diethylpropion	Tenuate	Sympathomimetics and Related Drugs	32
Disulfiram	Antabuse	Disulfiram	16
Diphenhydramine	Benadryl	Antihistamines	6
Divalproex	Depakote	Valproate	36
Donepezil	Aricept	Cholinesterase Inhibitors	14
Doxepin	Adapin, Sinequan	Tricyclics and Tetracyclics	35
Droperidol	Inapsine	Dopamine Receptor Antagonists	18
Estazolam	ProSom	Benzodiazepines	8
Ethopropazine	Parsidol	Anticholinergics	5

continues

TABLE A *continued*

Generic Name	Brand Name	Section Title	Chapter Number
Ethchlorvynol	Placidyl	Barbiturates and Similarly Acting Substances	7
Flumazenil	Romazicon	Benzodiazepines	8
Fluoxetine	Prozac, Sarafem	Selective Serotonin Reuptake Inhibitors	28
Fluphenazine	Prolixin, Permitil	Dopamine Receptor Antagonists	18
Flurazepam	Dalmane	Benzodiazepines	8
Fluvoxamine	Luvox	Selective Serotonin Reuptake Inhibitors	28
Gabapentin	Neurontin	Other Anticonvulsants	26
Galanthamine	Reminyl	Cholinesterase Inhibitors	14
Glutethimide	Doriden	Barbiturates and Similarly Acting Substance	7
Guanfacine	Tenex	α_2-Adrenergic Receptor Agonists	2
Halazepam	Paxipam	Benzodiazepines	8
Haloperidol	Haldol	Dopamine Receptor Antagonists	18
Hydroxyzine	Atarax, Vistaril	Antihistamines	6
Imipramine	Tofranil	Tricyclics and Tetracyclics	35
Isocarboxazid	Marplan	Monoamine Oxidase Inhibitors	21
Isradipine	DynaCirc	Calcium Channel Inhibitors	11
Labetalol	Normodyne, Trandate	β-Adrenergic Receptor Antagonists	3
Lamotrigine	Lamictal	Other Anticonvulsants	26
Levodopa	Larodopa	Dopamine Receptor Agonists	17
Levomethadyl	ORLAAM	Opioid Receptor Agonists	24
Levothyroxine	Levoxine, Levothroid, Synthroid	Thyroid Hormones	33
Liothyronine	Cytomel	Thyroid Hormones	33
Lithium	Eskalith, Lithobid, Lithonate	Lithium	19
Lorazepam	Ativan	Benzodiazepines	8
Loxapine	Loxitane	Dopamine Receptor Antagonists	18
Mazindol	Mazanor, Sanorex	Sympathomimetics and Related Drugs	32
Mephobarbital	Mebaral	Barbiturates and Similarly Acting Substances	7
Meprobamate	Miltown	Barbiturates and Similarly Acting Substances	7
Mesoridazine	Serentil	Dopamine Receptor Antagonists	18
Methadone	Dolophine, Methadose	Opioid Receptor Antagonists	24
Methamphetamine	Desoxyn	Sympathomimetics and Related Drugs	32
Methohexital	Brevital	Barbituates and Similarly Acting Substances	7
Methylphenidate	Ritalin	Sympathomimetics and Related Drugs	32
Metoprolol	Lopressor, Toprol	β-Adrenergic Receptor Antagonists	3
Midazolam	Versed	Benzodiazepine Receptor Agonists	8
Mirtazapine	Remeron	Mirtazapine	20
Moclobemide	Manerix[a]	Monoamine Oxidase Inhibitors	21
Modafinil	Provigil	Sympathomimetics and Related Drugs	32
Molindone	Moban	Dopamine Receptor Antagonists	18
Nadolol	Corgard	β-Adrenergic Receptor Antagonists	3
Nalmefene	Revex	Naltrexone	22
Naltrexone	ReVia	Naltrexone	22
Nefazodone	Serzone	Nefazodone	23
Nifedipine	Adalat, Procardia	Calcium Channel Inhibitors	11
Nimodipine	Nimotop	Calcium Channel Inhibitors	11
Nortriptyline	Pamelor, Aventyl	Tricyclics and Tetracyclics	35
Olanzapine	Zyprexa	Serotonin Dopamine Antagonists	29
Orlistat	Xenical	Orlistat	25
Orphenadrine	Norflex, Dispal	Anticholinergics	5

continues

TABLE A *continued*

Generic Name	Brand Name	Section Title	Chapter Number
Oxazepam	Serax	Benzodiazepine Receptor Agonists	8
Paraldehyde	—	Barbiturates and Similarly Acting Substances	7
Paroxetine	Paxil	Selective Serotonin Reuptake Inhibitors	28
Pemoline	Cylert	Sympathomimetics and Related Drugs	32
Phenelzine	Nardil	Monoamine Oxidase Inhibitors	21
Pentobarbital	Nembutal	Barbiturates and Similarly Acting Substances	7
Pergolide	Permax	Dopamine Receptor Agonists	17
Perphenazine	Trilafon	Dopamine Receptor Antagonists	18
Phenelzine	Nardil	Monoamine Oxidase Inhibitors	21
Phendimetrazine	Adipost, Bontril	Sympathomimetics and Related Drugs	32
Phenmetrazine	Prelude	Sympathomimetics and Related Drugs	32
Phenobarbital	Solfoton, Luminal	Barbiturates and Similarly Acting Substances	7
Phentermine	Adipex-P, Fastin, Ionamine	Sympathomimetics and Related Drugs	32
Pimozide	Orap	Dopamine Receptor Antagonists	18
Pindolol	Visken	β-Adrenergic Receptor Antagonists	3
Piperacetazine	Quide	Dopamine Receptor Antagonists	18
Pramipexole	Mirapex	Dopamine Receptor Agonists	17
Prazepam	Centrax	Benzodiazepines	8
Prochlorperazine	Compazine	Dopamine Receptor Antagonists	18
Procyclidine	Kemadrin	Anticholinergics	5
Promazine	Sparine	Dopamine Receptor Antagonists	18
Promethazine	Phenergan	Antihistamines	6
Propranolol	Inderal	β-Adrenergic Receptor Antagonists	3
Protriptyline	Vivactil	Tricyclics and Tetracyclics	35
Quazepam	Doral	Benzodiazepines	8
Quetiapine	Seroquel	Serotonin-Dopamine Antagonists	29
Reboxetine	Vestra	Reboxetine	27
Reserpine	Diupres	Dopamine Receptor Antagonists	18
Risperidone	Risperdal	Serotonin-Dopamine Antagonists	29
Rivastigmine	Exelon	Cholinesterase Inhibitors	14
Ropinirole	Requip	Dopamine Receptor Agonists	17
Secobarbital	Seconal	Barbiturates and Similarly Acting Substances	7
Selegiline	Eldepryl	Monoamine Oxidase Inhibitors	21
Sertraline	Zoloft	Selective Serotonin Reuptake Inhibitors	28
Sibutramine	Meridia	Sibutramine	30
Sildenafil	Viagra	Sildenafil	31
Tacrine	Cognex	Cholinesterase Inhibitors	14
Temazepam	Restoril	Benzodiazepines	8
Thiopental	Pentothal	Barbiturates and Similarly Acting Substances	7
Thioridazine	Mellaril	Dopamine Receptor Antagonists	18
Thiothixene	Navane	Dopamine Receptor Antagonists	18
Topiramate	Topamax	Other Anticonvulsants	26
Tranylcypromine	Parnate	Monoamine Oxidase Inhibitors	21
Trazodone	Desyrel	Trazodone	34
Triazolam	Halcion	Benzodiazepines	8
Trihexyphenidyl	Artane	Anticholinergics	5
Trifluoperazine	Stelazine	Dopamine Receptor Antagonists	18
Triflupromazine	Vesprin	Dopamine Receptor Antagonists	18
Trimipramine	Surmontil	Tricyclics and Tetracyclics	35
Valproate	Depakene	Valproate	36
Valproic Acid	Depakene	Valproate	36
Venlafaxine	Effexor	Venlafaxine	37
Verapamil	Calan, Isoptin	Calcium Channel Inhibitors	11
Yohimbine	Yocon	Yohimbine	38
Ziprasidone[b]	Zeldox	Serotonin-Dopamine Antagonists	29
Zaleplon	Sonata	Benzodiazepines	8
Zolpiderm	Ambien	Benzodiazepines	8

[a] No longer manufactured.   [b] Not sold in U.S.

MAJOR MENTAL DISORDERS AND COMMON DRUGS AND CLASSES OF DRUGS USED IN THEIR TREATMENT

Disorder	Chapter Number
Aggression and agitation (see Intermittent explosive disorder)	
Akathisia (see Medication-induced movement disorders)	
Alcohol dependence and withdrawal	
α_2-Adrenergic receptor antagonists	2
β-Adrenergic receptor antagonists	3
Benzodiazepines	8
Carbamazepine	12
Disulfiram	16
Naltrexone	22
Other anticonvulsants (gabapentin)	26
Valproate	36
Anorexia nervosa (see Eating disorders)	
Anxiety (see also specific anxiety disorders)	
Antihistamines	6
Benzodiazepines	8
Buspirone	10
Selective serotonin reuptake inhibitors	28
Tricyclics and tetracyclics	35
Venlafaxine	39
Attention-deficit disorders	
α_2-Adrenergic receptor antagonists	2
Bupropion	9
Buspirone	10
Selective serotonin reuptake inhibitors	28
Sympathomimetics	32
Tricyclics and tetracyclics	35
Benzodiazepine dependence and withdrawal (see Sedative, hypnotic, and anxiolytic dependence and withdrawal)	
Bipolar disorders	
Benzodiazepines (especially clonazepam, lorazepam and alprazolam)	8
Calcium channel inhibitors	11
Dopamine receptor antagonists	18
Other anticonvulsants	26
Lithium	19
Serotonin-dopamine antagonists	29
Valproate	36
Bulimia nervosa (see Easting disorders)	
Cocaine dependence and withdrawal	
Bupropion	9
Other anticonvulsants (gabapentin)	26
Valproate	36
Cyclothymic disorder (see Bipolar disorders)	
Delusional disorder (see Schizophrenia)	
Dementia	
Cholinesterase inhibitors	14
Dopamine receptor antagonists	18
Serotonin-dopamine antagonists	29
Depression	
Benzodiazepines (especially alprazolam)	8
Dopamine receptor agonists (bromocriptine)	17
Bupropion	9
Calcium channel inhibitors	11
Carbamazepine	12
Lithium	19
Mirtazapine	20
Monoamine oxidase inhibitors	21
Nefazodone	23
Reboxetine	27

continues

TABLE B   *continued*

Disorder	Chapter Number
Selective serotonin reuptake inhibitors	28
Sympathomimetics	32
Thyroid hormones	33
Trazodone	34
Tricyclics and tetracyclics	35
Valproate	36
Venlafaxine	39
Dysthymic disorder (see Depression)	
Dystonia (see Medication-induced movement disorders)	
Eating disorders and obesity	
Antihistamines (cyproheptadine)	6
Lithium	19
Monoamine oxidase inhibitors	21
Orlistat	25
Other anticonvulsants (topiramate)	26
Selective serotonin reuptake inhibitors	28
Sibutramine	30
Sympathomimetics	32
Trazodone	34
Tricyclics and tetracyclics	35
Valproate	36
Generalized anxiety disorder	
α_2-Adrenergic receptor antagonists	2
Barbiturates and similarly acting drugs	7
Benzodiazepines	8
Buspirone	10
Nefazodone	23
Selective serotonin reuptake inhibitors	28
Trazodone	34
Tricyclics and tetracyclics	35
Venlafaxine	36
Intermittent explosive disorder	
β-Adrenergic receptor antagonists	3
Carbamazepine	12
Buspirone	10
Calcium channel inhibitors	11
Dopamine receptor antagonists	18
Lithium	19
Other Anticonvulsants	26
Serotonin-dopamine antagonists	29
Valproate	36
Medication-induced movement disorders (see Neuroleptic malignant syndrome)	
β-Adrenergic receptor antagonists	3
Amantadine	4
Anticholinergics	5
Antihistamines	6
Benzodiazepines	8
Dopamine receptor antagonists	17
Other anticonvulsants (gabapentin)	26
Serotonin-dopamine antagonists	29
Neuroleptic malignant syndrome	
Dopamine receptor agonists (bromocriptine)	17
Dantrolene	15
Nicotine dependence and withdrawal	
α_2-Adrenergic receptor antagonists	2
Bupropion	9
Obsessive-compulsive disorder	
α_2-Adrenergic receptor antagonists	2
Selective serotonin reuptake inhibitors	28
Trazodone	34

continues

TABLE B   *continued*

Disorder	Chapter Number
Tricyclics and tetracyclics	35
Valproate	36
Opioid dependence and withdrawal	
α_2-Adrenergic receptor antagonists	2
Naltrexone	22
Opioid receptor agonists	24
Other anticonvulsants (gabapentin)	26
Panic disorder (with or without agoraphobia)	
α_2-Adrenergic receptor antagonists	2
β-Adrenergic receptor antagonists	3
Benzodiazepines (especially alprazolam and clonazepam)	8
Monoamine oxidase inhibitors	21
Nefazodone	23
Other anticonvulsants (gabapentin)	26
Selective serotonin reuptake inhibitors	28
Trazodone	34
Tricyclics and tetracyclics	35
Valproate	36
Parkinsonsim (see Medication-induced movement disorders)	
Phobias (see Panic disorder)	
α_2-Adrenergic receptor antagonists	2
β-Adrenergic receptor antagonists	3
Benzodiazepines	8
Monoamine oxidase inhibitors	21
Other anticonvulsants (gabapentin)	26
Reboxetine	27
Selective serotonin reuptake inhibitors	28
Posttraumatic stress disorder	
α_2-Adrenergic receptor antagonists	2
β-Adrenergic receptor antagonists	3
Antihistamines (cyproheptadine)	6
Benzodiazepines	8
Carbamazepine	12
Monoamine oxidase inhibitors	21
Nefazodone	23
Other anticonvulsants (lamotrigine)	26
Selective serotonin reuptake inhibitors	28
Tricyclics and tetracyclics	35
Valproate	36
Premenstrual dysphoric disorder and premenstrual syndrome	
Buspirone	10
Nefazodone	23
Selective serotonin reuptake inhibitors	28
Psychosis (see Schizophrenia)	
Rabbit syndrome (see Medication-induced movement disorders)	
Schizoaffective disorder (see Depression, Bipolar I disorder, and Schizophrenia)	
Schizophrenia	
Benzodiazepines	8
Carbamazepine	12
Dopamine receptor antagonists	18
Lithium	19
Other anticonvulsants (lamotrigine)	26
Serotonin-dopamine antagonists	29
Sedative, hypnotic, and anxiolytic dependence and withdrawal	
α_2-Adrenergic receptor antagonists	2
Barbiturates and similarly acting drugs	7
Carbamazepine	12
Other anticonvulsants (gabapentin)	26
Valproate	36

continues

TABLE B *continued*

Disorder	Chapter Number
Sexual dysfunctions	
Amantadine	4
Antihistamines (cyproheptadine)	6
Bupropion	9
Buspirone	10
Dopamine receptor agonists	17
Selective serotonin reuptake inhibitors	28
Sildenafil	31
Sympathomimetics	32
Trazodone	34
Tricyclics and tetracyclics (clomipramine)	35
Yohimbine	38
Sleep disorders	
Antihistamines	6
Barbiturates and similarly acting drugs	7
Benzodiazepines	8
Chloral hydrate	13
Sympathomimetics	32
Trazodone	34
Tricyclics and tetracyclics	35
Tourette's and other tic disorders	
α_2-Adrenergic receptor antagonists	2
Calcium channel inhibitors	11
Dopamine receptor antagonists	18
Violence (see Intermittent explosive disorder)	

1

General Principles of Psychopharmacology

The numerous pharmacological agents used to treat psychiatric disorders are referred to by three general terms that are used interchangeably: psychotropic drugs, psychoactive drugs, and psychotherapeutic drugs. Traditionally, those agents were divided into four categories: (1) antipsychotic drugs or neuroleptics used to treat psychosis, (2) antidepressant drugs used to treat depression, (3) antimanic drugs or mood stabilizers used to treat bipolar disorder, and (4) antianxiety drugs or anxiolytics used to treat anxious states (which were also effective as hypnotics in high dosages). That division, however, is less valid now than it was in the past for the following reasons: (1) Many drugs of one class are used to treat disorders previously assigned to another class. For example, many antidepressant drugs are used to treat anxiety disorders; and some antianxiety drugs are used to treat psychoses, depressive disorders, and bipolar disorders. (2) Drugs from all four categories are used to treat disorders not previously treatable by drugs—for example, eating disorders, panic disorder, and impulse-control disorders. (3) Drugs such as clonidine (Catapres), propranolol (Inderal), verapamil (Isoptin, Calan), and gabapentin (Neurontin) can effectively treat a variety of psychiatric disorders and do not fit easily into the traditional classification of drugs. (4) Some descriptive psychopharmacological terms overlap in meaning. For example, anxiolytics decrease anxiety, sedatives produce a calming or relaxing effect, and hypnotics produce sleep. However, most anxiolytics function as sedatives and at high doses can be used as hypnotics, and all hypnotics at low doses can be used for daytime sedation.

For these reasons this book uses a classification in which each drug is discussed according to its pharmacological category. Each drug is described in terms of its pharmacological actions, including pharmacodynamics and pharmacokinetics. Indications, contraindications, drug-drug interactions, and adverse side effects are also discussed.

GUIDE TO USE

Table A (see p. xv) lists the psychotherapeutic drugs according to the generic name, the trade name, and the chapter title and number in which it is discussed. Table B (see p. xviii) lists the major drugs used in the various psychiatric disorders.

PHARMACOLOGICAL ACTIONS

Pharmacological actions are divided into two categories, pharmacokinetic and pharmacodynamic. In simple terms, pharmacokinetics describes *what the body does to the drug*, and pharmacodynamics describes *what the drug does to the body*. Pharmacokinetic data trace the *absorption, distribution, metabolism,* and *excretion* of the drug in the body. Pharmacodynamic data measure the *effects* of the drug on cells in the brain and other tissues of the body.

Pharmacokinetics

Absorption.   Psychotherapeutic drugs reach the brain through the bloodstream. Orally administered drugs dissolve in the fluid of the gastrointestinal (GI) tract, depending on their lipid solubility and the GI tract's local pH, motility, and surface area and are then absorbed into the blood.

Stomach acidity may be reduced by gastric ion pump inhibitors, such as omeprazole (Prilosec) and lansoprazole (Prevacid); by histamine H_2 receptor blockers, such as cimetidine (Tagamet), famotidine (Pepcid), nizatidine (Axid), and ranitidine (Zantac); or by antacids. Gastric and intestinal motility may be either slowed by anticholinergic drugs or increased by dopamine receptor antagonists, such as metoclopramide (Reglan).

Under favorable conditions, parenteral administration can achieve therapeutic plasma concentrations more rapidly than can oral administration. However, if a drug is emulsified in an insoluble carrier matrix, intramuscular administration can sustain the drug's gradual release for several weeks. Such formulations are called *depot* preparations. Intravenous administration is the quickest route for achieving therapeutic blood concentrations, but it also carries the highest risk of sudden and life-threatening adverse effects.

Distribution and Bioavailability.   Drugs that circulate bound to plasma proteins are called *protein bound,* and those that circulate unbound are called *free.* Only the free fraction can pass through the blood–brain barrier.

The *distribution* of a drug to the brain is governed by the brain's regional blood flow, the blood–brain barrier, and the drug's affinity with its receptors in the brain. High cerebral blood flow, high lipid solubility, and high receptor affinity promote the therapeutic actions of the drug.

A drug's *volume of distribution* is a measure of the apparent space in the body available to contain the drug, which can vary with age, sex, adipose tissue content, and disease state.

Bioavailability refers to the fraction of the total amount of administered drug that can subsequently be recovered from the bloodstream. Bioavailability is an important variable, because Food and Drug Administration (FDA) regulations specify that the bioavailability of a generic formulation can differ from that of the brand-name formulation by no more than 30 percent.

Metabolism and Excretion

Metabolic Routes.   The four major metabolic routes for drugs are *oxidation, reduction, hydrolysis,* and *conjugation.* Metabolism usually yields inactive metabolites that are more polar and therefore more readily excreted. However, metabolism also transforms many inactive prodrugs into therapeutically active metabolites.

The liver is the principal site of *metabolism,* and bile, feces, and urine are the major routes of *excretion.* Psychotherapeutic drugs are also excreted in sweat, saliva, tears, and breast milk.

Quantitation of Metabolism and Excretion. Four important quantities regarding metabolism and excretion are time of *peak plasma concentration, half-life, first-pass effect,* and *clearance.*

The time between the administration of a drug and the appearance of *peak plasma concentrations* varies according to the route of administration and rate of absorption.

A drug's *half-life* is the amount of time it takes for metabolism and excretion to reduce a particular plasma concentration by half. A drug administered steadily at time intervals shorter than its half-life will reach 97 percent of its steady-state plasma concentration after five half-lives.

The *first-pass effect* refers to the initial metabolism of orally administered drugs within the portal circulation of the liver and is quantitated as the fraction of absorbed drug reaching the systemic circulation unmetabolized.

Clearance is a measure of the amount of the drug excreted from the body in a specific period of time.

Cytochrome P450 Enzymes. Most psychotherapeutic drugs are oxidized by the hepatic cytochrome P450 (CYP) enzyme system, which is so named because it strongly absorbs light at a wavelength of 450 nm.

The human CYP enzymes comprise several distinct families and subfamilies. In the CYP nomenclature, the family is denoted by a numeral, the subfamily by a capital letter, and the individual member of the subfamily by a second numeral (for example, 2D6). Persons with genetic polymorphisms in the CYP genes that encode inefficient versions of CYP enzymes are considered "poor metabolizers" (Table 1–1).

The CYP enzymes are responsible for the inactivation of most psychotherapeutic drugs. These enzymes act primarily in the endoplasmic reticulum of the hepatocytes and the cells of the intestine. Thus, cellular pathophysiology, such as that caused by viral hepatitis or cirrhosis, may affect the efficiency of drug metabolism by the CYP enzymes.

There are three ways in which drug interactions influence the CYP system (Table 1–2):

Induction. Expression of the CYP genes may be induced by alcohol, by certain drugs (barbiturates, anticonvulsants), or by smoking. For example, an inducer of CYP 3A4, such as cimetidine, may increase the metabolism and decrease the plasma concentrations of a substrate of 3A4, such as alprazolam (Xanax).

Noncompetitive inhibition. Certain drugs that are not substrates for a particular enzyme may nonetheless indirectly inhibit the enzyme and slow its metabolism of other drug substrates. For example, concurrent administration of a CYP 2D6 inhibitor, such as fluoxetine (Prozac), may inhibit the metabolism and thus raise the

TABLE 1–1
GENETIC POLYMORPHISMS

P450 Isoenzymes	Percentage of Poor Metabolizers
2C19	3–5% of whites, 15–20% of Asians
2C9	1–3% of whites
2D6	5–10% of whites

TABLE 1–2
CYTOCHROME P450 DRUG INTERACTIONS

Substrates		Inhibitors
1A2	Fluoxetine	**1A2**
Amitriptyline	Fluvoxamine	Fluvoxamine
Clomipramine	Methoxyamphetamine	**2C19**
Clozapine	Nortriptyline	Fluoxetine
Fluvoxamine	Paroxetine	Fluvoxamine
Haloperidol	Propranolol	Paroxetine
Imipramine	Venlafaxine	Topiramate
Propranolol	**3A3,4,5,7**	**2C9**
Tacrine	Alprazolam	Fluvoxamine
Verapamil	Amitriptyline	Paroxetine
2C19	Carbamazepine	**2D6**
Amitriptyline	Clomipramine	Chlorpheniramine
Citalopram	Clonazepam	Cimetidine
Clomipramine	Clozapine	Clomipramine
Diazepam	Diazepam	Fluoxetine
Hexobarbital	Imipramine	Haloperidol
Imipramine	Midazolam	Methadone
Mephobarbital	Triazolam	Moclobemide
Moclobemide	Astemizole	Paroxetine
Propranolol	Chlorpheniramine	**2E1**
2C9	Diltiazem	Disulfiram
Amitriptyline	Loratadine	**3A3,4,5,7**
Fluoxetine	Nefazodone	Fluvoxamine
2D6	Nifedipine	Grapefruit juice
Metoprolol	Nisoldipine	Nefazodone
Timolol	Nitrendipine	Norfluoxetine
Amitriptyline	Verapamil	**Inducers**
Clomipramine	Haloperidol	**2C19**
Desipramine	Methadone	Carbamazepine
Imipramine	Sertraline	**2C9**
Haloperidol	Sildenafil	Secobarbital
Perphenazine	Terfenadine	**3A3,4,5,7**
Risperidone	Trazodone	Barbiturates
Thioridazine	Verapamil	Carbamazepine
Amphetamine	Zaleplon	Phenobarbital
	Zolpidem	

plasma concentrations of CYP 2D6 substrates, including amitriptyline (Elavil). If one CYP enzyme is inhibited, then its substrate accumulates until it is metabolized by an alternate CYP enzyme.

Competitive inhibition. Concurrent administration of two or more substrates for a particular enzyme may produce competitive inhibition of the enzyme, but such interactions are not usually clinically relevant. For example, clomipramine (Anafranil) and theophylline (Theo-Dur, Slo-bid) are both substrates of CYP 1A2, but their concurrent administration has little effect on their respective plasma concentrations.

Clinically Relevant Pharmacokinetic Drug Interactions. With respect to CYP 2D6, tricyclic and tetracyclic drugs, dopamine receptor antagonists, and type 1C antiarrhythmic drugs should be used cautiously or avoided with certain selective serotonin reuptake inhibitors (SSRIs).

Because of inhibition of CYP 3A4, fluvoxamine (Luvox), nefazodone (Serzone), and fluoxetine should not be used together with alprazolam, triazolam (Halcion), or carbamazepine (Tegretol).

Due to interactions with CYP 1A2, fluvoxamine should not be used with theophylline or clozapine (Clozaril).

Inhibition of CYP 2C9/10 and CYP 2C19 warrants caution for the following combinations: fluoxetine plus phenytoin (Dilantin), sertraline (Zoloft) plus tolbutamide (Orinase), and fluvoxamine plus warfarin (Coumadin).

It is also important to consider that the long half-lives of certain psychotherapeutic drugs, especially fluoxetine, may prolong their inhibition of the CYP enzymes.

Pharmacodynamics

The major pharmacodynamic considerations include *molecular site of action*; the *dosage-response curve*; the *therapeutic index*; and the development of *tolerance, dependence, and withdrawal symptoms*.

Molecular Site of Action. Psychotherapeutic drugs may act at any of several molecular sites in brain cells. Some activate (agonists) or inactivate (antagonists) receptors for a specific neurotransmitter. Other drugs, particularly antidepressant drugs, bind to and block transporters that normally take up serotonin or norepinephrine from the synaptic cleft into the presynaptic nerve ending (reuptake inhibitors).

Some drugs block the passage of cations or anions through ion channels embedded in cellular membranes (channel inhibitors or blockers). Other drugs bind to and inhibit catabolic enzymes that normally inactivate neurotransmitters, which prolongs the lifespan of the active neurotransmitters (for example, monoamine oxidase inhibitors). Orlistat (Xenical) binds to an enzyme not directly involved with neurotransmitter metabolism.

Finally, several drugs have numerous molecular sites of action, although which sites are therapeutically relevant may remain unknown.

Dosage-Response Curves. The dosage-response curve plots the clinical response to the drug as a function of drug concentration (Figure 1–1). *Potency* refers to comparisons of the dosages of different drugs required to achieve a certain effect.

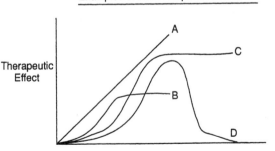

Examples of Dose-Response Curves

Figure 1-1. These dose-response curves plot the therapeutic effect as a function of increasing dose, often calculated as the log of the dose. Drug A has a linear dose response, drugs B and C have sigmoidal curves, and drug D has a curvilinear dose-response curve. Although smaller doses of drug B are more potent than are equal doses of drug C, drug C has a higher maximum efficacy than does drug B. Drug D has a therapeutic window such that both low and high doses are less effective than are midrange doses.

For example, haloperidol (Haldol) is more potent than is chlorpromazine (Thorazine), because about 5 mg of haloperidol is required to achieve the same therapeutic effect achieved by 100 mg of chlorpromazine. However, haloperidol and chlorpromazine are equal in their *clinical efficacy*—that is, the maximum achievable clinical response.

Therapeutic Index.   The *therapeutic index* is a relative measure of a drug's toxicity or safety. It is defined as the ratio of the median toxic dosage (TD_{50})—the dosage at which 50 percent of persons experience toxic effects—to the median effective dosage (ED_{50})—the dosage at which 50 percent of persons experience therapeutic effects. For example, haloperidol has a high therapeutic index, as evidenced by the wide range of dosages in which it is prescribed without monitoring of plasma concentrations. Conversely, lithium (Eskalith, Lithobid, Lithonate) has a low therapeutic index, thereby requiring the close monitoring of plasma concentrations to avoid toxicity.

Persons exhibit both interindividual and intraindividual variation in their responses to a specific drug. An individual may be hyporeactive, normally reactive, or hyperreactive to a particular drug. For example, some persons require 50 mg a day of sertraline, whereas other persons require 200 mg a day for control of their symptoms. An unpredictable, non-dosage-related drug response is called *idiosyncratic.* For example, diazepam (Valium) administered as a sedative paradoxically causes agitation in some persons.

Tolerance, Dependence, and Withdrawal Symptoms.   A person who becomes less responsive to a particular drug over time is said to develop *tolerance* to the effects of the drug. The development of tolerance can be associated with the appearance of physical *dependence,* which is the necessity to continue administering the drug to prevent the appearance of *withdrawal symptoms.*

THERAPEUTIC INDICATIONS

A therapeutic indication is a psychiatric diagnosis, as defined in the 10th revision of *International Statistical Classification of Diseases and Related Health Problems* (ICD-10) or the fourth edition text revision of *Diagnostic and Statistical Manual of Mental Disorders* (DSM-IV-TR), for which a specific drug ameliorates symptoms. The principal challenge to showing that a drug benefits a particular therapeutic indication is proving that clinical improvement is due to the drug and not to the placebo effect. Drug manufacturers attack this problem with carefully designed large-scale clinical trials supervised by a small army of clinical researchers. With a successful series of such trials, the FDA may grant the manufacturer the official right to advertise the drug as safe and effective for that therapeutic indication.

Clinicians must distinguish between official and unofficial therapeutic indications. This is necessary because every drug is in fact safe and effective for treating not only those indications proven in FDA-scale trials, but also for treating a much broader range of indications described in smaller trials.

Drug Approval Process in the United States

Under the federal Food, Drug, and Cosmetic (FDC) Act, initially passed in 1938 and subsequently heavily amended, the FDA has the authority (1) to control the initial availability of a drug by approving only those new drugs that demonstrate both safety and effectiveness and (2) to ensure that the drug's proposed labeling is truthful and contains all pertinent information for the safe and effective use of that drug. An additional concentration of government regulation is directed by the Drug Enforcement Agency (DEA), which classifies drugs according to their abuse potential (Table 1–3). Clinicians are advised to exercise increased caution when prescribing controlled substances.

In general, the FDA not only ensures that new medications are safe and effective, but also that new medication compares favorably with existing agents used for the same indications. The new agent is usually not approvable unless it is at least equivalent in safety and efficacy to existing agents, if not superior.

Off-Label Uses

According to the Medical Liability Mutual Insurance Company of New York State, once a drug is approved for commercial use, the clinician may, as part of the practice of medicine, lawfully prescribe a different dosage for a person or otherwise vary the conditions of use from what is approved in the package labeling, without notifying the FDA or obtaining its approval. In other words, the FDC Act does not limit the manner in which a clinician may use an approved drug.

TABLE 1–3
CHARACTERISTICS OF DRUGS AT EACH DEA LEVEL

Schedule (Control Level)	Characteristics of Drug at Each Schedule	Examples of Drugs at Each Schedule
I	High abuse potential No accepted use in medical treatment in the United States at the present time and, therefore, not for prescription use Can be used for research	Lysergic acid diethylamide (LSD), heroin, marijuana, peyote, phencyclidine (PCP), mescaline, psilocybin, nicocodeine, nicomorphine
II	High abuse potential Severe physical dependence liability Severe psychological dependence liability No refills; no telephone prescriptions	Amphetamine, opium, morphine, codeine, hydromorphone, phenmetrazine, amobarbital, secobarbital, pentobarbital, ketamine, methylphenidate
III	Abuse potential lower than levels I and II Moderate or low physical dependence liability High psychological liability Prescriptions must be rewritten after 6 months or five refills	Glutethimide; methyprylon; nalorphine; sulfonmethane; benzphetamine; phendimetrazine; chlorphentermine; compounds containing codeine, morphine, opium, hydrocodone, dihydrocodeine; diethylpropion; dronabinol
IV	Low abuse potential Limited physical dependence liability Limited psychological dependence liability Prescriptions must be rewritten after 6 months or five refills	Phenobarbital, benzodiazepines,[a] chloral hydrate, ethchlorvynol, ethinamate, meprobamate, paraldehyde
V	Lowest abuse potential of all controlled substances	Narcotic preparations containing limited amounts of nonnarcotic active medicinal ingredients

[a] In New York State benzodiazepines are treated as schedule II substances, which require a triplicate prescription for a maximum of 3 month's supply.

However, although clinicians may treat persons with an approved drug for unapproved purposes—that is, for indications not included on the drug's official labeling—without violating the FDC Act, this practice exposes the clinician to increased risk of medical malpractice liability. This is a significant concern, because the failure to follow the FDA-approved label may create an inference that the clinician is varying from the prevailing standard of care.

In summary, clinicians may prescribe medication for any reason they believe to be medically indicated for the welfare of the person. This clarification is important in view of the increasing regulation of clinicians by federal, state, and local governmental agencies.

When using a drug for an unapproved indication or in a dosage outside the usual range, the clinician should document the reason for these treatment decisions in the person's chart. If clinicians are in doubt about a treatment plan, they should consult a colleague or suggest that the person under treatment obtain a second opinion.

PRECAUTIONS AND ADVERSE EFFECTS

Precautions

Prior to use of a drug, it is important to be prepared to manage any expected adverse effects safely. The clinician should be fully aware of any warnings and precautions in the product literature and should anticipate how to respond at least to the more common adverse effects listed.

Adverse Effects

Many psychotherapeutic drugs affect several neurotransmitter systems, both in the brain and in the periphery, and thus cause a wide range of adverse effects. For example, older psychotherapeutic drugs commonly cause anticholinergic effects (Table 1–4). Many older psychotherapeutic drugs also bind to dopaminergic, histaminergic, and adrenergic receptors, resulting in the adverse effects listed in Table 1–5.

Newer agents tend to have fewer nontherapeutic neurotransmitter activities than do older agents. However, the SSRIs in particular cause a set of adverse effects thought to be directly due to their serotonergic actions. It is usually not possible to

TABLE 1–4
POTENTIAL ADVERSE EFFECTS CAUSED BY BLOCKADE OF MUSCARINIC ACETYLCHOLINE RECEPTORS

Blurred vision
Constipation
Decreased salivation
Decreased sweating
Delayed or retrograde ejaculation
Delirium
Exacerbation of asthma (through decreased bronchial secretions)
Hyperthermia (through decreased sweating)
Memory problems
Narrow-angle glaucoma
Photophobia
Sinus tachycardia
Urinary retention

TABLE 1–5
POTENTIAL ADVERSE EFFECTS OF PSYCHOTHERAPEUTIC DRUGS AND ASSOCIATED NEUROTRANSMITTER SYSTEMS

Antidopaminergic
  Endocrine dysfunction
    Hyperprolactinemia
    Menstrual dysfunction
    Sexual dysfunction
  Movement disorders
    Akathisia
    Dystonia
    Parkinsonism
    Tardive dyskinesia
Antiadrenergic (primarily α)
  Dizziness
  Postural hypotension
  Reflex tachycardia
Antihistaminergic
  Hypotension
  Sedation
  Weight gain
Multiple neurotransmitter systems
  Agranulocytosis (and other blood dyscrasias)
  Allergic reactions
  Anorexia
  Cardiac conduction abnormalities
  Nausea and vomiting
  Seizures

predict which persons will not tolerate a serotonergic agent. A history of poor tolerance of a previous antidepressant or paranoid features may predict a poor response to a serotonergic drug.

Persons generally have decreased trouble with adverse effects if they have been warned to expect them. Clinicians should distinguish between probable or expected adverse effects and rare or unexpected adverse effects.

The FDA requires that the product literature contains exhaustive reporting of the results of clinical trials, and careful reading will show that many of the listed adverse effects are in fact not causally associated with use of the drug. The product information must therefore be carefully analyzed to isolate those adverse effects seen more frequently in the treatment group than in the placebo group.

Treatment of Common Adverse Effects

Psychotherapeutic drugs may cause any of a range of adverse effects. The management of a particular adverse effect is similar, regardless of which psychotherapeutic drug the person is taking. If possible, another drug with similar benefits but fewer adverse effects should be used instead.

Sexual Dysfunction. Psychotherapeutic drug use can be associated with sexual dysfunction, specifically, decreased libido, impaired ejaculation and erection, and inhibition of female orgasm. This is by far the most common adverse effect associated with use of SSRIs. Fifty to 80 percent of persons taking an SSRI experience some sexual dysfunction, although few complain of severe dysfunction.

The pharmacological management of sexual dysfunction involves either switching from the SSRI to nefazodone or bupropion (Wellbutrin), which are much less likely than SSRIs to cause sexual dysfunction, or adding a prosexual agent. Merely administering bupropion concurrently may be enough to reverse the sexual inhibition caused by SSRIs.

Specific pharmacological strategies are available for treating dysfunctions of each stage of the sexual response cycle, but improvement of any stage of sexual function can be very reassuring and may stimulate full endogenous sexual functioning.

The best tolerated and most potent prosexual drug currently available is sildenafil (Viagra). Taken 1 hour before intercourse, it increases blood flow to the genital erectile tissues equally well in both men and women. In men, it improves erectile function and in women it promotes engorgement of the clitoris and labia minora. Sildenafil not only improves the arousal phase of the sexual response cycle, but it may also stimulate the desire and orgasm phases in both men and women.

Alprostadil (Muse, Caverject) is an alternative treatment for male erectile dysfunction. Alprostadil improves the arousal phase of the sexual response cycle and may also stimulate the desire and orgasm phases in men.

Other, less effective prosexual agents include neostigmine (Prostigmin) for impaired ejaculation, 7.5 to 15 mg taken orally 30 minutes before sexual intercourse. Erectile function may be improved with bethanechol (Urecholine), dopamine receptor agonists, amantadine (Symmetrel), or yohimbine (Yocon). Cyproheptadine (Periactin) can be used for inhibited female orgasm, 4 mg every morning; and for inhibited male orgasm secondary to serotonergic agents, 4 to 8 mg orally taken 1 to 2 hours before anticipated sexual activity.

Anxiety, Akathisia, Agitation, and Insomnia.   As many as one-quarter of persons initiating treatment with serotonergic antidepressants, especially fluoxetine, transiently experience an increase in psychomotor activation in the first 2 to 3 weeks of use.

The agitating effects of SSRIs modestly increase the risk of acting out suicidal impulses in persons at risk for suicide. During the initial period of SSRI treatment, persons at risk for self-injury should maintain close contact with the clinician or should be hospitalized, depending on the clinician's assessment of the risk for suicide.

The insomnia and anxiety associated with use of serotonergic drugs may be counteracted by administration of a benzodiazepine or trazodone (Desyrel) for the first several weeks. A small number of persons will experience persistent increased anxiety beyond the initial 3-week period, and these persons may require a nonserotonergic antidepressant drug.

GI Upset and Diarrhea.   Most of the body's serotonin is in the GI tract, and serotonergic drugs, particularly sertraline and fluvoxamine, may therefore produce mildly to moderately severe stomach pain, nausea, and diarrhea, usually only for the first few weeks of therapy. Sertraline is most likely to cause loose stools and fluvoxamine is most likely to cause nausea.

These symptoms may be minimized by initiating treatment with a very small dosage and administering the drug after eating. Dietary alteration, such as the BRAT diet (*b*ananas, *r*ice, *a*pples, and *t*oast), may reduce loose stools. These symptoms usually abate over time, but some persons never accommodate and must switch to another drug.

Headache.   A small fraction of persons initiating therapy with an SSRI experience mildly to moderately severe headache. SSRI-associated headaches often respond to over-the-counter analgesics, but it may be necessary for some persons to switch to another antidepressant.

Despite the fact that SSRIs may cause headache, however, SSRIs much more commonly provide relief from headache. SSRIs are an effective treatment for chronic tension-type headache and for migraine headache.

Anorexia.   SSRI-associated appetite suppression is more pronounced in obese persons and persons with carbohydrate craving and may therefore be desirable. However, other persons may gain weight while taking SSRIs. Clinicians can reassure persons who experience SSRI-associated weight changes that most persons return to their pretreatment weight by the end of the first year.

Fluoxetine (60 mg per day) in the context of a comprehensive program of behavioral management is an approved treatment for bulimia and is also useful for treatment of anorexia nervosa. However, fluoxetine may be abused by persons with eating disorders if used in an unmonitored fashion. Unless a comprehensive therapeutic program is available, SSRIs should be used cautiously by persons with eating disorders.

Weight Gain.   Many psychotherapeutic drugs cause weight gain as a result of either fluid retention or increased caloric intake.

Edema can be treated by elevating the affected body parts or by administering a diuretic. If the person adds a diuretic to a regimen of lithium or cardiac medications, the clinician must monitor blood concentrations, blood chemistries, and vital signs.

Increased caloric intake is safely managed only through dietary regulation. No drug has yet been shown to suppress the appetite safely in all persons. The most effective appetite suppressants, the amphetamines, are not used generally because of concerns about abuse.

Sibutramine (Meridia) causes modest weight loss in some persons through inhibition of reuptake of serotonin and norepinephrine. Thus, it should not be used by persons taking any type of antidepressant drug, including SSRIs, bupropion, venlafaxine (Effexor), nefazodone, trazodone, mirtazapine (Remeron), reboxetine (Vestra), tricyclic and tetracyclic drugs, and monoamine oxidase inhibitors.

Orlistat does not suppress the appetite; instead it blocks absorption of fat from the intestine. Thus, it reduces caloric intake from fatty foods but not from carbohydrates or proteins. Because orlistat causes retention of dietary fats in the intestines, it frequently causes excessive flatulence.

Most overweight persons misperceive their daily caloric intake as considerably lower than it actually is. Persons wishing to lose weight must adhere strictly to a reduced-calorie diet and must assiduously document every calorie of food they consume.

Somnolence.   Many psychotropic drugs cause sedation. Some persons may self-medicate this adverse effect with caffeine, but this practice may worsen orthostatic hypotension.

It is important for the clinician to alert the person to the possibility of sedation and to document that the person was advised not to drive or operate dangerous equipment if sedated by medications. Fortunately, newer generations of antidepressant and antipsychotic drugs are much less likely to cause sedation than were their predecessors, and the newer drugs should be substituted for the sedating medications when possible.

Dry Mouth. Dry mouth is caused by the blockade of muscarinic acetylcholine receptors. When persons attempt to relieve the dry mouth by constantly sucking on sugar-containing hard candies, they increase their risk for dental caries. They can avoid the problem by chewing sugarless gum or sucking on sugarless hard candies.

Some clinicians recommend the use of a 1 percent solution of pilocarpine (Salagen), a cholinergic agonist, as a mouth wash three times daily. Other clinicians suggest bethanechol tablets, another cholinergic agonist, 10 to 30 mg, once or twice daily. It is best to start with 10 mg once a day and to increase the dosage slowly. Adverse effects of cholinomimetic drugs, such as bethanechol, include tremor, diarrhea, abdominal cramps, and excessive eye watering.

Most newer drugs are free of anticholinergic effects.

Blurred Vision. The blockage of muscarinic acetylcholine receptors causes mydriasis (pupillary dilation) and cycloplegia (ciliary muscle paresis), resulting in blurred vision. The symptom can be relieved by cholinomimetic eyedrops. A 1 percent solution of pilocarpine can be prescribed as one drop four times daily. Alternatively, bethanecol can be used as it is used for dry mouth.

Urinary Retention. The anticholinergic activity of many psychotherapeutic drugs can lead to urinary hesitation, dribbling, urinary retention, and increased urinary tract infections. Elderly persons with prostatic enlargement are at increased risk for these adverse effects. Ten to 30 mg of bethanechol three to four times daily is usually effective in the treatment of the urological adverse effects.

Constipation. The anticholinergic activity of psychotherapeutic drugs can cause constipation. The first line of treatment involves the prescribing of bulk laxatives, such as Citrucel, FiberCon, Konsyl, Metamucil, Perdiem, and Unifiber. If this treatment fails, cathartic laxatives, such as milk of magnesia, or other laxative preparations can be tried. Prolonged use of cathartic laxatives can result in a loss of their effectiveness. Bethanechol, 10 to 30 mg three to four times daily, can also be used.

Orthostatic Hypotension. Orthostatic hypotension is caused by the blockade of α_1-adrenergic receptors. The elderly are at particular risk for development of orthostatic hypotension. The risk of hip fractures from falls is significantly elevated in persons who are taking psychotherapeutic drugs.

Most simply, the person can be instructed to get up slowly and to sit down immediately if dizziness is experienced. Treatments for orthostatic hypotension include avoidance of caffeine, intake of at least 2 L of fluid per day, addition of salt to food (unless proscribed by a physician), reassessment of the dosages of any antihypertensive medications, and wearing support hose. Fludrocortisone (Florinef) is rarely needed.

Overdosages

An extreme adverse effect of drug treatment is an attempt by a person to commit suicide by overdosing on a psychotherapeutic drug. Clinicians should be aware of the risk and attempt to prescribe the safest possible drugs.

It is good clinical practice to write nonrefillable prescriptions for small quantities of drugs when suicide is a consideration. In extreme cases, an attempt should be made to verify that persons are taking the medication and not hoarding the pills for a later overdosage attempt. Persons may attempt suicide just as they are beginning to get better. Clinicians, therefore, should continue to be careful about prescribing large quantities of medication until the person has almost completely recovered.

Another consideration for clinicians is the possibility of an accidental overdosage, particularly by children in the household. Persons should be advised to keep psychotherapeutic medications in a safe place. A guide to the signs and symptoms and the treatment of overdosages with psychotherapeutic drugs is contained in Table 43–1 in Chapter 43.

Discontinuation Syndromes

The transient emergence of mild serotonergic symptoms upon discontinuation or reduction of dosage is associated with a number of drugs, including paroxetine (Paxil), venlafaxine, sertraline, fluvoxamine, and the tricyclic and tetracyclic drugs. More-severe discontinuation symptoms are associated with lithium (rebound mania), dopamine-receptor antagonists (tardive dyskinesias), and benzodiazepines (anxiety and insomnia).

There is a spectrum of severity of the serotonin discontinuation syndrome, which consists of agitation, nausea, dysequilibrium, and dysphoria. The syndrome is more likely to occur if the plasma half-life of the agent is brief, if the drug is taken for at least 2 months, or if higher dosages are used. The symptoms are time limited and can be minimized by a gradual reduction of the dosage.

DRUG INTERACTIONS

Drug interactions may be either pharmacokinetic or pharmacodynamic, and they vary greatly in their potential to cause serious problems. Pharmacokinetic drug interactions concern the effects of drugs on their respective plasma concentrations, and pharmacodynamic drug interactions concern the effects of drugs on their respective receptor activities.

Pharmacodynamic drug-drug interactions causing additive biochemical changes may trigger toxic adverse effects. For example, monoamine oxidase inhibitors, when coadministered with either tricyclic antidepressants or SSRIs, may precipitate a serotonin syndrome in which serotonin is metabolized slowly and thus accumulates in excessive concentrations. The interaction of disulfiram (Antabuse) and alcohol is another example of toxicity due to pharmacodynamic drug interactions.

Some clinically important drug interactions are well studied and well proven, other interactions are well documented but have only modest effects, and still other interactions are true but unproved, although reasonably plausible. Clinicians must remember that (1) animal pharmacokinetic data are not always readily generalizable to humans; (2) in vitro data do not necessarily replicate the results obtained under in vivo conditions; (3) single-case reports can contain misleading information; and (4) studies of acute conditions should not be uncritically regarded as relevant to chronic, steady-state conditions.

An additional consideration is one of phantom drug interactions. The person may be taking only drug A and then later receive both drug A and drug B. The clinician may then notice some effect and attribute it to the induction of metabolism. In fact, what may have occurred is that the person was more compliant at one point in the observation period than in another, or there may have been some other effect of which the clinician was unaware. The clinical literature may contain reports of phantom drug interactions that are rare or nonexistent.

The informed clinician needs to keep these considerations in mind and to focus on the clinically important interactions, not on the ones that may be mild, unproved, or entirely phantom. At the same time, the clinician should maintain an open and receptive attitude toward the possibility of pharmacokinetic and pharmacodynamic drug interactions.

DOSAGE AND CLINICAL GUIDELINES

Diagnosis and the Identification of Target Symptoms

Treatment with psychotherapeutic drugs begins with formation of a therapeutic bond between the doctor and the person seeking treatment. The initial interview is devoted to defining the clinical problem as comprehensively as possible, with special attention paid to the identification of specific target symptoms whose improvement will indicate that the drug therapy is effective.

Medication History.   Past and present medication history discusses the use of all prescription, nonprescription, herbal, and illicit drugs ever taken, including caffeine, ethanol, and nicotine; the sequence in which the drugs were used; the dosages used; the therapeutic effects; the adverse effects; details of any overdosages; and the reasons for discontinuing any drug.

Persons and their families are often ignorant about what drugs have been used before, in what dosages, and for how long. This ignorance may reflect the tendency of clinicians not to explain drug trials before writing the prescriptions. Clinicians should provide written records of drug trials for each person to present to future caregivers.

A caveat to obtaining a history of drug response from persons is that, because of their mental disorders, they may inaccurately report the effects of a previous drug trial. If possible, therefore, the persons' medical records should be obtained to confirm their reports.

Explaining Rationale, Risks, Benefits, and Treatment Alternatives

The use of psychotherapeutic drugs should not be oversimplified into a one diagnosis–one pill approach. Many variables impinge on a person's psychodynamic response to drug treatment. Some persons may view a drug as a panacea, and other persons may view a drug as an assault. Expert psychopharmacologists must often work inventively to assimilate any distorted perceptions into a person's overall treatment plan.

Clinicians should resist the temptation to use the simplicity of prescription of current psychotherapeutic drugs as a time-saving convenience. The discussion of the rationale of treatment, the risks and benefits of drug therapy, and full enumeration of the treatment alternatives should be conducted on an appropriate intellectual and emotional plane. Tapping into a person's innate curiosity about drug treatment frequently evokes a positive therapeutic transference toward the psychopharmacologist.

Compliance with the dosing regimen is improved by providing a person ample opportunities to ask questions at the time of prescription, distributing written material that reinforces proper use of the medication, streamlining the medication regimen as much as possible, and ensuring that office visits begin at the scheduled appointment time.

The theoretical biases of the treating clinician are critical to the success of drug treatment. A psychopharmacologist's unambiguous endorsement of a particular drug therapy can allay a person's doubts and optimize future evaluations of the treatment.

Choice of Drug

Previous Drug History.   From among the drugs appropriate to a particular diagnosis, the specific drug should be selected according to the person's history of drug response (compliance, therapeutic response, and adverse effects), the person's family history of drug response, the profile of adverse effects expected for that particular person, and the clinician's usual practice. If a drug has previously been effective in treating a person or a family member, the same drug should be used again unless there is some specific reason not to use the drug. A history of severe adverse effects from a specific drug is a strong indicator that the person would again not be compliant with that particular drug regimen.

Adverse Effect Profile.   Most psychotherapeutic drugs of a single class are equally efficacious; however, the drugs do differ in their adverse effects on individual persons. A drug should be selected that minimally exacerbates any preexisting medical problems.

Assessment of Outcome

Any clinical improvements that occur during the course of drug treatment may or may not be specifically related to use of the drug. For example, psychological distress often improves with the simple reassurances of a medical caregiver. Therefore, it is important to identify unambiguously those clinical improvements caused by the pharmacological effects of the medications.

In clinical practice, a person's subjective impression of a beneficial drug effect is the single most consistent indicator of future response to that drug. In contrast, assessments of clinical outcome in randomized, double-blind, placebo-controlled clinical trials necessarily rely on quantitative psychiatric rating scales, such as the Brief Psychiatric Rating Scale, the Positive and Negative Syndrome Scale, the Beck Depression Scale, the Hamilton Rating Scale for Depression, the Hamilton Anxiety Rating Scale, or the Global Assessment of Functioning Scale.

Therapeutic Trials.   A drug's therapeutic trial in a particular person should last for a previously determined length of time. Because behavioral symptoms are more difficult to assess than are other physiological symptoms, such as hypertension, it is particularly important to identify specific target symptoms at the initiation of a drug trial. The clinician and the person can then assess the target symptom over the course of the drug trial to help determine whether the drug has been effective.

If a drug has not been effective in reducing target symptoms within the specified length of time and if other reasons for the lack of response can be eliminated, the drug should be tapered and stopped.

The addition of new medications without the discontinuation of a prior drug is a common but problematic practice. Although indicated in specific circumstances, such as lithium potentiation of an unsuccessful trial of antidepressants, it often results in increased noncompliance and adverse effects and the clinician's not knowing whether it was the second drug alone or the combination of drugs that resulted in a therapeutic success or adverse effect.

Possible Reasons for Therapeutic Failures

The failure of a specific drug trial should prompt the clinician to reconsider a number of possibilities.

First, did the person take the drug as directed?

Second, was the drug administered in sufficient dosage for an appropriate period of time? Persons can have varying drug absorption and metabolic rates for the same drug, and, if available, plasma drug concentrations should be obtained to assess this variable.

Third, was the original diagnosis correct? This reconsideration should include the possibility of an undiagnosed cognitive disorder, including illicit drug abuse.

Fourth, are the observed remaining symptoms the drug's adverse effects and not related to the original disease? Antipsychotic drugs, for example, can produce akinesia, which resembles psychotic withdrawal; akathisia and neuroleptic malignant syndrome resemble increased psychotic agitation.

Fifth, did a pharmacokinetic or pharmacodynamic interaction with another drug the person was taking reduce the efficacy of the psychotherapeutic drug?

Strategies for Increasing Efficacy

The most fruitful initial strategy for increasing the efficacy of a psychotherapeutic drug is to review whether the drug is being taken correctly. A fresh clinical evaluation of the psychiatric symptoms and the rationale of the drug therapy is one of the psychopharmacologist's most valuable tools for revealing previously unappreciated impediments to drug efficacy.

In general, adherence to the prescribed medication regimen is maximized by administration of the drug in the fewest daily dosages; by administration immediately before retiring to sleep; and by the use of cues in the person's home environment, such as strategically posted written reminders, timely reminding by a significant other, and incorporation of drug administration into a preexisting routine, such as daily dental hygiene.

If target symptoms do not respond to the highest tolerated dosage, then drug augmentation strategies should be considered. The potential benefit of the augmenting agent must be weighed against the increased risk of drug interactions and the person's psychodynamic reaction to additional medication.

Duration of Treatment

Use of the Correct Dosage.   Subtherapeutic dosages and incomplete trials should not be prescribed solely to assuage the clinician's anxiety about the development of adverse effects. The prescription of drugs for mental disorders must be made by a knowledgeable practitioner and requires continuous clinical observation. Treatment response and the emergence of adverse effects must be monitored closely. The dosage of the drug must be adjusted accordingly, and appropriate treatments for emergent adverse effects must be instituted as quickly as possible.

Long-Term Maintenance Therapy.   Psychotherapeutic drugs should be taken at effective dosages for sufficient time periods, as determined by previous clinical investigations and personal experience. It is important to recognize that persons with mood, anxiety, and thought disorders live with an increased risk for relapse into illness at virtually any phase of their lives.

Clinicians should anticipate and alert persons to the natural variations of psychiatric illnesses. For example, a person who has taken medication to treat an acute psychotic episode may soon thereafter experience a relatively symptom-free period and may then impulsively discontinue taking the medication without seeking psychopharmacological advice. If, in fact, the acute illness had run its natural course and cycled into a more benign phase, then the person would have mistaken an upturn in the natural history of the illness for a medical "cure."

The impulse to discontinue psychotherapeutic drugs is perilous, because long-term data show that persons who stop their medications after resolution of an acute episode of mental illness markedly increase their risk of relapse during the subsequent year, compared with persons who remain on maintenance drug therapy. This is especially important for persons who experience a psychotic episode, a manic episode, or a suicidal depression, because the risk of permanent disability in these disorders increases with each additional acute relapse.

Continuous educational review and reinforcement of the role of psychotherapeutic drugs in the management of psychiatric symptoms is an essential duty of the treating clinician. Comparing psychiatric illnesses with common chronic medical conditions, such as hypertension and diabetes mellitus, is often instructive.

Special Populations

Children.   Special care must be given when administering psychotherapeutic drugs to children. Although the smaller volume of distribution suggests the use of lower dosages than in adults, children's higher rate of metabolism indicates that higher ratios of milligrams of drug to kilograms of body weight should be used. General dosage guidelines for various drugs used to treat children and adolescents are provided in Tables 1–6 through 1–10. Table 1–11 summarizes adverse effects and their management in children and adolescents.

In practice, it is best to begin with a small dosage and to increase the dosage

TABLE 1–6
SYMPATHOMIMETICS USED FOR ATTENTION-DEFICIT HYPERACTIVITY DISORDER IN CHILDREN AND ADOLESCENTS

Drug[a]	Oral Dosage Range (mg/day)
Methylphenidate (Ritalin)	2.5–60
Dextroamphetamine (Dexedrine)	2.5–30
Dextroamphetamine-amphetamine (Adderall)	2.5–40
Pemoline (Cylert)	18.75–112.5

[a] All cause weight loss with extended use.
Table by Barbara J. Coffey, M.D.

TABLE 1-7
ANTIPSYCHOTICS FOR USE IN CHILDREN AND ADOLESCENTS

Drug	Indications	Oral Dosage Range (mg)	Common Adverse Effects	
			Short-Term	Long-Term
Dopamine-receptor antagonists				
Phenothiazines				
Chlorpromazine (Thorazine)	Childhood-onset psychoses, acute or chronic; acute agitation	10–300	Autonomic nervous system: sedation, dry mouth, orthostatic hypotension, urinary retention, blurring of vision	Withdrawal and tardive dyskinesia
Thioridazine (Mellaril)		10–300		Cognitive blunting
Trifluoperazine (Stelazine)		1–20	EPS: acute dystonic reaction, akathisia, parkinsonism	Weight gain
Fluphenazine (Prolixin)		1–10	Endocrine: prolactin, menstrual irregularities	
Perphenazine (Trilafon)		2–24		
Butyrophenones				
Haloperidol (Haldol)	Tourette's disorder; childhood-onset psychoses	1–16		Same as phenothiazines
Thioxanthenes				
Thiothixene (Navane)	Same as phenothiazines	1–5	Hypersensitivity: rash, blood dyscrasias, elevated liver function	Same as phenothiazines
Dibenzoxazepines				
Loxapine (Loxitane)	Same as phenothiazines	5–60	CNS: seizures, behavioral reactions	Same as phenothiazines
Dihydroindolones				
Molindone (Moban)	Same as phenothiazines	10–50	EPS	Same as phenothiazines

Drug	Indication	Dose range (mg)	Adverse effects	
Diphenylbutylpiperidines				
Pimozide (Orap)	Tourette's disorder	1–10	EPS: ECG changes	Same as phenothiazines
Serotonin–dopamine antagonists				
Dibenzodiazepines				
Clozapine (Clozaril)	Treatment-refractory psychosis	25–300	Agranulocytosis; salivation	
Olanzapine (Zyprexa)	Childhood-onset psychosis	2.5–10	Fatigue	Weight gain
Quetiapine (Seroquel)	Childhood-onset psychosis	25–500	Fatigue, dizziness	
Benzisoxazole				
Risperidone (Risperdal)	Childhood-onset psychosis; Tourette's disorder	1–6	Fatigue, ECG changes	Weight gain
Benzisothiazolylpiperazine				
Ziprasidone (Zeldox)	Childhood-onset psychosis	40–160	Fatigue, dizziness	

Suggested treatment regimen for psychosis and autistic spectrum disorders
Risperidone
  Start with 0.25 mg for 1 week; increase by 0.25 mg every week
  Daily maintenance dose range: 0.5–3.0 mg
Olanzapine
  Start with 2.5 mg for 3–4 days; increase by 2.5 mg every 5–7 days
  Daily maintenance dosage range: 5–10 mg
Suggested treatment regimen for Tourette's disorder
Risperidone
  Start with 0.25 mg for 1 week; increase by 0.25 mg every week
  Daily maintenance dosage range 0.5–3.0 mg

EPS, extrapyramidal adverse effects; CNS, central nervous system; ECG, electrocardiogram.
Adapted from Barbara J. Coffey, M.D.

TABLE 1-8
ANTIDEPRESSANTS FOR USE IN CHILDREN AND ADOLESCENTS

Drug	Indications	Oral Dosage Range (mg a day)	Common Adverse Effects Short-Term	Long-Term
Imipramine (Tofranil)	Enuresis	25–125	Autonomic nervous system: dry mouth, orthostatic hypotension, blurring vision	Same as short term
Desipramine (Norpramin)	Attention-deficit/hyperactivity disorder[a,b]	25–200	Cardiovascular: alterations in conduction, pulse, blood pressure; prolonged PR, QTc; arrhythmias	
	Major depressive disorder[a,b]	100–300		
	Separation anxiety[a] (school refusal)	100–200		
Nortriptyline (Aventyl)	Major depressive disorder	50–100	Same as imipramine	
Clomipramine (Anafranil)	Obsessive-compulsive disorder	25–200		
Fluoxetine (Prozac)	Obsessive-compulsive disorder[b]	10–40	Sedation, gastrointestinal effects, insomnia, activation, sexual dysfunction	Weight changes
	Major depressive disorder			
	Selective mutism?			
Sertraline (Zoloft)	Obsessive-compulsive disorder, depressive disorders	50–300	Same as fluoxetine	
Paroxetine (Paxil)	Obsessive-compulsive disorder, panic disorder, depressive disorders	10–50	Same as fluoxetine	
Fluvoxamine (Luvox)	Obsessive-compulsive disorder, depressive disorders	25–200	Same as fluoxetine	
Bupropion (Wellbutrin)	Attention-deficit/hyperactivity disorder	50–300	Insomnia	

Suggested treatment regimen for enuresis
Start with 0.5 mg/kg of imipramine at nighttime for 2–3 nights
Increase by 25 mg or 0.5 mg/kg every 2–3 nights until therapeutic response
Daily maintenance dosage range: 0.5–2.5 mg/kg

Suggested treatment regimen for attention-deficit/hyperactivity disorder
Start with 0.5 mg/kg bupropion
Increase by 25 mg or 0.5 mg/kg every 5–7 days until therapeutic response or adverse effects
Daily maintenance dosage range: 1–5 mg/kg

Suggested treatment regimen for childhood major depressive disorder
Start with fluoxetine (or equivalent) 5–10 mg for 5–7 days
Increase by 5–10 mg every week
Daily maintenance dose range: 10–40 mg or equivalent

a Also responsive to imipramine.
b Based on plasma concentrations: 150–250 ng/mL.
Adapted from Barbara J. Coffey, M.D.

TABLE 1-9
ANXIOLYTICS AND SEDATIVE-HYPNOTIC DRUGS FOR USE IN CHILDREN AND ADOLESCENTS

Drug	Indications	Oral Dosage Range (mg a day)	Common Adverse Effects	
			Short-Term	Long-Term
Benzodiazepines				
Diazepam (Valium)	Night terrors	1–10	Drowsiness	Cognitive effects
	Anxiety disorders	2–10	Paradoxical agitation or excitement	Cognitive effects
Lorazepam (Ativan)	Anxiety, acute or chronic	0.5–6	Sedation	
Chlordiazepoxide (Librium)	Anxiety disorders	10–100	Sedation	
Alprazolam (Xanax)	Separation anxiety; panic	0.25–4	Disinhibition	
Flurazepam (Dalmane)	Bedtime sedation	15–30	Daytime sedation	Withdrawal reaction
Clonazepam (Klonopin)	Anxiety, panic	0.25–3	Daytime sedation	
Antihistamines				
Diphenhydramine (Benadryl)	Bedtime sedation	25–300	Oversedation; hypersensitivity; rash, dryness of mucous membranes	
Hydroxyzine (Vistaril or Atarax)	Anxiety states, agitation, bedtime sedation	25–300	Same as diphenhydramine	
Other				
Buspirone (BuSpar)	Anxiety disorders	5–30	Sedation; headache, dizziness	
Chloral hydrate (Noctec)	Bedtime sedation	500–1000		

Table by Barbara J. Coffey, M.D.

TABLE 1-10
MOOD STABILIZERS FOR USE IN CHILDREN AND ADOLESCENTS

Generic Name (Trade Name)	Indications	Dosage (mg/kg a day)	Therapeutic Serum Concentration	Common Adverse Effects
Valproate (Depakene) Valproic acid (Depakene) Divalproex (Depakote)	Bipolar and some recurrent depressive disorders; some behavior disorders with aggressivity; augmentation for refractory major depressive disorder	30–60	50–100 µg/mL	Dose-related: sedation, elevation of liver enzymes Other: nausea, vomiting, tremor, transient hair loss, leukopenia, thrombocytopenia, pancreatitis, hepatotoxicity[a]
Carbamazepine (Tegretol) Lithium (Eskalith, Lithobid)		10–20 150–1800 (blood concentrations; 0.6–1.2 mEq/L)	8–12 µg/mL 0.6–1.2 mEq/L	Sedation, tremor, ataxia, rash Short-term Gastrointestinal: nausea, vomiting, diarrhea, abdominal distress CNS: tremor, memory lapses, fatigue Renal: polyuria, polydipsia Hematological: leukocytosis Long-term Weight gain Cognitive blunting Tubular changes Endocrine: goiter

Suggested treatment regimen for childhood and adolescent bipolar disorders (children over age 6 years)

Lithium
 Start with 150 mg in the PM then increase by 150 mg every 3–5 days until blood concentration is 0.6–1.5 mEq/L
 Daily maintenance dosage range: 300–2400 mg daily (0.6–1.2 mEq/L)
Valproate
 Start with 125–250 mg in the PM and increase by 125–250 mg every 1–3 days to blood level concentration 50–100 ng/mL
 Daily maintenance dosage range: 250–1500 mg
Carbamazepine
 Start with 100–200 mg daily and increase by 100 mg every 3–7 days to blood concentration 8–12 ng/mL
 Daily maintenance dosage range: 300–1200 mg

CNS, central nervous system.
[a] Hypersensitivity and drug allergy may occur with any anticonvulsant.
Table by Barbara J. Coffey, M.D.

TABLE 1–11
ADVERSE EFFECTS AND THEIR MANAGEMENT IN CHILDREN AND ADOLESCENTS

Drug Category	Common Adverse Effects	Clinical Management
Antipsychotics (dopamine receptor antagonists and serotonin-dopamine antagonists)	Short-term Autonomic nervous system Dry mouth	 In general, lower dosage if possible or switch drug if persistent; child may equilibrate after several weeks
	Urinary retention	Bethanechol (Urecholine) only if severe and persistent
	Constipation	Docusate (Colace) tablets or bisacodyl (Dulcolax) suppositories
	Orthostatic hypotension	Avoid sudden postural changes; dosage reduction if severe
	Extrapyramidal Acute dystonia	 Diphenhydramine (Benadryl) or benztropine (Cogentin) intramuscularly, then switch to oral form
	Parkinsonism	Anticholinergic or antiparkinsonian medication p.r.n.
	Akathisia	Lower dosage; sometimes a β-adrenergic receptor antagonist can help
	Other Hypersensitivity or rash	 Discontinue use
	Drowsiness	Child usually becomes tolerant; if persistent switch to less-sedating class
	Photosensitivity	Avoid sun exposure
	LFTs	May not have clinical significance; follow-up indicated
	Blood dyscrasias	Hematology consultation
	Long-term Weight gain	 Lower dosage; consider switch to another class
	Dyskinesias (tardive and withdrawal)	Prevention is best; use lowest possible dose for maintenance
Sympathomimetics	Short-term Anorexia, nausea, abdominal pain	 Reduce dosage; give dosage after eating; consider switch
	Insomnia	Move PM dose to earlier in the day; reduce dosage then reintroduce
	Dysphoria	Consider another sympathomimetic if persistent or bupronin
	Long-term Weight loss	 Supplement diet, institute drug holidays, or change drug
	Tics	Discontinue, if stimulant is effective consider rechallenge; consider bupronin
Tricyclic drugs	Autonomic nervous system	See antipsychotic agents
	Cardiovascular (blood pressure, HR, PR, T-wave changes, ↑ QTc, and arrhythmias)	Monitor ECGs serially; most changes have little clinical significance in healthy child
	CNS (seizures)	Discontinue medication gradually; EEG; may need anticonvulsant
Anxiolytics and sedative-hypnotic agents		
Antihistamines	Oversedation	Decrease total dosage; administer most at bedtime
	Rash	Discontinue medication
Benzodiazepines	Disinhibition	Discontinue medication
	Cognitive decrements	Reduce dosage or discontinue
Lithium	Gastrointestinal: nausea, vomiting, abdominal pain, diarrhea, metallic taste	Consider dosage reduction if persistent
	CNS: tremor, memory lapses, fatigue	Consider dosage reduction if persistent
	Endocrine: goiter	Discontinue medication and follow with laboratory studies
	Renal: polyuria, polydipsia	Monitor BUN, creatinine, electrolytes, and urinalysis on a regular basis (every 2–3 months)
	Hematological: leukocytosis	Monitor; may not be of clinical significance

LFTs, liver function tests; TCA, tricyclic antidepressant; ECG, electrocardiogram; CNS, central nervous system; EEG, electroencephalogram; BUN, blood urea nitrogen.
Adapted from Barbara J. Coffey, M.D.

until clinical effects are observed. The clinician, however, should not hesitate to use adult dosages in children if the dosages are effective and the adverse effects are acceptable.

Geriatric Patients. The two major concerns when treating geriatric persons with psychotherapeutic drugs are that elderly persons may be especially susceptible to adverse effects (particularly cardiac effects) and that they may metabolize drugs slowly (Table 1–12) and thus require low dosages of medication. Another concern is that geriatric persons are often taking other medications, thereby requiring the clinician to consider the possible drug interactions.

In practice, clinicians should begin treating geriatric persons with a low dosage, usually about one half the usual dosage. The dosage should be raised in small amounts more slowly than for middle-aged adults until either a clinical benefit is achieved or unacceptable adverse effects appear. Although many geriatric persons require a low dosage of medication, many others require the usual adult dosage. Tables 1–13 through 1–20 provide clinical information on commonly used drugs in geropsychiatry.

Pregnant and Nursing Women. The basic rule is to avoid administering any drug to a woman who is pregnant (particularly during the first trimester) or who is breast-feeding a child. This rule, however, occasionally needs to be broken when the mother's mental disorder is severe.

If a potentially teratogenic psychotherapeutic medication needs to be administered during pregnancy, the risks and benefits of therapeutic abortion should be discussed. The most teratogenic drugs in the psychopharmacopeia are valproate (Depakene), carbamazepine, and lithium. Valproate exposure is associated with spina bifida or midline craniofacial abnormalities in up to 10 percent of pregnancies, and carbamazepine exposure causes similar midline defects in up to 5 percent of pregnancies. Prophylactic folic acid supplementation may reduce the risk of spina bifida. Lithium exposure during pregnancy is associated with birth anomalies in 4 percent

TABLE 1–12
PHARMACOKINETICS AND AGING

Phase	Change	Effect
Absorption	Gastric pH increases Decreased surface villi Decreased gastric motility and delayed gastric emptying Intestinal perfusion decreases	Absorption is slowed but just as complete
Distribution	Total body water and lean body mass decrease Increased total body fat, more marked in women than in men	Volume of distribution (Vd) increases for lipid-soluble drugs, decreases for water-soluble drugs
	Albumin decreased, gamma globulin increased, alpha, acid glycoprotein unchanged	The free or unbound percentage of albumin-bound drugs increases
Metabolism	Renal: renal blood flow and glomerular filtration rates decrease Hepatic: decreased enzyme activity and perfusion	Decreased metabolism leads to prolonged half-lives, if Vd remains the same
Total body weight	Decreases	Think on a mg-per-kg basis
Receptor sensitivity	May increase	Increased effect

From Guttmacher LB: *Concise Guide to Somatic Therapies in Psychiatry,* American Psychiatric Press, Washington, DC, 1988:126, with permission.

TABLE 1-13
PHARMACOKINETICS AND AVERAGE DAILY GERIATRIC DOSAGE OF COMMONLY USED BENZODIAZEPINES

Drug	Half-Life (h)	Active Metabolites	Average Daily Dosage (mg)	
			Adult	Elderly
Alprazolam	12–15	Yes (minor)	0.5–6	0.25–3
Chlordiazepoxide	7–28	Yes (many)	25–100	5–50
Clonazepam	18–56	Yes	1–8	0.5–4
Clorazepate	30–200	Yes	15–60	7.5–30
Diazepam	20–60	Yes	5–30	2–15
Halazepam	15–50	Yes	20–160	20–80
Lorazepam	10–20	None	1–6	0.5–3
Oxazepam	5–15	None	15–90	10–45
Prazepam	25–200	Yes	20–60	10–20

From Sheikh JI. Anxiety disorders. In: *Textbook of Geriatric Neuropsychiatry*, Coffey CE, Cummings JL. American Psychiatric Press, Washington, DC, 1994, with permission.

of pregnancies. In particular, lithium exposure is associated in 0.1 percent of pregnancies with Ebstein's anomaly, a serious abnormality in cardiac development.

Other psychotherapeutic drugs (antidepressants, antipsychotics, and anxiolytics), although less clearly associated with birth defects, should also be avoided during pregnancy if at all possible. When a pregnant woman becomes psychotic, serotonin-dopamine antagonists, dopamine-receptor antagonists, or electroconvulsive therapy (ECT) is preferable to valproate, carbamazepine, or lithium.

The administration of psychotherapeutic drugs at or near delivery may cause neonatal sedation and respiratory depression, possibly requiring mechanical ventilatory support, or physical dependence on the drug, requiring detoxification and the treatment of a withdrawal syndrome.

Virtually all psychotherapeutic drugs are secreted in the milk of a nursing mother; therefore, mothers taking these agents should not breast-feed their infants.

Persons with Hepatic or Renal Insufficiency.   Drugs that are metabolized in the liver may accumulate to toxic concentrations in persons with hepatocellular insufficiency of any cause, including cirrhosis, hepatitis, metabolic disorders, and bile duct obstruction. Drugs that are excreted by the kidneys may accumulate to toxic concentrations in persons with renal insufficiency of any cause, including atherosclerosis, nephrosis, nephritis, infiltrative disorders, and outflow obstruction. Presence of hepatocellular or renal insufficiency requires administration of a reduced dosage, usually half of the recommended dosage for healthy persons. Clini-

TABLE 1-14
GERIATRIC DOSAGES OF NONBENZODIAZEPINE DRUGS USED TO TREAT ANXIETY AND INSOMNIA

Generic Name	Trade Name	Geriatric Dosage Range (mg a day)
Buspirone	BuSpar	5–60
Secobarbital	Seconal	50–300
Meprobamate	Miltown	400–800
Chloral hydrate	Noctec	500–1000
Zolpidem	Ambien	2.5–10
Zaleplon	Sonata	5–20
Propranolol	Inderal	40–160
Atenolol	Tenormin	25–100

TABLE 1–15
GERIATRIC DOSAGES AND ADVERSE EFFECTS OF ANTIPSYCHOTICS

Medication	Brand Name	Dosage Range in Elderly Patients (mg a day)[a]	Adverse Effects[b]			Receptor Affinity In Vitro	
			Anticholinergic Effects	Extrapyramidal Effects	Hypotensive Effects	Dopamine Receptor (D₂)	Serotonin Receptor (5-HT₂ₐ)
Chlorpromazine	Thorazine	10–300	+++	+	+++	++	++
Thioridazine	Mellaril	10–300	+++	+	+++	++	+
Loxapine	Loxitane	5–75	++	++	++	++	++
Molindone	Moban	5–75	++	++	+	++	+
Perphenazine	Trilafon	2–32	++	++	++	++	+
Thiothixene	Navane	1–15	++	+++	++	+++	+
Fluphenazine	Prolixin	0.5–5	+	+++	+	+++	+
Haloperidol	Haldol	0.5–5	+	+++	+	+++	+
Clozapine[c]	Clozaril	12.5–200	+++	−	+++	+	++
Risperidone[c]	Risperdal	0.5–6	+	+	+	+++	+++
Olanzapine[c]	Zyprexa	2.5–20	++	−	+	++	++
Quetiapine[c]	Seroquel	25–500	+	−	+	+	+

[a] Routine clinical dosage ranges are listed. Higher or lower dosages may be indicated in some cases.
[b] Medication effects: −, none; +, mild; ++, moderate; +++, marked.
[c] Optimal dosage ranges and adverse effects listed are based on limited experience.
Table by David L. Sultzer, M.D., and Helen Lavretsky, M.D.

TABLE 1–16
ADVERSE EFFECTS OF ANTIPSYCHOTIC MEDICATIONS IN ELDERLY PATIENTS

Anticholinergic effects	Cognitive impairment,[a] delirium,[a] dry mouth, blurred vision, constipation,[a] urinary retention,[a] tachycardia, exacerbation of narrow-angle glaucoma
Acute extrapyramidal effects	Rigidity,[a] bradykinesia,[a] tremor,[a] dystonia, akathisia
Tardive movement disorders	Tardive dyskinesia,[a] tardive dystonia, tardive akathisia
Cardiovascular effects	Hypotension,[a] tachycardia,[a] electrocardiogram changes (nonspecific T-wave changes, increased QT interval)
Other adverse effects	Sedation,[a] falls,[a] cognitive impairment,[a] elevated prolactin concentration, sexual dysfunction, weight gain, neuroleptic malignant syndrome, elevated hepatic enzyme values, jaundice, hyponatremia, seizure, skin photosensitivity, retinopathy, agranulocytosis, nasal congestion

[a] Effects due to dopamine receptor antagonists that are particularly common or severe among older patients, even with treatment at low dosages.
Table by David L. Sultzer, M.D., and Helen Lavretsky, M.D.

TABLE 1–17
GERIATRIC DOSAGES OF COMMONLY USED ANTIDEPRESSANTS

Generic Name	Trade Name	Geriatric Dosage Range (mg a day)
Tricyclics		
Imipramine	Tofranil	25–300
Desipramine	Norpramin, Pertofrane	10–300
Trimipramine	Surmontil	25–300
Amitriptyline	Elavil	25–300
Nortriptyline	Pamelor, Aventyl	10–150
Protriptyline	Vivactil	10–40
Doxepin	Adapin, Sinequan	10–300
Tetracyclic		
Maprotiline	Ludiomil	25–150
Serotonin-selective reuptake inhibitors		
Citalopram	Celexa	10–60
Fluoxetine	Prozac	5–80
Fluvoxamine	Luvox	25–150
Paroxetine	Paxil	5–20
Sertraline	Zoloft	50–200
Trazodone	Desyrel	100–500
Bupropion	Wellbutrin	75–450
Nefazodone	Serzone	100–400
Monoamine oxidase inhibitors (MAOIs)[a]		
Phenelzine	Nardil	15–45
Tranylcypromine[b]	Parnate	10–20

[a] Persons taking MAOIs should be on a tyramine-free diet.
[b] Not recommended in persons older than age 60 because of pressor effects.

TABLE 1–18
DRUGS USED TO TREAT BIPOLAR DISORDER IN THE ELDERLY

Generic Name	Trade Name	Geriatric Dosage Range (mg a day)
Lithium carbonate	Eskalith, Lithane, Lithotabs	75–900
Carbamazepine	Tegretol	200–1200
Valproate, divalproex	Depakote, Depakene	250–1000
Clonazepam	Klonopin	0.5–1.5
Olanzapine	Zyprexa	2.5–20

TABLE 1-19
MEDICATIONS FOR DEMENTIA IN THE ELDERLY

Cholinesterase inhibitors
  Donepezil
  Rivastigmine
  Tacrine
Other medications available on the U.S. market
  Nonsteroidal anti-inflammatory drugs (e.g., ibuprofen)
  Estrogens
    Conjugated estrogens (Premarin)
    Estradiol
  Vitamin E

TABLE 1-20
GERIATRIC DOSAGES OF PSYCHOSTIMULANTS

Generic Name	Trade Name	Generic Dosage Range (mg a day)
Dextroamphetamine	Dexedrine	2.5-10
Pemoline	Cylert	18.75-37.5
Methylphenidate	Ritalin	2.5-40

cians should be particularly alert to signs and symptoms of adverse drug effects in persons with hepatic or renal disorders. If available, monitoring of plasma drug concentrations may help guide dosage adjustments.

Persons with Other Medical Illnesses.   Considerations in administering psychotherapeutic drugs to medically ill persons include a potentially increased sensitivity to the drug's adverse effects, either increased or decreased metabolism and excretion of the drug, and interactions with other medications. As with children and geriatric persons, the most reasonable clinical practice is to begin with a low dosage, increase it slowly, and watch for both clinical and adverse effects.

Laboratory Monitoring

The risk of an adverse reaction to certain drugs can sometimes be predicted through laboratory monitoring of either the plasma drug concentrations or blood indicators of organ dysfunction, such as hepatic transaminases.

For a more detailed discussion of this topic, see Grebb JA: General Principles of Psychopharmacology, Sec 31.1, p 2235, and Janicak PG, Davis JM: Pharmacokinetics and Drug Interactions, Sec 31.2, p 2250, in CTP/VII.

2

α_2-Adrenergic Receptor Agonists: Clonidine and Guanfacine

Clonidine (Catapres) and guanfacine (Tenex) are α_2-adrenergic receptor agonists used in psychiatry for control of the withdrawal symptoms from opiates and opioids, treatment of Tourette's disorder, suppression of agitation in posttraumatic stress disorder, and control of aggressive or hyperactive behavior in children, especially those with autistic features.

CHEMISTRY

The molecular structures of clonidine and guanfacine are shown in Figure 2–1.

PHARMACOLOGICAL ACTIONS

Clonidine and guanfacine are well absorbed from the gastrointestinal (GI) tract and reach peak plasma levels 1 to 3 hours after oral administration. The half-life of clonidine is 6 to 20 hours and that of guanfacine is 10 to 30 hours.

The agonist effects of clonidine and guanfacine on presynaptic α_2-adrenergic receptors in the sympathetic nuclei of the brain result in a decrease in the amount of norepinephrine released from the presynaptic nerve terminals. This serves generally to reset the body's sympathetic tone at a lower level and decrease arousal.

THERAPEUTIC INDICATIONS

There is considerably more experience in clinical psychiatry with clonidine than with guanfacine. Recent interest in the use of guanfacine for the same indications that respond to clonidine centers on guanfacine's longer half-life and relative lack of sedative effects.

Withdrawal from Opioids, Alcohol, Benzodiazepines, or Nicotine

Clonidine and guanfacine are effective in reducing the autonomic symptoms of rapid opioid withdrawal (for example, hypertension, tachycardia, dilated pupils, sweating, lacrimation, and rhinorrhea) but not the associated subjective sensations. Clonidine administration (0.1 to 0.2 mg two to four times a day) is initiated prior to detoxification and is then tapered off over 1 to 2 weeks (Table 2–1).

Clonidine and guanfacine can reduce symptoms of alcohol and benzodiazepine withdrawal, including anxiety, diarrhea, and tachycardia. Clonidine and guanfacine can reduce craving, anxiety, and irritability symptoms of nicotine withdrawal. The

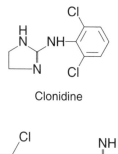

Clonidine

Guanfacine

Figure 2-1. Molecular structures of clonidine and guanfacine.

transdermal patch formulation of clonidine is associated with better long-term compliance for purposes of detoxification than is the tablet formulation.

Tourette's Disorder

Clonidine and guanfacine are effective drugs for the treatment of Tourette's disorder. Most clinicians begin treatment for Tourette's disorder with the standard

TABLE 2-1
ORAL CLONIDINE PROTOCOLS FOR OPIOID DETOXIFICATION

Clonidine 0.1–0.2 mg p.o. 4 times a day; hold for systolic blood pressure <90 mm Hg or bradycardia; stabilize for 2–3 days, then taper over 5–10 days
OR
Clonidine 0.1–0.2 mg p.o. q4–6h as needed for withdrawal signs or symptoms; stabilize for 2–3 days, then taper over 5–10 days
OR
Test dose with clonidine 0.1–0.2 mg p.o. or sublingually (for patients weighing over 200 lb) check blood pressure after 1 h. If diastolic BP >70 mm Hg and no symptoms of hypotension, begin treatment as follows

Weight (lb)	Number of clonidine patches
<110	2-3 TTS-1 patches
110–160	1 TTS-2 and 2 TTS-1 patches
160–200	2 TTS-2 patches
>200	2-3 TTS-2 patches

OR
Test dose of oral clonidine 0.1 mg; check BP after 1 h (if systolic blood pressure <90, do not give patch)
Place 2 TTS-2 clonidine patches (or 3 patches if patient weighs >150 lb) on hairless area of upper body; then
For first 23 h after patch application, give oral clonidine 0.2 mg q6h; then
For next 24 h, give oral clonidine 0.1 mg q6h
Change patches weekly
After 2 weeks of 2 patches, switch to 1 TTS-2 patch (or 2 TTS-2 patches if patient weighs >150 lb)
After 1 week of 1patch, discontinue patches

From American Society of Addiction Medicine: Detoxification: Principle and Protocols. In: *The Principles Update Series: Topics in Addiction Medicine,* section 11. American Society of Addiction, 1997, with permission.

dopamine receptor antagonists, haloperidol (Haldol) and pimozide (Orap), and the serotonin-dopamine antagonists, risperidone (Risperdal) and olanzapine (Zyprexa). However, if concerned about the adverse effects of these drugs, the clinician may begin treatment with clonidine or guanfacine. The starting child dosage of clonidine is 0.05 mg a day; it can be raised to 0.3 mg a day in divided doses. Three months are needed before the beneficial effects of clonidine can be seen in Tourette's disorder. The response rate has been reported to be in the range of 0 to 70 percent.

Other Tic Disorders

Clonidine and guanfacine reduce the frequency and severity of tics in persons with tic disorder with or without comorbid attention-deficit/hyperactivity symptoms.

Hyperactivity and Aggression in Children

Clonidine and guanfacine can be useful alternatives for the treatment of attention-deficit/hyperactivity disorder. They are used in place of sympathomimetics and antidepressants, which may produce paradoxical worsening of hyperactivity in some children with mental retardation, aggression, or features on the spectrum of autism. Clonidine and guanfacine can improve mood, reduce activity level, and improve social adaptation. Some multiply-impaired children may respond favorably to clonidine, while others may simply become sedated. The starting dosage is 0.05 mg a day; it can be raised to 0.3 mg a day in divided doses. The efficacy of clonidine and guanfacine for control of hyperactivity and aggression often diminishes over several months of use.

Clonidine or guanfacine can be combined with methylphenidate (Ritalin) or dextroamphetamine (Dexedrine, Dextrostat) to treat hyperactivity and inattentiveness, respectively. A small number of cases have been reported of sudden death of children taking clonidine together with methylphenidate; however, it has not been conclusively demonstrated that these medications contributed to these deaths. The clinician should explain to the family that the efficacy and safety of this combination have not been investigated in controlled trials. Periodic cardiovascular assessments, including vital signs and electrocardiograms, are warranted if this combination is used.

Posttraumatic Stress Disorder

Acute exacerbations of posttraumatic stress disorder may be associated with hyperadrenergic symptoms, such as hyperarousal, exaggerated startle response, insomnia, vivid nightmares, tachycardia, agitation, hypertension, and perspiration. These symptoms may respond to the use of clonidine or, especially for overnight benefit, to the use of guanfacine.

Other Disorders

Other potential indications for clonidine include other anxiety disorders (panic disorder, phobias, obsessive-compulsive disorder, and generalized anxiety disorder) and mania, in which it may be synergistic with lithium (Eskalith) or carbamazepine (Tegretol). Anecdotal reports have noted the efficacy of clonidine in schizrenia and tardive dyskinesia. A clonidine patch can reduce the hypersalivation and dysphagia caused by clozapine (Clozaril).

PRECAUTIONS AND ADVERSE REACTIONS

The most common adverse effects associated with clonidine are dry mouth and eyes, fatigue, sedation, dizziness, nausea, hypotension, and constipation, which result in discontinuation of therapy by about 10 percent of all persons taking the drug. Some persons also experience sexual dysfunction. Tolerance may develop to these adverse effects. A similar but milder adverse effect profile is seen with guanfacine, especially at doses of 3 mg or more per day. Clonidine and guanfacine should not be taken by adults with blood pressure below 90/60 or with cardiac arrhythmias, especially bradycardia. Development of bradycardia warrants gradual, tapered discontinuation of the drug. Clonidine in particular is associated with sedation, and tolerance does not usually develop to this adverse effect. Uncommon central nervous system (CNS) adverse effects of clonidine include insomnia, anxiety, and depression; rare CNS adverse effects include vivid dreams, nightmares, and hallucinations. Fluid retention associated with clonidine treatment can be treated with diuretics.

The transdermal patch formulation of clonidine can cause local skin irritation, which can be minimized by rotating the sites of application.

Overdose

Persons who take an overdose of clonidine can present with coma and constricted pupils, symptoms similar to those of an opioid overdose. Other symptoms of overdose are decreased blood pressure, pulse, and respiratory rates. Guanfacine overdose produces a milder version of these symptoms. Clonidine and guanfacine should be used with caution in persons with heart disease, any type of vascular disease, renal disease, Raynaud's syndrome, or a history of depression. Clonidine and guanfacine should be avoided during pregnancy and by nursing mothers. Elderly persons are more sensitive to the drug than are younger adults. Children are susceptible to the same adverse effects as are adults.

Withdrawal

Abrupt discontinuation of clonidine can cause anxiety, restlessness, perspiration, tremor, abdominal pain, palpitations, headache, and a dramatic rise in blood pressure. These symptoms may appear about 20 hours after the last dose of clonidine and thus may be seen if one or two doses are skipped. A similar set of symptoms occasionally occurs 2 to 4 days after discontinuation of guanfacine, but the usual course

TABLE 2–2
α₂-ADRENERGIC RECEPTOR AGONISTS USED IN PSYCHIATRY[a]

Drug	Preparations	Usual Child Starting Dosage	Usual Child Dosage Range	Usual Starting Adult Dosage	Usual Adult Dosage
Clonidine tablets (Catapres)	0.1, 0.2, 0.3 mg	0.05 mg a day	Up to 0.3 mg a day tablets in divided doses	0.1–0.2 mg 2–4 times a day (0.2–0.8 mg a day)	0.3–1.2 mg a day, 2–3 times a day (1.2 mg a day maximal dosage)
Clonidine transdermal system (Catapres-TTS)	0.1, 0.2, 0.3 mg a day	0.05 mg a day	Up to 0.3 mg a day patch every 5 days (0.5 mg a day every 5 days maximal dosage)	0.1 mg a day every 7 days	0.1 mg a day patch per week 0.6 mg a day every 7 days)
Guanfacine (Tenex)	1, 2 mg tablets	1 mg a day at bedtime	1–2 mg a day at bedtime (3 mg a day maximal dosage)	1 mg a day at bedtime	1–2 mg at bedtime (3 mg a day maximal dosage)

[a] Dosages for medical indications, such as hypertension, vary.

is a gradual return to baseline blood pressure over 2 to 4 days. Because of the possibility of discontinuation symptoms, dosages of clonidine and guanfacine should be tapered down slowly.

DRUG INTERACTIONS

Coadministration of clonidine and tricyclic drugs can reduce the hypotensive effects of clonidine. Clonidine and guanfacine may enhance the CNS depressive effects of barbiturates, alcohol, other sedative-hypnotics, and trazodone (Desyrel). Clonidine and guanfacine may have an unwanted synergistic hypotensive effect if coadministered with other antihypertensive drugs. The α_2-adrenergic receptor antagonist yohimbine (Yocon) blocks the effects of clonidine and guanfacine. The concomitant use of β-adrenergic receptor antagonists can increase the severity of rebound phenomena when clonidine and guanfacine are discontinued.

LABORATORY INTERFERENCES

No known laboratory interferences are associated with the use of clonidine or guanfacine.

DOSAGE AND CLINICAL GUIDELINES

Clonidine is available in 0.1-, 0.2-, and 0.3-mg tablets. The usual starting dosage is 0.1 mg orally twice a day; the dosage can be raised by 0.1 mg a day to an appropriate level (up to 1.2 mg per day). Clonidine must always be tapered when it is discontinued, to avoid rebound hypertension, which may occur about 20 hours after the last clonidine dose. A weekly transdermal formulation of clonidine is available at doses of 0.1, 0.2, and 0.3 mg per day. The usual starting dosage is the 0.1-mg/day patch, which is changed each week for adults and every 5 days for children; the dosage can be increased as needed every 1 to 2 weeks. Transition from the oral to the transdermal formulations should be accomplished gradually, by overlapping them for 3 to 4 days.

Guanfacine is available in 1- and 2-mg tablets. The usual starting dose is 1 mg before sleep, and this may be increased to 2 mg before sleep after 3 to 4 weeks, if necessary. Regardless of the indication for which clonidine or guanfacine is being used, the drug should be withheld if a person becomes hypotensive (blood pressure below 90/60).

Table 2–2 provides a summary of the α_2-adrenergic receptor agonists used in psychiatry.

For a more detailed discussion of this topic, see Sussman N: Clonidine, Sec 31.16, p 2352, in CTP/VII.

3

β-Adrenergic Receptor Antagonists

β-Adrenergic receptor antagonists (also known as beta-blockers and β-adrenergic drugs) are peripherally and centrally acting agents for the treatment of social phobia (for example, performance anxiety), lithium (Eskalith)-induced postural tremor, neuroleptic-induced acute akathisia, and for the control of aggressive behavior (Table 3–1).

CHEMISTRY

The β-receptor antagonists most commonly used in psychiatry are propranolol (Inderal), nadolol (Corgard), pindolol (Visken), labetalol (Normodyne, Trandate), atenolol (Tenormin), metoprolol (Lopressor, Toprol), and acebutolol (Sectral). The molecular structures of these drugs are shown in Figure 3–1.

PHARMACOLOGICAL ACTIONS

The β-receptor antagonists differ with regard to lipophilicities, metabolic routes, β-receptor selectivity, and half-lives (Table 3–2). The absorption of the β-receptor antagonists from the gastrointestinal tract is variable. The agents that are most soluble in lipids (that is, are lipophilic) are likely to cross the blood–brain barrier and enter the brain; those agents that are least lipophilic are less likely to enter the brain. When central nervous system (CNS) effects are desired, a lipophilic drug may be preferred; when only peripheral effects are desired, a less lipophilic drug may be indicated.

Propranolol, nadolol, pindolol, and labetalol have essentially equal potency at both the β_1- and β_2-receptors, whereas metoprolol, atenolol, and acebutolol have greater affinity for the β_1-receptor than for the β_2-receptor. Relative β_1 selectivity confers few pulmonary and vascular effects on these drugs, although they must be used with caution in asthmatic persons, because the drugs retain some activity at the β_2-receptors.

Pindolol has sympathomimetic effects in addition to its β-antagonist effects, which has permitted its use for augmentation of antidepressant drugs. Pindolol, propranolol, and nadolol possess some antagonist activity at the serotonin 5-HT$_{1A}$ receptors.

THERAPEUTIC INDICATIONS

Anxiety Disorders

Propranolol is useful for the treatment of social phobia, primarily of the performance type (for example, disabling anxiety before a musical performance). Data are

TABLE 3–1
PSYCHIATRIC USES FOR β-ADRENERGIC RECEPTOR ANTAGONISTS

Definitely effective
  Performance anxiety
  Lithium-induced tremor
  Neuroleptic-induced akathisia
Probably effective
  Adjunctive therapy for alcohol withdrawal and other substance-related disorders
  Adjunctive therapy for aggressive or violent behavior
Possibly effective
  Antipsychotic augmentation
  Antidepressant augmentation

Non – β_1 – selective β_1 – selective

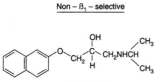

Propranolol

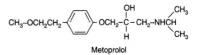

Metoprolol

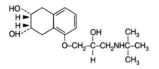

Nadolol

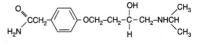

Atenolol

Pindolol

Acebutolol

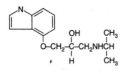

Labetalol

Figure 3–1. Molecular structures of β-adrenergic receptor antagonists.

TABLE 3–2
β-ADRENERGIC DRUGS USED IN PSYCHIATRY

Generic Name	Trade Name	Lipophilic	Metabolism	Receptor Selectivity	Half-Life (h)	Usual Starting Dosage (mg)	Usual Maximum Dosage (mg)
Propranolol	Inderal	Yes	Hepatic	$\beta_1 = \beta_2$	3–6	10–20 two or three times a day	30–140 three times a day
Nadolol	Corgard	No	Renal	$\beta_1 = \beta_2$	14–24	40 once daily	30–240 once daily
Pindolol	Visken	Intermediate	Hepatic	$\beta_1 = \beta_2$	3–4	5 two times a day	30 two times a day
Labetalol	Normodyne, Trandate	Intermediate	Hepatic	$\beta_1 = \beta_2$	4–6	100 two times a day	400–800 three times a day
Metoprolol	Lopressor	Yes	Hepatic	$\beta_1 > \beta_2$	3–4	50 two times a day	75–150 two times a day
Atenolol	Tenormin	No	Renal	$\beta_1 > \beta_2$	5–8	50 once daily	50–100 once daily
Acebutolol	Sectral	No	Hepatic	$\beta_1 > \beta_2$	3–4	400 once daily	600 two times a day

also available for its use in treatment of panic disorder, posttraumatic stress disorder, and generalized anxiety disorder. In social phobia, the common treatment approach is to take 10 to 40 mg of propranolol 20 to 30 minutes before the anxiety-provoking situation. Persons may try a test run of the β-receptor antagonist before using it before an anxiety-provoking situation to be sure that they do not experience any adverse effects from the drug or the dosage. β-Receptor antagonists may blunt cognition in some people. β-Receptor antagonists are less effective for the treatment of panic disorder than are benzodiazepines or selective serotonin reuptake inhibitors (SSRIs).

Lithium-Induced Postural Tremor

β-Receptor antagonists are beneficial for lithium-induced postural tremor and other medication-induced postural tremors—for example, those induced by tricyclic drugs and valproate (Depakene). The initial approach to this movement disorder includes lowering the dose of lithium, eliminating aggravating factors such as caffeine, and administration of lithium at bedtime. However, if these interventions are inadequate, propranolol in the range of 20 to 160 mg a day, given two or three times daily, is generally effective for the treatment of lithium-induced postural tremor.

Neuroleptic-Induced Acute Akathisia

Many studies have shown that β-receptor antagonists can be effective in the treatment of neuroleptic-induced acute akathisia. Most clinicians believe that β-receptor antagonists are more effective for this indication than are anticholinergics and benzodiazepines. β-receptor antagonists are not effective in the treatment of such neuroleptic-induced movement disorders as acute dystonia and parkinsonism.

Aggression and Violent Behavior

β-Receptor antagonists may be effective in reducing the number of aggressive and violent outbursts in persons with impulse disorders, schizophrenia, and aggression associated with brain injuries such as trauma, tumors, anoxic injury, encephalitis, alcohol dependence, and degenerative disorders (for example, Huntington's disease). Many studies have added a β-receptor antagonist to the ongoing therapy (for example, antipsychotics, anticonvulsants, lithium); therefore, it is difficult to distinguish additive effects from independent effects. Propranolol dosages for this indication range from 50 to 800 mg a day.

Alcohol Withdrawal

Propranolol has been reported to be useful as an adjuvant to benzodiazepines but not as a sole agent in the treatment of alcohol withdrawal. The following dose schedule is suggested: no propranolol for a pulse rate below 50; 50 mg propranolol for a pulse rate between 50 and 79; and 100 mg propranolol for a pulse rate of 80 or above.

Antidepressant Augmentation

Pindolol has been used to augment and hasten the antidepressant effects of SS-RIs, tricyclic drugs, and electroconvulsive therapy. Small studies have shown that pindolol administered at the onset of antidepressant therapy may shorten the usual 2- to 4-week latency of antidepressant response by several days. Because of the possibility that the β-receptor antagonists may induce depression in some persons, augmentation strategies with these drugs need to be further clarified in controlled trials.

Other Disorders

A number of case reports and controlled studies have reported data indicating that β-receptor antagonists may be of modest benefit for persons with schizophrenia and with manic symptoms. It has also been used in some cases of stuttering.

PRECAUTIONS AND ADVERSE REACTIONS

The β-receptor antagonists are contraindicated for use in people with asthma, insulin-dependent diabetes, congestive heart failure, significant vascular disease, persistent angina, and hyperthyroidism. The contraindication in diabetic persons is due to the drugs' antagonizing the normal physiological response to hypoglycemia. The β-receptor antagonists can worsen atrioventricular (A-V) conduction defects and lead to complete A-V heart block and death. If the clinician decides that the risk-benefit ratio warrants a trial of a β-receptor antagonist in a person with one of these coexisting medical conditions, a β_1-selective agent should be the first choice. All currently available β-receptor antagonists are excreted in breast milk and should be administered with caution to nursing women.

The most common adverse effects of β-receptor antagonists are hypotension and bradycardia. In persons at risk for these adverse effects, a test dosage of 20 mg a day of propranolol can be given to assess reaction to the drug. Depression has been associated with lipophilic β-receptor antagonists such as propranolol, but it is probably rare. Nausea, vomiting, diarrhea, and constipation may also be caused by treatment with these agents. Serious CNS adverse effects (for example, agitation, confusion, and hallucinations) are rare. Table 3–3 lists the possible adverse affects of β-receptor antagonists.

DRUG INTERACTIONS

Concomitant administration of propranolol results in increases in plasma concentrations of antipsychotics, anticonvulsants, theophylline (Theo-Dur, Slo-Bid), and levothyroxine (Synthroid). Other β-receptor antagonists possibly have similar effects. The β-receptor antagonists that are eliminated by the kidneys may have similar effects on drugs that are also eliminated by the renal route. Barbiturates, phenytoin (Dilantin), and cigarette smoking increase the elimination of β-receptor antagonists that are metabolized by the liver. Several reports have associated hypertensive crises and bradycardia with the coadministration of β-receptor antagonists and monoamine oxidase inhibitors. Depressed myocardial contractility and A-V nodal conduction may occur from concomitant administration of a β-receptor antagonist and calcium channel inhibitors.

LABORATORY INTERFERENCES

The β-receptor antagonists do not interfere with standard laboratory tests.

Dosage and Clinical Guidelines

Propranolol is available in 10-, 20-, 40-, 60-, 80-, and 90-mg tablets; 4-, 8-, and 80-mg/mL solutions; and 60-, 80-, 120-, and 160-mg sustained-release capsules. Nadolol is available in 20-, 40-, 80-, 120-, and 160-mg tablets. Pindolol is available in 5- and 10-mg tablets. Labetalol is available in 100-, 200-, and 300-mg tablets. Metoprolol is available in 50- and 100-mg tablets; and in 50-, 100-, and 200-mg sustained-release tablets. Atenolol is available in 25-, 50-, and 100-mg tablets. Acebutolol is available in 200- and 400-mg capsules.

For the treatment of chronic disorders, propranolol administration is usually initiated at 10 mg by mouth three times a day or 20 mg by mouth twice daily. The dosage can be raised by 20 to 30 mg a day until a therapeutic effect begins to emerge. The dosage should be leveled off at the appropriate range for the disorder under treatment. The treatment of aggressive behavior sometimes requires dosages up to

TABLE 3–3
ADVERSE EFFECTS AND TOXICITY OF β-ADRENERGIC RECEPTOR ANTAGONISTS

Cardiovascular
  Hypotension
  Bradycardia
  Dizziness
  Congestive failure (in patients with compromised myocardial function)
Respiratory
  Asthma (less risk with β_1-selective drugs)
Metabolic
  Worsened hypoglycemia in diabetic patients on insulin or oral agents
Gastrointestinal
  Nausea
  Diarrhea
  Abdominal pain
Sexual Function
  Impotence
Neuropsychiatric
  Lassitude
  Fatigue
  Dysphoria
  Insomnia
  Vivid nightmares
  Depression (rare)
  Psychosis (rare)
Other (rare)
  Raynaud's phenomenon
  Peyronie's disease
Withdrawal syndrome
  Rebound worsening of preexisting angina pectoris when β-adrenergic receptor antagonists are
    discontinued

800 mg a day, and therapeutic effects may not be seen until the person has been receiving the maximal dosage for 4 to 8 weeks. For the treatment of social phobia, primarily the performance type, the patient should take 10 to 40 mg of propranolol 20 to 30 minutes before the performance.

Pulse and blood pressure readings should be taken regularly, and the drug should be withheld if the pulse rate is below 50 or the systolic blood pressure is below 90. The drug should be temporarily discontinued if it produces severe dizziness, ataxia, or wheezing. Treatment with β-receptor antagonists should never be discontinued abruptly. Propranolol should be tapered by 60 mg a day until a dosage of 60 mg a day is reached, after which the drug should be tapered by 10 to 20 mg a day every 3 or 4 days.

For a more detailed discussion of this topic, see Simpson GM, Flowers CJ: β-Adrenergic Receptor Antagonists, Sec 31.5, p 2271 in CTP/VII.

4

Amantadine

Amantadine (Symmetrel) is used primarily for the treatment of medication-induced movement disorders, such as neuroleptic-induced parkinsonism. It is also used as an antiviral agent for the prophylaxis and treatment of influenza A infection.

CHEMISTRY

Amantadine's molecular structure is given in Figure 4–1.

PHARMACOLOGICAL ACTIONS

Amantadine is well absorbed from the gastrointestinal (GI) tract after oral administration, reaches peak plasma concentrations in approximately 2 to 3 hours, has a half-life of about 12 to 18 hours, and attains steady-state concentrations after approximately 4 to 5 days of therapy. Amantadine is excreted unmetabolized in the urine. Amantadine plasma concentrations can be as much as twice as high in elderly persons as in younger adults. Patients with renal failure accumulate amantadine in their bodies.

Amantadine augments dopaminergic neurotransmission in the central nervous system (CNS); however, the precise mechanism for the effect is unknown. The mechanism may involve dopamine release from presynaptic vesicles, blocking reuptake of dopamine into presynaptic nerve terminals, or an agonist effect on post synaptic dopamine receptors.

THERAPEUTIC INDICATIONS

The primary indication for amantadine in psychiatry is for the treatment of extrapyramidal signs and symptoms, such as parkinsonism, akinesia, and so-called rabbit syndrome (focal perioral tremor of the choreoathetoid type) caused by the administration of dopamine receptor antagonist drugs (e.g., haloperidol [Haldol]). Amantadine is as effective as the anticholinergics (e.g., benztropine [Cogentin]) for these indications and results in improvement in approximately one half of all persons who take it. However, amantadine is not generally considered as effective as the anticholinergics for the treatment of acute dystonic reactions and is not effective in treating tardive dyskinesia and akathisia.

Amantadine is a reasonable compromise for persons with extrapyramidal symptoms who would be sensitive to additional anticholinergic effects, particularly those taking a low-potency dopamine receptor antagonist or the elderly. Elderly persons are prone to anticholinergic adverse effects in both the CNS, such as anticholinergic delirium, and in the peripheral nervous system, such as urinary reten-

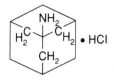

Figure 4-1. Molecular structure of amantadine.

tion. Amantadine is associated with less memory impairment than the anticholinergics are.

Amantadine has been reported to be of benefit in treating some selective serotonin reuptake inhibitor–associated side effects, such as lethargy, fatigue, anorgasmia, and ejaculatory inhibition.

Amantadine is used in general medical practice for the treatment of parkinsonism of all causes, including idiopathic parkinsonism.

PRECAUTIONS AND ADVERSE EFFECTS

The most common CNS effects are mild dizziness, insomnia, and impaired concentration (dosage related), which occur in 5 to 10 percent of all persons. Irritability, depression, anxiety, dysarthria, and ataxia occur in 1 to 5 percent of persons. More-severe CNS adverse effects, including seizures and psychotic symptoms, have been reported. Nausea is the most common peripheral adverse effect of amantadine. Headache, loss of appetite, and blotchy spots on the skin have also been reported.

Livedo reticularis of the legs (a purple discoloration of the skin, caused by dilation of blood vessels) has been reported in up to 5 percent of persons who take the drug for over a month. It usually diminishes with elevation of the legs and resolves in almost all cases when drug use is terminated.

Amantadine is relatively contraindicated in persons with renal disease or a seizure disorder. Amantadine should be used with caution in persons with edema or cardiovascular disease. Some evidence indicates that amantadine is teratogenic and, therefore, should not be taken by pregnant women. Because amantadine is excreted in milk, women who are breast-feeding should not take the drug.

Suicide attempts with amantadine overdosages are life threatening. Symptoms can include toxic psychoses (confusion, hallucinations, aggressiveness) and cardiopulmonary arrest. Emergency treatment beginning with gastric lavage is indicated.

DRUG INTERACTIONS

Coadministration of amantadine with phenelzine (Nardil) or other monoamine oxidase inhibitors (MAOIs) may result in a significant increase in resting blood pressure. The coadministration of amantadine with CNS stimulants can result in insomnia, irritability, nervousness, and possibly seizures or irregular heartbeat. Amantadine should not be coadministered with anticholinergics because unwanted side effects—such as confusion, hallucinations, nightmares, dryness of mouth, and blurred vision—may be exacerbated.

DOSAGE AND CLINICAL GUIDELINES

Amantadine is available in 100-mg capsules and as a 50 mg/5 mL syrup. The usual starting dosage of amantadine is 100 mg given orally twice a day, although the dosage can be cautiously increased up to 200 mg given orally twice a day if indicated. Amantadine should be used in persons with renal impairment only in consultation with the physician treating the renal condition. If amantadine is successful in the treatment of the drug-induced extrapyramidal symptoms, it should be continued for 4 to 6 weeks and then discontinued to see whether the person has become tolerant to the neurological adverse effects of the antipsychotic medication. Amantadine should be tapered over 1 to 2 weeks once a decision has been made to discontinue the drug. Persons taking amantadine should not drink alcoholic beverages.

For a more detailed discussion of this topic, see Meyer JM, Simpson GM: Anticholinergics and Amantadine, Sec 31.6, p 1919, in CTP/VII.

5

Anticholinergics

In the clinical practice of psychiatry, the anticholinergic drugs are primarily used for the treatment of medication-induced movement disorders, particularly neuroleptic-induced parkinsonism, neuroleptic-induced acute dystonia, and medication-induced postural tremor.

CHEMISTRY

The molecular structures of representative anticholinergic drugs are shown in Figure 5–1.

PHARMACOLOGICAL ACTIONS

All anticholinergic drugs are well absorbed from the gastrointestinal tract after oral administration, and all are lipophilic enough to enter the central nervous system (CNS). Trihexyphenidyl (Artane) and benztropine (Cogentin) reach peak plasma concentrations in 2 to 3 hours after oral administration and have a duration of action of 1 to 12 hours. Benztropine is absorbed equally rapidly by intramuscular (i.m.) and intravenous (i.v.) administration; intramuscular administration is preferred because of its low risk for adverse effects.

All six anticholinergic drugs listed in this chapter block muscarinic acetylcholine receptors, and benztropine and ethopropazine (Parsidol) also have some antihistaminergic effects. None of the available anticholinergic drugs has any effects on the nicotinic acetylcholine receptors. Of the six drugs, trihexyphenidyl is the most stimulating agent, perhaps acting through dopaminergic neurons, and benztropine is the least stimulating and, thus, is least associated with abuse potential.

THERAPEUTIC INDICATIONS

The primary indication for the use of anticholinergics in psychiatric practice is for the treatment of *neuroleptic-induced parkinsonism*, characterized by tremor, rigidity, cogwheeling, bradykinesia, sialorrhea, stooped posture, and festination. All the available anticholinergics are equally effective in the treatment of parkinsonian symptoms. Neuroleptic-induced parkinsonism is most common in the elderly and is most frequently seen with high-potency dopamine receptor antagonists, for example, haloperidol (Haldol). The onset of symptoms usually occurs after 2 or 3 weeks of treatment. The incidence of neuroleptic-induced parkinsonism is significantly lower with the newer antipsychotic drugs of the serotonin-dopamine antagonist (SDA) class.

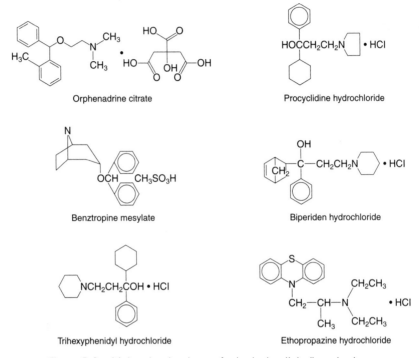

Figure 5-1. Molecular structures of selected anticholinergic drugs.

Another indication is for the treatment of *neuroleptic-induced acute dystonia*, which is most common in young men. The syndrome often occurs early in the course of treatment, is commonly associated with high-potency dopamine receptor antagonists (e.g., haloperidol), and most commonly affects the muscles of the neck, the tongue, the face, and the back. Anticholinergic drugs are effective both in the short-term treatment of dystonias and in prophylaxis against neuroleptic-induced acute dystonias.

Akathisia is characterized by a subjective and objective sense of restlessness, anxiety, and agitation. Although a trial of anticholinergics for the treatment of neuroleptic-induced acute akathisia is reasonable, these drugs are not generally considered as effective as the β-adrenergic receptor antagonists, the benzodiazepines, and clonidine (Catapres).

PRECAUTIONS AND ADVERSE REACTIONS

The adverse effects of the anticholinergic drugs result from blockade of muscarinic acetylcholine receptors. Anticholinergic drugs should be used cautiously, if at all, by persons with prostatic hypertrophy, urinary retention, and narrow-angle glaucoma. The anticholinergics are occasionally used as drugs of abuse because of their mild mood-elevating properties.

The most serious adverse effect associated with anticholinergic toxicity is anticholinergic intoxication, which can be characterized by delirium, coma, seizures, agitation, hallucinations, severe hypotension, supraventricular tachycardia, and peripheral manifestations—flushing, mydriasis, dry skin, hyperthermia, and decreased bowel sounds. Treatment should begin with the immediate discontinuation of all anticholinergic drugs. The syndrome of anticholinergic intoxication can be diagnosed and treated with physostigmine (Antilirium, Eserine), an inhibitor of anticholinesterase, 1 to 2 mg i.v. (1 mg every 2 minutes) or i.m. every 30 or 60 minutes. Treatment with physostigmine should be used only in severe cases and only when emergency cardiac monitoring and life-support services are available, because physostigmine can lead to severe hypotension and bronchial constriction.

DRUG INTERACTIONS

The most common drug-drug interactions with the anticholinergics occur when they are coadministered with psychotropics that also have high anticholinergic activity, such as dopamine receptor antagonists, tricyclic and tetracyclic drugs, and monoamine oxidase inhibitors (MAOIs). Many other prescription drugs and over-the-counter cold preparations also induce significant anticholinergic activity. The coadministration of those drugs can result in a life-threatening anticholinergic intoxication syndrome. Anticholinergic drugs can also delay gastric emptying, thereby decreasing the absorption of drugs that are broken down in the stomach and usually absorbed in the duodenum (e.g., levodopa [Larodopa] and dopamine receptor antagonists).

LABORATORY INTERFERENCES

No known laboratory interferences have been associated with anticholinergics.

DOSAGE AND CLINICAL GUIDELINES

The six anticholinergic drugs discussed in this chapter are available in a range of preparations (Table 5–1).

Neuroleptic-Induced Parkinsonism

For the treatment of neuroleptic-induced parkinsonism, the equivalent of 1 to 4 mg benztropine should be given one to four times daily. The anticholinergic drug should be administered for 4 to 8 weeks, then it should be discontinued to assess whether the person still requires the drug. Anticholinergic drugs should be tapered over a period of 1 to 2 weeks.

Treatment with anticholinergics as prophylaxis against the development of neuroleptic-induced parkinsonism is usually not indicated, since the symptoms of neuroleptic-induced parkinsonism are usually mild enough and gradual enough in onset to allow the clinician to initiate treatment only after it is clearly indicated. However,

TABLE 5–1
ANTICHOLINERGIC DRUGS

Generic Name	Brand Name	Tablet Size	Injectable	Usual Daily Oral Dose	Short-Term Intramuscular or Intravenous Dose
Benztropine	Cogentin	0.5, 1, 2 mg	1 mg/mL	1–4 mg one to three times	1–2 mg
Biperiden	Akineton	2 mg	5 mg/mL	2 mg one to three times	2 mg
Ethopropazine	Parsidol	10, 50 mg	—	50–100 mg one to three times	—
Orphenadrine	Norflex, Dispal	100 mg	30 mg/mL	50–100 mg three times	60 mg IV given over 5 min
Procyclidine	Kemadrin	5 mg	—	2.5–5 mg three times	—
Trihexyphenidyl	Artane, Trihexane, Trihexy-5	2, 5 mg elixir 2 mg per 5 mL	—	2–5 mg two to four times	—

in young men, prophylaxis may be indicated, especially if a high-potency dopamine receptor antagonist is being used. The clinician should attempt to discontinue the antiparkinsonian agent in 4 to 6 weeks to assess whether its continued use is necessary.

Neuroleptic-Induced Acute Dystonia

For the short-term treatment and prophylaxis of neuroleptic-induced acute dystonia, 1 to 2 mg of benztropine or its equivalent in another drug should be given i.m.. The dose can be repeated in 20 to 30 minutes as needed. If the person still does not improve in another 20 to 30 minutes, a benzodiazepine (for example, 1 mg i.m. or i.v. lorazepam [Ativan]) should be given. Laryngeal dystonia is a medical emergency and should be treated with benztropine, up to 4 mg in a 10-minute period, followed by 1 to 2 mg of lorazepam, administered slowly by the i.v. route.

Prophylaxis against dystonias is indicated in persons who have had one episode or in persons at high risk (young men taking high-potency dopamine receptor antagonists). Prophylactic treatment is given for 4 to 8 weeks and then gradually tapered over 1 to 2 weeks to allow assessment of its continued need. The prophylactic use of anticholinergics in persons requiring antipsychotic drugs has largely become a moot issue because of the availability of serotonin-dopamine antagonists, which are relatively free of parkinsonian effects.

Akathisia

As mentioned above, anticholinergics are not the first drugs of choice for this syndrome. The β-adrenergic receptor antagonists (Chapter 3) and perhaps the benzodiazepines (Chapter 8) and clonidine (Chapter 2) are preferable drugs to try initially.

For a more detailed discussion of this topic, see Meyer JM, Simpson GM: Anticholinergics and Amantadine, Sec 31.6, p 2276, in CTP/VII.

6

Antihistamines

Certain antihistamines (antagonists of histamine H_1 receptors) are used in clinical psychiatry to treat neuroleptic-induced parkinsonism and neuroleptic-induced acute dystonia and also as hypnotics and anxiolytics. Diphenhydramine (Benadryl) is used to treat neuroleptic-induced parkinsonism and neuroleptic-induced acute dystonia and sometimes as a hypnotic. Hydroxyzine hydrochloride (Atarax) and hydroxyzine pamoate (Vistaril) are used as anxiolytics. Promethazine (Phenergan) is used for its sedative and anxiolytic effects. Cyproheptadine (Periactin) has been used for the treatment of anorexia nervosa and inhibited male and female orgasm caused by serotonergic agents.

So-called second-generation H_1 receptor antagonists fexofenadine (Allegra), loratadine (Claritin), and cetirizine (Zyrtec) are not used in psychiatry. Terfenadine (Seldane) and astemizole (Hismanal) have been withdrawn from commercial availability because they are associated with serious cardiac arrhythmias when coadministered with some drugs (e.g., nefazodone [Serzone], selective serotonin reuptake inhibitors [SSRIs]); these drugs can cause serious and life-threatening cardiac toxicity.

Table 6–1 lists antihistaminic drugs not used in psychiatry but which may have psychiatric adverse effects or drug-drug interactions.

CHEMISTRY

The molecular structures of representative first-generation antihistamines used in psychiatry are shown in Figure 6–1.

PHARMACOLOGICAL ACTIONS

The H_1 antagonists used in psychiatry are well absorbed from the gastrointestinal (GI) tract. The antiparkinsonian effects of intramuscular (i.m.) diphenhydramine have their onset in 15 to 30 minutes, and the sedative effects of diphenhydramine peak in 1 to 3 hours. The sedative effects of hydroxyzine and promethazine begin after 20 to 60 minutes and last for 4 to 6 hours. Because all three drugs are metabolized in the liver, persons with hepatic disease, such as cirrhosis, may attain high plasma concentrations with long-term administration. Cyproheptadine is well absorbed after oral administration, and its metabolites are excreted in the urine.

Activation of H_1 receptors stimulates wakefulness; therefore, receptor antagonism causes sedation. All four agents also possess some antimuscarinic cholinergic activity. Cyproheptadine is unique among the drugs, since it has both potent antihistamine and serotonin 5-HT$_2$ receptor antagonist properties.

THERAPEUTIC INDICATIONS

Antihistamines are useful as a treatment for neuroleptic-induced parkinsonism, neuroleptic-induced acute dystonia, and neuroleptic-induced akathisia. They are an alternative to anticholinergics and amantadine for these purposes. The antihistamines are relatively safe hypnotics, but they are not superior to the benzodiazepines, which have been much better studied in terms of efficacy and safety. The antihistamines have not been proved effective for long-term anxiolytic therapy; therefore, either the benzodiazepines, buspirone (BuSpar), or SSRIs are preferable for such treatment. Cyproheptadine is sometimes used to treat impaired orgasms, especially delayed orgasm resulting from treatment with serotonergic drugs.

Because it promotes weight gain, cyproheptadine may be of some use in the treatment of eating disorders, such as anorexia nervosa. Cyproheptadine can reduce recurrent nightmares with posttraumatic themes. The antiserotonergic activity of cyproheptadine may counteract the serotonin syndrome caused by concomitant use of multiple serotonin-activating drugs, such as SSRIs and monoamine oxidase inhibitors.

PRECAUTIONS AND ADVERSE REACTIONS

Antihistamines are commonly associated with sedation, dizziness, and hypotension, all of which can be severe in elderly persons, who are also likely to suffer from the anticholinergic effects of those drugs. Paradoxical excitement and agitation is an adverse effect seen in a small number of persons. Poor motor coordination can result in accidents; therefore, persons should be warned about driving and operating dangerous machinery. Other common adverse effects include epigastric distress, nausea, vomiting, diarrhea, and constipation. Because of mild anticholinergic activity, some people experience dry mouth, urinary retention, blurred vision, and constipation. For this reason also, antihistamines should be used only at very low doses, if at all, by persons with narrow-angle glaucoma or obstructive GI, prostate, or bladder conditions. A central anticholinergic syndrome with psychosis may be induced by either cyproheptadine or diphenhydramine. The use of cyproheptadine in some persons has been associated with weight gain, which may contribute to its reported efficacy in some persons with anorexia nervosa.

TABLE 6–1
OTHER ANTIHISTAMINES WITH RELEVANCE TO PSYCHIATRY

Class	Generic Name	Brand Name	Comments
H₂ receptor antagonist	Cimetidine Ranitidine Famotidine Nizatidine	Tagamet Zantac Pepcid Axid	Widely prescribed for treatment of ulcers and gastroesophageal reflux. All have the potential for CNS toxicities, including psychosis and delirium
Second-generation (nonsedating) H₁ receptor antagonists	Lorazadine Catirizine Fexofenadine	Claritin Zyrtec Allegra	No apparent cardiotoxicity, but increased levels can occur when administered with CYP 3A4 inhibitors

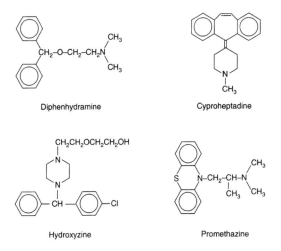

Figure 6-1. Molecular structures of antihistamines used in psychiatry.

In addition to the above adverse effects, antihistamines have some potential for abuse. The coadministration of antihistamines and opioids can increase the euphoria experienced by persons with substance dependence. Overdoses of antihistamines can be fatal. Antihistamines are excreted in breast milk, so their use should be avoided by nursing mothers. Because of some potential for teratogenicity, the use of antihistamines should also be avoided by pregnant women.

DRUG INTERACTIONS

The sedative property of antihistamines can be additive with other central nervous system (CNS) depressants, such as alcohol, other sedative-hypnotic drugs, and many psychotropic drugs, including tricyclic drugs and dopamine receptor antagonists. The anticholinergic activity can also be additive with that of other anticholinergic drugs and can sometimes result in severe anticholinergic symptoms or intoxication. The beneficial effects of SSRIs can be antagonized by cyproheptadine.

LABORATORY INTERFERENCES

H_1 antagonists may eliminate the wheal and induration that form the basis of allergy skin tests. Promethazine may interfere with pregnancy tests and may increase blood glucose concentrations. Diphenhydramine may yield a false-positive urine test result for phencyclidine (PCP). Hydroxyzine use can falsely elevate the results of certain tests for urinary 17-hydroxycorticosteroids.

DOSAGE AND CLINICAL GUIDELINES

The antihistamines are available in a variety of preparations (Table 6–2). Intramuscular injections should be deep, since superficial administration can cause local irritation.

Intravenous (i.v.) administration of 25 to 50 mg of diphenhydramine is an effective treatment for neuroleptic-induced acute dystonia, which may immediately disappear. Treatment with 25 mg three times a day—up to 50 mg four times a day if

TABLE 6–2
DOSAGE AND ADMINISTRATION OF TRADITIONAL ANTIHISTAMINES USED IN PSYCHIATRY

Drugs	Route	Preparation	Dosage
Diphenhydramine (Benadryl)	p.o.	Capsules and tablets: 25 mg, SO mg elixir and syrup: 12.5 mg/5 mL	Adults: 25–50 mg 3–4 times daily Usual sleep-aid dose: 50 mg at bedtime Children: 5 mg/kg/24 h in 4 divided dose, not to exceed 300 mg/day
	i.m. (deep)	Solution: 10 mg/mL, 50 mg/mL	Adults: 10–50 mg i.v. or deep i.m. may use 100 mg if required, maximum daily dose 400 mg: for dystonic reactions, 50 mg i.v. over 2–3 min Children: 5 mg/kg/24 h (maximum 300 mg/day)
Hydroxyzine (Atarax, Vistaril)	p.o.	Hydrochloride syrup: 10 mg/5 mL Tablets:10 mg, 25 mg, 50 mg, 100 mg Pamoate suspension: 25 mg/5 mL Capsules: 25 mg, 50 mg, 100 mg	Adults: 25–100 mg q.i.d. Children: under 6: 50 mg/24 h in 3–4 divided doses over 6: 50–100 mg/day in 3–4 divided doses
	i.m.	Hydrochloride solution: 25 mg/mL, 50 mg/mL	Adults: 50–100 mg q4–6h p.r.n. for sedation Children: 0.5 mg/lb to body weight
Promethazine (Phenergan)	p.o.	Syrup: 6.25 mg/5 mL, 25 mg/5 mL Tablets: 12.5 mg, 25 mg, 50 mg	Adults: 25–50 mg for sedation Children: 12.5–25 mg at bedtime for nighttime and preoperative sedation
	p.r.	Suppositories: 50 mg, 25 mg, 12.5 mg	
	i.m.	Solution: 25 mg/mL and 50 mg/mL	
Cyproheptadine (Periactin)	p.o.	Tablets: 4 mg Syrup: 2 mg/5 mL	Adult: usually 4–20 mg/day (may require up to 32 mg/day) for allergies, not to exceed 0.5 mg/kg/day; for antidepressants-induced anorgasmia: 4–16 mg, either in divided daily doses or approximately 1–2 h prior to coitus Children: for allergies, approximately 0.25 mg/kg/day 2–6 yr old: 2 mg p.o. 2–3 times daily; maximum 12 mg/day 7–14 yr old: 4 mg p.o. 2–3 times daily; maximum 16 mg/day

necessary—can be used to treat neuroleptic-induced parkinsonism, akinesia, and buccal movements. Diphenhydramine can be used as a hypnotic at a 50-mg dose for mild transient insomnia. Doses of 100 mg have not been shown to be superior to doses of 50 mg, but they produce more anticholinergic effects than doses of 50 mg.

Hydroxyzine is most commonly used as a short-term anxiolytic. Hydroxyzine should not be given i.v., since it is irritating to the blood vessels. Dosages of 50 to 100 mg given orally four times a day for long-term treatment or 50 to 100 mg i.m. every 4 to 6 hours for short-term treatment are usually effective.

SSRI-induced anorgasmia may be reversed with 4 to 16 mg a day of cyproheptadine taken by mouth 1 or 2 hours before anticipated sexual activity. A number of case reports and small studies have also reported that cyproheptadine may be of some use in the treatment of eating disorders, such as anorexia nervosa. Cyproheptadine is available in 4-mg tablets and a 2 mg/5 mL solution. Children and elderly patients are more sensitive to the effects of antihistamines than are young adults.

For a more detailed discussion of this topic, see Labbate LA, Arana GW, Ballenger JC: Antihistamines, Sec 31.8, p 2304, in CTP/VII.

7

Barbiturates and Similarly Acting Drugs

Benzodiazepines, other anxiolytics such as buspirone (BuSpar), and the hypnotics zolpidem (Ambien) and zaleplon (Sonata) have practically eliminated the use of the barbiturates and similar compounds, such as meprobamate (Miltown). The newer agents have a lower abuse potential and a higher therapeutic index than the barbiturates; nevertheless, the barbiturates and similarly acting drugs still have a role in the treatment of certain mental disorders.

CHEMISTRY

The various clinically available barbiturates are derived from the same barbituric acid substrate and differ primarily in their substitutions at the C_5 position of the parent molecule. The molecular structures of the various barbiturates are shown in Figure 7–1.

PHARMACOLOGICAL ACTIONS

The barbiturates are well absorbed after oral administration. The binding of barbiturates to plasma proteins is high, but lipid solubility varies. The individual barbiturates are metabolized by the liver and excreted by the kidneys. The half-lives of specific barbiturates range from 1 to 120 hours. Barbiturates may also induce hepatic enzymes (cytochrome P450) thereby reducing the levels of both the barbiturate and any other concurrently administered drugs metabolized by the liver. The mechanism of action of barbiturates involves the γ-aminobutyric acid (GABA) receptor–benzodiazepine receptor–chloride ion channel complex.

THERAPEUTIC INDICATIONS

Electroconvulsive Therapy

Methohexital (Brevital) is commonly used as an anesthetic agent for electroconvulsive therapy (ECT). It has lower cardiac risks than other barbiturate anesthetics. Used intravenously, methohexital produces rapid unconsciousness and because of rapid redistribution has a brief duration of action (5 to 7 minutes). Typical dosing for ECT is 0.7 to 1.2 mg/kg. Methohexital may also be used to abort prolonged seizures in ECT or to limit postictal agitation.

Seizures

Phenobarbital (Solfoton, Luminal), the most commonly used barbiturate for treatment of seizures, has indications for the treatment of generalized tonic-clonic

General Formula:

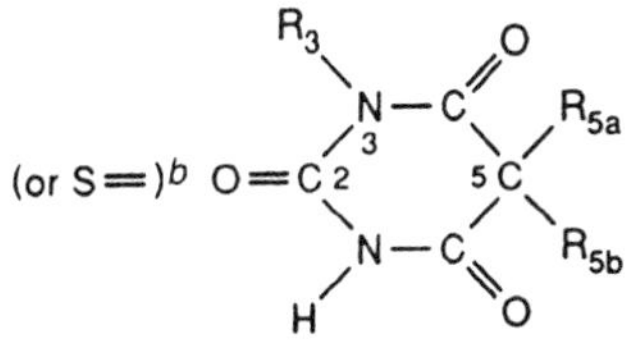

Barbiturate	R_{5a}	R_{5b}
Amobarbital	Ethyl	Isopentyl
Aprobarbital	Allyl	Isopropyl
Butabarbital	Ethyl	Sec-Butyl
Butalbital	Allyl	Isobutyl
Mephobarbital[a]	Ethyl	Phenyl
Methohexital[a]	Allyl	1-Methyl-2-Pentynyl
Pentobarbital	Ethyl	1-Methylbutyl
Phenobarbital	Ethyl	Phenyl
Secobarbital	Allyl	1-Methylbutyl
Thiamylal[b]	Allyl	1-Methylbutyl
Thiopental[b]	Ethyl	1-Methylbutyl

[a] $R_3 = H_1$ except in mephobarbital and methohexital, where it is replaced by CH_3.
[b] O, except in thiamylal and thiopental, where it is replaced by S.

Figure 7–1. Molecular structures and names of barbiturates available in the United States. (From Rall TW. Hypnotics and Sedatives; Ethanol. In: *Goodman and Gilman's The Pharmacological Basis of Therapeutics*, 8th ed. Goodman A, Gilman AG, Rall TW, et al., editors. New York: McGraw–Hill, 1990, with permission.)

and simple partial seizures. Parenteral barbiturates are used in the emergency management of seizures independent of cause. Intravenous phenobarbital should be administered slowly, 10 to 20 mg/kg for status epilepticus.

Narcoanalysis

Amobarbital (Amytal) has been used historically as a diagnostic aid in a number of clinical conditions, including conversion reactions, catatonia, hysterical stupor, and unexplained muteness, and to differentiate stupor of depression, schizophrenia, and structural brain lesions.

The "Amytal interview" is performed by placing the patient in a reclining position and administering amobarbital intravenously, 50 mg a minute. Infusion is continued until lateral nystagmus is sustained or drowsiness is noted, usually at 75 to 150 mg. Following this, 25 to 50 mg may be administered every 5 minutes to maintain narcosis. The patient should be allowed to rest for 15 to 30 minutes after the interview before attempting to walk.

Sleep

The barbiturates reduce sleep latency and the number of awakenings during sleep, though tolerance to these effects generally develops within 2 weeks. Discontinuation of barbiturates often leads to rebound increases on electroencephalogram (EEG) measures of sleep and a worsening of the insomnia.

Withdrawal from Sedative Hypnotics

Barbiturates are sometimes used to determine extent of tolerance to barbiturates or other hypnotics to guide detoxification. Once intoxication has resolved, a test dose of pentobarbital (200 mg) is given orally. An hour later the patient is examined. Tolerance and dose requirements are determined by the degree to which the patient is affected. If the patient is not sedated, another 100 mg of pentobarbital may be administered every 2 hours, up to three times (maximum, 500 mg over 6 hours). The amount needed for mild intoxication corresponds to the approximate daily dose of barbiturate used. Phenobarbital (30 mg) may then be substituted for each 100 mg of pentobarbital. This daily dose requirement may be administered in divided doses and gradually tapered by 10 percent a day, with adjustments made according to withdrawal signs (Table 7–1).

PRECAUTIONS AND ADVERSE REACTIONS

Some adverse effects of barbiturates are similar to those of benzodiazepines, including paradoxical dysphoria, hyperactivity, and cognitive disorganization. Rare adverse effects associated with barbiturate use include the development of Stevens-Johnson syndrome, megaloblastic anemia, and neutropenia.

A major difference between the barbiturates and the benzodiazepines is the low therapeutic index of the barbiturates. An overdose of barbiturates can easily prove fatal. In addition to narrow therapeutic indexes, the barbiturates are associated with a significant risk of abuse potential and the development of tolerance and dependence. Barbiturate intoxication is manifested by confusion, drowsiness, irritability, hyporeflexia or areflexia, ataxia, and nystagmus. The symptoms of barbiturate withdrawal are similar to, but more marked than, those of benzodiazepine withdrawal.

Because of some evidence of teratogenicity, barbiturates should not be used by pregnant women or women who are breast-feeding. Barbiturates should be used with

TABLE 7–1
PENTOBARBITAL CHALLENGE TEST

1. Give pentobarbital 200 mg orally.
2. Observe for intoxication after 1 h (e.g., sleepiness, slurred speech, or nystagmus).
3. If patient is not intoxicated, give another 100 mg of pentobarbital every 2 h (maximum 500 mg over 6 h).
4. Total dose given to produce mild intoxication is equivalent to daily abuse level of barbiturates.
5. Substitute phenobarbital 30 mg (longer half-life) for each 100 mg of pentobarbital.
6. Dosage by about 10% a day.
7. Adjust rate if signs of intoxication or withdrawal are present.

caution by patients with a history of substance abuse, depression, diabetes, hepatic impairment, renal disease, severe anemia, pain, hyperthyroidism, or hypoadrenalism. Barbiturates are also contraindicated in patients with acute intermittent porphyria, impaired respiratory drive, or limited respiratory reserve.

DRUG INTERACTIONS

The primary area for concern about drug interactions is the potentially additive effects of respiratory depression. Barbiturates should be used with great caution with other prescribed CNS drugs (including antipsychotic and antidepressant drugs) and nonprescribed CNS agents (e.g., alcohol). Caution must also be exercised when prescribing barbiturates to patients who are taking other drugs that are metabolized in the liver, especially cardiac drugs and anticonvulsants. Because individual patients have a wide range of sensitivities to barbiturate-induced enzyme induction, it is not possible to predict the degree to which the metabolism of concurrently administered medications are affected. Drugs that may have their metabolism enhanced by barbiturate administration include opioids, antiarrhythmic agents, antibiotics, anticoagulants, anticonvulsants, antidepressants, β-adrenergic receptor antagonists, dopamine receptor antagonists, contraceptives, and immunosuppressants (Table 7–2).

LABORATORY INTERFERENCES

No known laboratory interferences are associated with the administration of barbiturates.

DOSAGE AND CLINICAL GUIDELINES

Barbiturates and other drugs described below begin to act within 1 to 2 hours of administration. The dosages of barbiturates vary (Table 7–3), and treatment should begin with low dosages that are increased to achieve a clinical effect. Children and older people are more sensitive to the effects of the barbiturates than are young adults. The most commonly used barbiturates are available in a variety of dose

TABLE 7–2
DRUG INTERACTIONS

The metabolism of the following drugs has been reported to be increased with long-term use of barbiturates. Others unlisted may also be affected
Analgesics—acetaminophen, fenoprofen
Antiarrhythmics—digitalis, lidocaine, mexiletine
Antibiotics—chloramphenicol, metronidazol, rifampin, tetracycline, griseofulvin
Anticoagulants—warfarin
Anticonvulsants—carbamazepine, phenytoin
Antidepressants—amitriptyline, desipramine, paroxetine, protriptyline
Antihypertensives—methyldopa
Antipsychotics—haloperidol, thioridazine, loxapine
β-Adrenergic receptor antagonists—labetalol, propranolol, metoprolol
Benzodiazepines—clonazepam, diazepam
Contraceptives—all containing estrogens
Immunosuppresants—corticosteroids, cyclophosphamide, cyclosporine, decarbazine
Xanthines—aminophylline, caffeine, theophylline

TABLE 7–3
BARBITURATE DOSAGES

Drug	Selected Preparations[a]	Daily Dosage Range[b] (sedative[c]/hypnotic)	Anticonvulsant	Pediatric
Amobarbital	30, 200 mg	100–200 mg[c]/ 50–300 mg	65–500 mg (i.v.)	2–6 mg/kg up to 100 mg
Aprobarbital	40 mg/5mL (e)	40–160 mg[c]/ 40–120 mg	Not established	Not established
Butabarbital	30 mg/5 mL (e) 15, 30, 50, 100 mg	45–120 mg[c]/ 50–100 mg	Not established	2–6 mg/kg (max 100 mg)
Mephobarbital	32, 50, 100 mg	66–300 mg[c]/ 100 mg	200–600 mg	16–32 mg three to four times daily (≤ age 5) 32–64 mg three to four times daily (> age 5)
Methohexital	500 mg/50 mL (1)	0.7–1.2 mg/kg for ECT	Not established	Not established
Pentobarbital	50, 100 mg 50 mg/mL (1) 20 mg/mL (e) 30, 60, 120, 200 mg (r)	60–100 mg[c]/ 100–150 mg	100 mg i.v. at 1-min intervals up to 500 mg	2–6 mg/kg up to 100 mg
Phenobarbital	8, 15, 30, 60, 100 mg 30, 60, 65, 130 mg/mL (l) 20 mg/5 mL (e)	30–120 mg[c]/ 100–300 mg	100–300 mg i.v., up to 600 mg/day 60–250 mg/day oral	1–3 mg/kg
Secobarbital	100 mg 50 mg/mL (l)	100–300 mg[c]/ 100 mg	5.5 mg/kg intravenous, may repeat every 3–4 hours	3–5 mg/kg

[a] Other preparations are available.
[b] Dosages are oral form (tablets or capsules) unless specified: i, injection; r, rectal suppository.
[c] Sedative dosage is equal to the hypnotic dosage, but should be split 3 to 4 times daily.

forms. Barbiturates with half-lives in the 15- to 40-hour range are preferable, because long-acting drugs tend to accumulate in the body. Clinicians should instruct patients clearly about the adverse effects and the potential for dependence associated with barbiturates.

Although determining plasma concentrations of barbiturates is rarely necessary in psychiatry, monitoring of phenobarbital concentrations is standard practice when the drug is used as an anticonvulsant. The therapeutic blood concentrations for phenobarbital in this indication range from 15 to 40 mg/L, although some patients may experience significant adverse effects in that range.

Barbiturates are contained in combination products with which the clinician should be familiar (Table 7–4).

OTHER SIMILARLY ACTING DRUGS

A number of agents that act similarly to the barbiturates are used in the treatment of anxiety and insomnia. Four such available drugs are paraldehyde (Paral),

TABLE 7–4
BARBITURATES CONTAINED IN COMBINATION PRODUCTS

Product Name	Barbiturate	Other Content
Floricet with Codeine	Butalbital, 50 mg	Caffeine, 40 mg; codeine, 30 mg; acetaminophen, 325 mg
Florinal with Codeine	Butalbital, 50 mg	Caffeine, 40 mg; codeine, 30 mg, aspirin, 325 mg
Cafatine-PB	Phenobarbital, 30 mg	Caffeine, 100 mg; engotamine tartate, 1 mg; alkaloid of belladona, 0.125 mg
Barbidonna	Phenobarbital, 32 mg	Atropine sulfate 0.025 mg; scopolamine, 0.0074 mg; hyoscyamine, 0.1286 mg
Butibel	Butabarbital, 15 mg	Belladonna extract, 15 mg
Donnatal Extentabs	Phenobarbital, 48.6 mg	Atropine sulfate 0.0582 mg; scopolamine, 0.0195 mg; hyoscyamine, 0.311 mg
Phenerbel-S	Phenobarbital, 40 mg	Alkaloid of belladona, 0.2 mg ergotamine tartate, 0.6 mg

ethchlorvynol (Placidyl), meprobamate, and glutethimide (Doriden). These drugs are rarely used because of their abuse potential and potential toxic effects.

Paraldehyde

Paraldehyde is a cyclic ether, first used in 1882 as a hypnotic. It has also been used to treat epilepsy, alcohol withdrawal symptoms, and delirium tremens. Because of its low therapeutic index it has been supplanted by the benzodiazepines and other anticonvulsants.

Chemistry.   The molecular structure of paraldehyde is shown in Figure 7–2.

Pharmacological Actions.   Paraldehyde is rapidly absorbed from the gastrointestinal (GI) tract and from intramuscular injections. It is primarily metabolized to acetaldehyde by the liver, and unmetabolized drug is expired by the lungs. Reported half-lives range from 3.4 to 9.8 hours. Onset of action is 15 to 30 minutes.

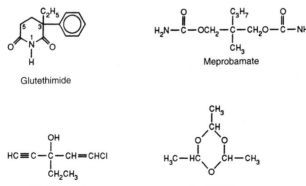

Glutethimide

Meprobamate

Ethchlorvynol

Paraldehyde

Figure 7-2.   Molecular structures of similarly acting drugs.

Therapeutic Indications. Paraldehyde is not indicated as an anxiolytic or hypnotic and has little place in current psychopharmacology.

Precautions and Adverse Reactions. Paraldehyde frequently causes foul breath because of expired unmetabolized drug. It may inflame pulmonary capillaries and cause coughing. It may also cause local thrombophlebitis with intravenous use. Patients may experience nausea and vomiting with oral use. Overdose leads to metabolic acidosis and decreased renal output. There is risk of abuse among drug addicts.

Drug Interactions. Disulfiram (Antabuse) inhibits acetaldehyde dehydrogenase and reduces metabolism of paraldehyde, leading to possible toxic concentration of paraldehyde. Paraldehyde has addictive sedating effects in combination with other CNS depressants such as alcohol or benzodiazepines.

Laboratory Interferences. Paraldehyde may interfere with the metyrapone, phentolamine, or urinary 17-hydroxycorticosteroid tests.

Dosage and Clinical Guidelines. Paraldehyde is available in 30-mL vials for oral, intravenous, or rectal use. For seizures in adults, up to 12 mL (diluted to a 10 percent solution) may be administered by gastric tube every 4 hours. For children the oral dose is 0.3 mg/kg.

Meprobamate

Meprobamate, a carbamate, was introduced shortly before the benzodiazepines, specifically to treat anxiety. It is also used for muscle relaxant effects.

Chemistry. The molecular structure of meprobamate is shown in Figure 7–2.

Pharmacological Actions. Meprobamate is rapidly absorbed from the GI tract and from intramuscular injections. It is primarily metabolized by the liver, and a small portion is excreted unchanged in urine. The plasma half-life is approximately 10 hours.

Therapeutic Indications. Meprobamate is indicated for short-term treatment of anxiety disorders. It has also been used as a hypnotic and is prescribed as a muscle relaxant.

Precautions and Adverse Reactions. Meprobamate may cause CNS depression and death in overdose and carries the risk of abuse by patients with drug or alcohol dependence. Abrupt cessation following long-term use may lead to withdrawal syndrome including seizures and hallucinations. Meprobamate may exacerbate acute intermittent porphyria. Other rare side effects include hypersensitivity reactions, wheezing, hives, paradoxical excitement, and leukopenia. It should not be used in patients with hepatic compromise.

Drug Interactions. Meprobamate has additive sedating effects in combination with other CNS depressants such as alcohol, barbiturates, or benzodiazepines.

Laboratory Interferences. Meprobamate may interfere with the metyrapone, phentolamine, or urinary 17-hydroxycorticosteroid tests.

Dosage and Clinical Guidelines. Meprobamate is available in 200-, 400-, and 600-mg tablets, 200- and 400-mg extended-release capsules, and various combinations, e.g., aspirin, 325 mg, and 200 mg of meprobamate (Equagesic) for oral use. For adults, the usual dosage is 400 to 800 mg twice daily. Elderly patients and children age 6 to 12 require half the adult dose.

Ethchlorvynol

Ethchlorvynol, a tertiary carbinol, was marketed to treat insomnia and anxiety. It has been replaced by the benzodiazepines and other safer agents in the treatment of anxiety and sleep disturbance. It has a low therapeutic index.

Chemistry.   The molecular structure of ethchlorvynol is shown in Figure 7–2.

Pharmacological Action.   Ethchlorvynol is rapidly absorbed from the GI tract. It is primarily metabolized by the liver, and a small portion is metabolized by the kidney. Metabolites are excreted in the urine. Elimination half-life is approximately 10 to 20 hours.

Therapeutic Indications.   Ethchlorvynol is indicated for up to 1-week treatment of insomnia.

Precautions and Adverse Reactions.   Ethchlorvynol may cause CNS depression, slurred speech, double vision, confusion, and death in overdose. There is risk of abuse by patients with drug or alcohol dependence. Abrupt cessation following long-term use may lead to a withdrawal syndrome including seizures and hallucinations. Ethchlorvynol may exacerbate acute intermittent porphyria or cause cholestatic jaundice. Hypersensitivity reactions are uncommon. Paradoxical excitement is rare. It should not be used in patients with hepatic compromise.

Drug Interactions.   In combination with other CNS drugs including tricyclic drugs, alcohol, barbiturates or benzodiazepines, ethchlorvynol has additive sedating effects. Ethchlorvynol stimulates hepatic microenzymes and may increase metabolism of many drugs, most notably warfarin (Coumadin).

Laboratory Interferences.   Ethchlorvynol may cause a false-positive phentolamine test result.

Dosage and Clinical Guidelines.   Ethchlorvynol is available in 200-, 500-, and 750-mg capsules. For adults, the usual dose is 500 to 750 mg at bedtime. It is best taken with food to limit rate of onset for patients in whom ataxia is of concern. Patients requiring withdrawal should be switched to a barbiturate such as phenobarbital and gradually tapered. Safety and efficacy in children or elderly patients has not been established.

Glutethimide

Chemistry.   The molecular structure of glutethimide is shown in Figure 7–2.

Pharmacological Action.   Glutethimide is absorbed erratically from the GI tract, is metabolized by the liver, and has an onset action of 30 minutes. Its elimination half-life is 10 to 12 hours, and it is known to induce hepatic microsomal enzymes. It has potent anticholinergic activity.

Therapeutic Indications.   Glutethimide has been used to treat insomnia.

Precautions and Adverse Reactions.   Glutethimide may cause CNS depression, slurred speech, double vision, confusion, and death in overdose. There is a risk of abuse by patients with drug or alcohol dependence. Abrupt cessation following long-term use may lead to a withdrawal syndrome including seizures and hallucinations. Glutethimide may exacerbate acute intermittent porphyria. Because of its potent anticholinergic effects it should be used cautiously in patients with prostatic hypertrophy or narrow-angle glaucoma. Hypersensitivity reactions are uncommon.

Paradoxical excitement is rare. It should not be used in patients with hepatic damage.

Drug Interactions.   Glutethimide has additive sedating effects in combination with other CNS drugs including alcohol, barbiturates, and benzodiazepines. Glutethimide induces hepatic microenzymes and may increase metabolism of many drugs, most notably warfarin.

Laboratory Interferences.   Glutethimide may cause a false-positive phentolamine test result or interfere with urine assays for 17-ketosteroids.

Dosage and Clinical Guidelines.   Glutethimide is available in 500-mg tablets. For adults, the usual dose for insomnia is 250 to 500 mg at bedtime. For elderly patients the recommended dose is 250 mg. Safety and efficacy in children has not been established. Patients requiring withdrawal should be switched to a barbiturate such as phenobarbital and gradually tapered.

For a more detailed discussion of this topic, see Labbate LA, Arana GW, Ballenger JC: Barbiturates and Similarly Acting Substances, Sec 31.9, p 2309, in CTP/VII.

8

Benzodiazepines

The benzodiazepine family of drugs and the nonbenzodiazepine agonists, zolpidem (Ambien) and zaleplon (Sonata), have rapid calming and sedative effects. Benzodiazepines are effective for immediate treatment of panic disorder, phobias, and agitation associated with bipolar I disorder. In addition, the benzodiazepines are used as anesthetics, anticonvulsants, and muscle relaxants.

Benzodiazepines are sometimes classified as sedative-hypnotics, although other drugs can also be classified in this group (e.g., barbiturates). A *sedative drug* reduces daytime anxiety, tempers excessive excitement, and generally quiets or calms the person. A *hypnotic drug* produces drowsiness and facilitates the onset and the maintenance of sleep. In general, benzodiazepines act as hypnotics in high doses and as anxiolytics or sedatives in low doses.

Benzodiazepines are the drugs of first choice for management of acute anxiety and agitation. Because of the risk of psychological dependence, long-term use of benzodiazepines should be reserved for those persons whose anxiety symptoms are not adequately controlled by selective serotonin reuptake inhibitors (SSRIs) or buspirone (BuSpar).

Zolpidem and zaleplon promote sleep for 4 to 5 hours with minimal residual cognitive or motor effects and without the agitation sometimes experienced as a withdrawal effect of benzodiazepines.

Flumazenil (Romazicon) is an effective benzodiazepine receptor antagonist used in emergency care of benzodiazepine overdosage.

CHEMISTRY

The structural formulas of the benzodiazepines are shown in Figure 8–1, zolpidem and zaleplon in Figure 8–2, and flumazenil in Figure 8–3.

PHARMACOLOGICAL ACTIONS

With the exception of clorazepate (Tranxene), all the benzodiazepines are completely absorbed unchanged from the gastrointestinal (GI) tract. The absorption, the attainment of peak concentrations, and the onset of action are quickest for diazepam (Valium), lorazepam (Ativan), alprazolam (Xanax), triazolam (Halcion), and estazolam (ProSom). The rapid onset of effects is important to persons who take a single dose of a benzodiazepine to calm an episodic burst of anxiety or to fall asleep rapidly. Several benzodiazepines are effective following intravenous (i.v.) injection, whereas only lorazepam and midazolam (Versed) have rapid and reliable absorption following intramuscular (i.m.) administration.

Diazepam, chlordiazepoxide, clonazepam (Klonopin), clorazepate, flurazepam (Dalmane), prazepam (Centrax), quazepam (Doral), and halazepam (Paxipam) have

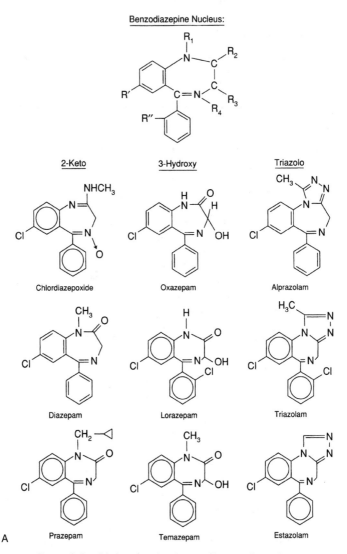

Figure 8–1. Molecular structures of benzodiazepines.

plasma half-lives of 30 to more than 100 hours and are, therefore, the longest-acting benzodiazepines. The plasma half-life of these compounds can be as high as 200 hours in persons whose metabolism is genetically slow. Because the attainment of steady-state plasma concentrations of the drugs can take up to 2 weeks, persons may experience symptoms and signs of toxicity after only 7 to 10 days of treatment with a dosage that seemed initially to be in the therapeutic range.

The half-lives of lorazepam, oxazepam (Serax), temazepam (Restoril), and estazolam are between 8 and 30 hours. Alprazolam has a half-life of 10 to 15 hours and

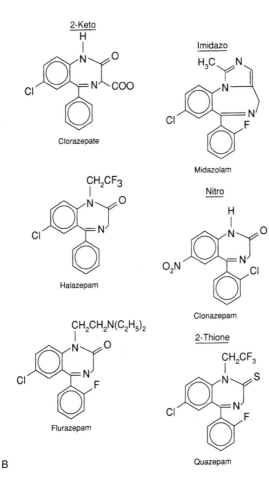

Figure 8-1. *Continued*

triazolam has the shortest half-life (2 to 3 hours) of all the orally administered benzodiazepines.

The advantages of long–half-life drugs over short–half-life drugs include less-frequent dosing, less variation in plasma concentration, and less-severe withdrawal phenomena. The disadvantages include drug accumulation, increased risk of daytime psychomotor impairment, and increased daytime sedation. The advantages of the short–half-life drugs over the long–half-life drugs include no drug accumulation and less daytime sedation. The disadvantages include more-frequent dosing and earlier and more-severe withdrawal syndromes. Rebound insomnia and anterograde amnesia are thought to be more of a problem with the short–half-life drugs than with the long–half-life drugs. (Table 8–1 lists the half-lives of the drugs.)

Zolpidem and zaleplon are rapidly and well absorbed after oral administration, though absorption can be delayed by as much as 1 hour if they are taken with food. Zolpidem reaches peak plasma concentrations in 1.6 hours and has a half-life of 2.6

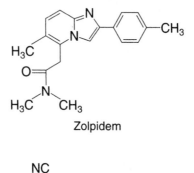

Zolpidem

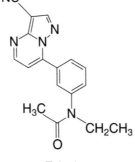

Zaleplon

Figure 8–2.   Molecular structures of zolpidem and zaleplon.

hours. Zaleplon reaches peak plasma concentrations in 1 hour and has a half-life of 1 hour. The rapid metabolism and lack of active metabolites of zolpidem and zaleplon avoid the accumulation of potentially toxic compounds often seen with long-term use of benzodiazepines.

Benzodiazepines activate all three specific γ-aminobutyric acid–benzodiazepine (GABA-BZ) binding sites of the $GABA_A$-receptor, which opens chloride channels and reduces the rate of neuronal and muscle firing. Because of the wide tissue distribution of $GABA_A$-receptors, benzodiazepines have sedative, muscle relaxant, and anticonvulsant effects. Zolpidem and zaleplon selectively activate only one of the benzodiazepine binding sites, which may account for their selective sedative effects and relative lack of muscle relaxant and anticonvulsant effects.

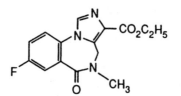

Figure 8–3.   Molecular structure of flumazenil.

HALF-LIVES, DOSES, AND PREPARATIONS OF BENZODIAZEPINE RECEPTOR AGONISTS AND ANTAGONISTS

Drug	Dose Equivalents	Half-Life (h)	Rate of Absorption	Usual Adult Dosage	Dose Preparations
Agonists					
Clonazepam	0.5	Long (metabolite, >20)	Rapid	1-6 mg/d b.i.d.	0.5-mg, 1.0-mg, and 2.0-mg tablets
Diazepam	5	Long (>20) Nordazepam—long, >20)	Rapid	4-40 mg/d b.i.d. to q.i.d.	2-mg, 5-mg, and 10-mg tablets (slow-release 15-mg capsules)
Alprazolam	0.25	Intermediate (6-20)	Medium	0.5-10 mg/d b.i.d. to q.i.d.	0.25-mg, 0.5-mg, 1.0-mg, and 2.0-mg tablets
Lorazepam	1	Intermediate (6-20)	Medium	1-6 mg/d t.i.d.	0.5-mg, 1.0-mg, and 2.0-mg tablets, 2 mg/mL 4 mg/mL parenteral
Oxazepam	15	Intermediate (6-20)	Slow	30-120 mg/d t.i.d. or q.i.d.	10-mg, 15-mg, and 30-mg capsules (15-mg tablets)
Temazepam	5	Intermediate (6-20)	Medium	7.5-30 mg/d h.s.	7.5-mg, 15-mg, and 30-mg capsules
Chlordiazepoxide	10	Intermediate (6-20) (Demethylchlordiazepoxide—intermediate, 6-20) (Demoxapam—long, >20) (Nordazepam—long, >20)	Medium	10-150 mg t.i.d. or q.i.d.	5-mg, 10-mg, and 25-mg tablets or capsules
Flurazepam	5	Short (<6) (N-hydroxyethylflurazepam—short, <6) (N-desalkylflurazepam—long, >20)	Rapid	15-30 h.s.	15-mg and 30-mg capsules
Triazolam	0.1-0.03	Short (<6)	Rapid	0.125 mg or 0.250 mg h.s.	0.125-mg or 0.250-mg tablets
Clorazepate	7.5	Short (<6) Nordazepam—long, >20)	Rapid	15-60 mg b.i.d. or q.i.d.	3.75-mg, 7.5-mg, and 15-mg tablets (slow release 11.25-mg and 22.5-mg tablets
Halazepam	20	Short (<6) (Nordazepam—long, >20)	Medium	60-160 mg/d t.i.d. or q.i.d.	20-mg and 40-mg tablets
Prazepam	10	Short (<6) (Nordazepam—long, >20)	Slow	30 mg/d (20-60 mg/d) q.i.d. or t.i.d.	5-mg, 10-mg, or 20-mg capsules
Estazolam	0.33	Intermediate (6-20) (4-hydroxyestazolam—intermediate 6-20)	Rapid	1.0 or 2.0 h.s.	1-mg and 2-mg tablets
Quazepam	5	Long (>20) (2-oxoquazepam-N-desalkylflurazepam—long, >20)	Rapid	7.5 or 15 mg h.s.	7.5-mg and 15-mg tablets
Midazolam	1.25-1.7	Short (<6)	Rapid	5 to 50 mg parenteral	5 mg/mL parenteral, 1-mL, 2-mL, 5-mL, and 10-mL vials
Zolpidem	2.5	Short (<6)	Rapid	5 mg or 10 mg h.s.	5-mg and 10-mg tablets
Zaleplon	?	Short (1)	Rapid	10 mg h.s.	5 mg and 10-mg capsules
Antagonist					
Flumazenil	0.05	Short (<6)	Rapid	0.2 to 0.5 mg/min injection over 3-10 min (total, 1-5 mg)	0.1 mg/mL (5 mL and 10-mL vials)

THERAPEUTIC INDICATIONS

Insomnia

Because insomnia may be a symptom of a physical or psychiatric disorder, hypnotics should not be used for more than 7 to 10 consecutive days without a thorough investigation of the cause of the insomnia.

The sole indication for zolpidem and zaleplon is insomnia, but the spectrum of their psychological effects closely resembles that of benzodiazepines. Zolpidem and particularly zaleplon are usually not associated with rebound insomnia after the discontinuation of their use for short periods. Use of zolpidem and zaleplon for periods longer than 1 month is not associated with the delayed emergence of adverse effects.

Flurazepam, temazepam, quazepam, estazolam, and triazolam are the benzodiazepines approved for use as hypnotics. The benzodiazepine hypnotics differ principally in their half-lives; flurazepam has the longest half-life, and triazolam has the shortest. Flurazepam may be associated with minor cognitive impairment on the day after its administration, and triazolam may be associated with mild rebound anxiety and anterograde amnesia. Quazepam may be associated with daytime impairment when used for a long time. Temazepam or estazolam may be a reasonable compromise for the usual adult person. Estazolam produces rapid onset of sleep and a hypnotic effect for 6 to 8 hours.

Anxiety Disorders

Generalized Anxiety Disorder. Benzodiazepines are highly effective for the relief of anxiety associated with generalized anxiety disorder. Most persons should be treated for a predetermined, specific, and relatively brief period. However, because generalized anxiety disorder is a chronic disorder with a high rate of recurrence, some persons with generalized anxiety disorder may warrant long-term maintenance treatment with benzodiazepines.

Panic Disorder. Two high-potency benzodiazepines, alprazolam and clonazepam, are effective for treatment of panic disorder with or without agoraphobia. The SSRIs sertraline (Zoloft) and paroxetine (Paxil) are also indicated for treatment of panic disorder. Benzodiazepines and SSRIs can be initiated together to treat acute panic symptoms, then use of the benzodiazepine can be tapered off after 3 to 4 weeks once the therapeutic benefits of the SSRI have emerged.

Social Phobia. Clonazepam has been shown to be an effective treatment for social phobia. In addition, several other benzodiazepines (e.g., diazepam) have been used as adjunctive medications for treatment of social phobia.

Other Anxiety Disorders. Benzodiazepines are used adjunctively for treatment of adjustment disorder with anxiety, pathological anxiety associated with life events (for example, after an accident), obsessive-compulsive disorder, and posttraumatic stress disorder.

Mixed Anxiety-Depressive Disorder

Alprazolam is indicated for the treatment of anxiety associated with depression. The availability of several antidepressant drugs with more favorable safety profiles makes alprazolam a second-line drug for this indication; however, some patients respond to this medication when other drugs have had minimal effect.

Bipolar I Disorder

Clonazepam, lorazepam, and alprazolam are effective in the management of acute manic episodes and as an adjuvant to maintenance therapy in lieu of antipsychotics. As an adjuvant to lithium (Eskalith), clonazepam may result in an increased time between cycles and fewer depressive episodes.

Akathisia

The first-line drug for akathisia is most commonly a β-adrenergic receptor antagonist. However, benzodiazepines are also effective in treating some patients with akathisia.

Parkinson's Disease

A small number of persons with idiopathic Parkinson's disease will respond to long-term use of zolpidem with reduced bradykinesia and rigidity. Zolpidem dosages of 10 mg four times daily may be tolerated without sedation for several years.

Other Psychiatric Indications

Clonazepam augmentation may accelerate but not potentiate the antidepressant effects of fluoxetine (Prozac). Chlordiazepoxide (Librium) clorazepate is used to manage the symptoms of alcohol withdrawal. The benzodiazepines (especially i.m. lorazepam) are used to manage agitation, both substance-induced (except amphetamine) and psychotic agitation in the emergency room. Benzodiazepines have been used instead of amobarbital (Amytal) for drug-assisted interviewing. Benzodiazepines have also been used in the treatment of catatonia.

Flumazenil for Benzodiazepine Overdosage

Flumazenil is used to reverse the adverse psychomotor, amnestic, and sedative effects of benzodiazepine receptor agonists, including benzodiazepines, zolpidem, and zaleplon. Flumazenil is administered i.v. and has a half-life of 7 to 15 minutes. The most common adverse effects of flumazenil are nausea, vomiting, dizziness, agitation, emotional lability, cutaneous vasodilation, injection-site pain, fatigue, impaired vision, and headache. The most common serious adverse effect associated with use of flumazenil is the precipitation of seizures, which is especially likely to occur in persons with seizure disorders, those who are physically dependent on benzodiazepines, or those who have ingested large quantities of benzodiazepines. Flumazenil alone may impair memory retrieval.

In mixed-drug overdosage the toxic effects (e.g., seizures and cardiac arrhythmias) of other drugs (e.g., tricyclic drugs) may emerge with the reversal of the benzodiazepine effects of flumazenil. For example, seizures caused by an overdosage of tricyclic drugs may have been partially treated in a person who had also taken an overdosage of benzodiazepines. With flumazenil treatment, the tricyclic-induced seizures or cardiac arrhythmias may appear and result in a fatal outcome. Flumazenil does not reverse the effects of ethanol, barbiturates, or opioids.

For the initial management of a known or suspected benzodiazepine overdosage, the recommended initial dosage of flumazenil is 0.2 mg (2 mL) administered i.v. over 30 seconds. If the desired consciousness is not obtained after 30 seconds, a further dose of 0.3 mg (3 mL) can be administered over 30 seconds. Further doses of 0.5 mg (5 mL) can be administered over 30 seconds at 1-minute intervals up to a cumulative dose of 3.0 mg. The clinician should not rush the administration of flumazenil. A secure airway and intravenous access should be established before the administration of the drug. Persons should be awakened gradually.

Most persons with a benzodiazepine overdosage respond to a cumulative dose of 1 to 3 mg of flumazenil; doses above 3 mg of flumazenil do not reliably produce additional effects. If a person has not responded 5 minutes after receiving a cumulative dose of 5 mg of flumazenil, the major cause of sedation is probably not benzodiazepine-receptor agonists, and additional flumazenil is unlikely to have an effect.

Sedation can return in 1 to 3 percent of persons treated with flumazenil. It can be prevented or treated by giving repeated dosages of flumazenil at 20-minute intervals. For repeat treatment, no more than 1 mg (given as 0.5 mg a minute) should be given at any one time, and no more than 3 mg should be given in any 1 hour.

PRECAUTIONS AND ADVERSE REACTIONS

The most common adverse effect of benzodiazepines is drowsiness, which occurs in about 10 percent of all persons. Because of this adverse effect, persons should be advised to be careful while driving or using dangerous machinery when taking the drugs. Drowsiness can be present during the day after the use of a benzodiazepine for insomnia the previous night, so-called residual daytime sedation. Some persons also experience ataxia (less than 2 percent) and dizziness (less than 1 percent). These symptoms can result in falls and hip fractures, especially in elderly persons. The most serious adverse effects of benzodiazepines occur when other sedative substances, such as alcohol, are taken concurrently. These combinations can result in marked drowsiness, disinhibition, or even respiratory depression. Infrequently, benzodiazepine receptor agonists cause mild cognitive deficits that may impair job performance. Persons taking benzodiazepine receptor agonists should be advised to exercise additional caution when driving or operating dangerous machinery.

High-potency benzodiazepines, especially triazolam, and zolpidem can cause anterograde amnesia. An unusual, paradoxical increase in aggression has been reported in persons given benzodiazepines, although this effect may be most common in persons with preexisting brain damage. Allergic reactions to the drugs are rare, but a few studies report maculopapular rashes and generalized itching. The symptoms of benzodiazepine intoxication include confusion, slurred speech, ataxia, drowsiness, dyspnea, and hyporeflexia.

Triazolam has received significant attention in the media because of an alleged association with serious aggressive behavioral manifestations. Therefore, the manufacturer recommends that the drug be used no more than 10 days for treatment of insomnia and that physicians should carefully evaluate the emergence of any abnormal thinking or behavioral changes in persons treated with triazolam, giving appropriate consideration to all potential causes. Triazolam was banned in Great Britain in 1991.

Persons with hepatic disease and elderly persons are particularly likely to have adverse effects and toxicity from the benzodiazepines, including hepatic coma, especially when the drugs are administered repeatedly or in high dosages. Benzodiazepines can produce clinically significant impairment of respiration in persons with chronic obstructive pulmonary disease and sleep apnea. Alprazolam may exert a direct appetite stimulant effect and may cause weight gain. Benzodiazepines should be used with caution by persons with a history of substance abuse, cognitive disorders, renal disease, hepatic disease, porphyria, CNS depression, or myasthenia gravis.

Some data indicate that benzodiazepines are teratogenic; therefore, their use during pregnancy is not advised. Moreover, the use of benzodiazepines in the third trimester can precipitate a withdrawal syndrome in the newborn. The drugs are secreted in the breast milk in sufficient concentrations to affect the newborn. Benzodiazepines may cause dyspnea, bradycardia, and drowsiness in nursing babies.

Zolpidem and zaleplon are generally well tolerated. At zolpidem dosages of 10 mg per day and zaleplon dosages above 10 mg per day, a small number of persons will experience dizziness, drowsiness, dyspepsia, or diarrhea. Zolpidem and zaleplon are secreted in breast milk and are, therefore, contraindicated for use by nursing mothers. The dosage of zolpidem and zaleplon should be reduced in the elderly and in persons with hepatic impairment. In rare cases, zolpidem may cause hallucinations, which can last up to 1 hour in some persons. The coadministration of zolpidem and SSRIs may extend the duration of hallucinations in susceptible patients to 1 to 7 hours.

Tolerance, Dependence, and Withdrawal

When benzodiazepines are used for short periods (1 to 2 weeks) in moderate dosages, they usually cause no significant tolerance, dependence, or withdrawal effects. The short-acting benzodiazepines (e.g., triazolam) may be an exception to this rule, as some persons have reported increased anxiety the day after taking a single dosage of the drug. Some persons also report a tolerance for the anxiolytic effects of benzodiazepines and require increased dosages to maintain the clinical remission of symptoms.

The appearance of a withdrawal syndrome, also called a discontinuation syndrome, depends on the length of time the person has taken a benzodiazepine, the dosage the person has been taking, the rate at which the drug is tapered, and the half-life of the compound. Benzodiazepine withdrawal syndrome consists of anxiety, nervousness, diaphoresis, restlessness, irritability, fatigue, light-headedness, tremor, insomnia, and weakness (Table 8–2). Abrupt discontinuation of benzodiazepines, particularly those with short half-lives, is associated with severe withdrawal symptoms, which may include depression, paranoia, delirium, and seizures. These severe symptoms are more likely to occur if flumazenil is used for rapid reversal of the benzodiazepine receptor agonist effects. Some features of the syndrome may occur in as many as 90 percent of the persons treated with the drugs. The development of a severe withdrawal syndrome is seen only in persons who have taken high dosages for long periods. The appearance of the syndrome may be delayed for 1 or 2 weeks in persons who had been taking benzodiazepines with long half-lives. Alprazolam seems to be particularly associated with an immediate and severe withdrawal syndrome and should be tapered gradually.

When the medication is to be discontinued, the drug must be tapered slowly (25 percent a week); otherwise, recurrence or rebound of symptoms is likely. Monitoring of any withdrawal symptoms (possibly with a standardized rating scale) and psychological support of the person are helpful in the successful accomplishment of benzodiazepine discontinuation. Concurrent use of carbamazepine (Tegretol) during benzodiazepine discontinuation has been reported to permit a more rapid and better-tolerated withdrawal than does a gradual taper alone. The dosage range of carbamazepine used to facilitate withdrawal is 400 to 500 mg a day. Some clinicians report particular difficulty in tapering and discontinuing alprazolam, especially in persons who have been receiving high dosages for long periods. There have been reports of successful discontinuation of alprazolam by switching to clonazepam, which is then gradually withdrawn.

Zolpidem and zaleplon can produce a mild withdrawal syndrome lasting 1 day after prolonged use at higher therapeutic dosages. Rarely, a person taking zolpidem has self-titrated up the daily dosage to 300 to 400 mg a day. Abrupt discontinuation of such a high dosage of zolpidem may cause withdrawal symptoms for 4 or more days. Tolerance does not develop to the sedative effects of zolpidem and zaleplon.

TABLE 8–2
COMMONLY OBSERVED SYMPTOMS OR BENZODIAZEPINE WITHDRAWAL SYNDROME

Anxiety
Irritability
Insomnia
Fatigue
Headache
Muscle twitching or aching
Tremor, shakiness
Sweating
Dizziness
Concentration difficulties
[a]Nausea, loss of appetite
[a]Observable depression
[a]Depersonalization, derealization
[a]Increased sensory perception (smell, light, taste, touch)
[a]Abnormal perception or sensation of movement

[a] Symptoms likely to represent true withdrawal, rather than an exacerbation or return of original anxiety. From Roy-Byrne PP, Hommer D: Benzodiazepine withdrawal: Overview and implications for the treatment of anxiety. *Am J Med* 1988;84:1041, with permission.

DRUG INTERACTIONS

The most common and potentially serious benzodiazepine receptor agonist interaction is excessive sedation and respiratory depression occurring when benzodiazepines, zolpidem, or zaleplon are administered concomitantly with other CNS depressants, such as alcohol, barbiturates, tricyclic and tetracyclic drugs, dopamine receptor antagonists, opioids, and antihistamines. Ataxia and dysarthria may be likely to occur when lithium, antipsychotics, and clonazepam are combined. The combination of benzodiazepines and clozapine (Clozaril) has been reported to cause delirium and should be avoided. Cimetidine (Tagamet), disulfiram (Antabuse), isoniazid (Nydrazid), estrogen, and oral contraceptives increase the plasma concentrations of diazepam, chlordiazepoxide, clorazepate, flurazepam, prazepam, and halazepam. Cimetidine increases the plasma concentrations of zaleplon. The plasma concentrations of triazolam and alprazolam are increased to potentially toxic concentrations by nefazodone (Serzone) and fluvoxamine (Luvox). The manufacturer of nefazodone recommends that the dosage of triazolam be lowered by 75 percent and the dosage of alprazolam lowered by 50 percent, when given concomitantly with nefazodone. Over-the-counter preparations of kava plant, advertised as a "natural tranquilizer," can potentiate the action of benzodiazepine receptor agonists through synergistic overactivation of GABA receptors. Carbamazepine can lower the plasma concentration of alprazolam. Antacids and food may decrease the plasma concentrations of benzodiazepines, and smoking may increase the metabolism of benzodiazepines. Rifampin (Rifadin), phenytoin (Dilantin), carbamazepine, and phenobarbital (Solfoton, Luminal) significantly increase the metabolism of zaleplon. The benzodiazepines may increase the plasma concentrations of phenytoin and digoxin (Lanoxin). SSRIs may prolong and exacerbate the severity of zolpidem-induced hallucinations.

LABORATORY INTERFERENCES

No known laboratory interferences are associated with the use of benzodiazepines, zolpidem, and zaleplon.

DOSAGE AND CLINICAL GUIDELINES

The clinical decision to treat an anxious person with a benzodiazepine should be carefully considered. Medical causes of anxiety (e.g., thyroid dysfunction, caffeinism, and prescription medications) should be ruled out. Benzodiazepine use should be started at a low dosage, and the person should be instructed regarding the drug's sedative properties and abuse potential. An estimated length of therapy should be decided at the beginning of therapy, and the need for continued therapy should be reevaluated at least monthly because of the problems associated with long-term use. However, certain persons with anxiety disorders are unresponsive to treatments other than benzodiazepines in long-term use.

Benzodiazepines are available in a wide range of formulations (Table 8–1). Some benzodiazepines are more potent than others in that one compound requires a relatively smaller dosage than another compound to achieve the same effect. For example, clonazepam requires 0.25 mg to achieve the same effect as 5 mg of diazepam; thus, clonazepam is considered a high-potency benzodiazepine. Conversely, oxazepam has an approximate dosage equivalence of 15 mg and is a low-potency drug. The four high-potency benzodiazepines—alprazolam, triazolam, estazolam, and clonazepam—are the drugs most likely to be effective for the treatment of bipolar I disorder, panic disorder, and the phobias.

Zolpidem is available in 5- and 10-mg tablets. A single 10-mg dose is the usual dose for the treatment of insomnia and is also the maximum daily dose. A single dose of zolpidem can be expected to provide 5 hours of sleep with minimal residual impairment. For persons over age 65 or persons with hepatic impairment, an initial dose of 5 mg is advised.

Zaleplon is available in 5- and 10-mg capsules. A single 10-mg dose is the usual adult dose. The dose can be increased to a maximum of 20 mg as tolerated. A single dose of zaleplon can be expected to provide 4 hours of sleep with minimal residual impairment. For persons over age 65 or persons with or hepatic impairment, an initial dose of 5 mg is advised.

For a more detailed discussion of this topic, see Ballenger JC: Benzodiazepine Receptor Agonists and Antagonists, Sec 31.10, p 2317, in CTP/VII.

9

Bupropion

Bupropion (Wellbutrin, Zyban) is a first-line agent for treatment of depression and smoking cessation. It generally is more effective against symptoms of depression than those of anxiety, and it is quite effective in combination with selective serotonin reuptake inhibitors (SSRIs). Despite early warnings that it could cause seizures, clinical experience shows that when used at recommended doses, bupropion is no more likely to cause seizures than is any other antidepressant drug. Smoking cessation is most successful when bupropion (called Zyban for this indication) is used in combination with behavioral modification techniques.

Bupropion is a unique antidepressant in the available armamentarium of drugs, with a highly favorable profile of adverse effects. Of particular note among antidepressants, it is associated with little inhibition of sexual function. It is also associated with a higher likelihood of weight loss than weight gain. It possesses some dopaminergic effects and may serve as a mild psychostimulant as well as an antidepressant.

CHEMISTRY

Bupropion is a unicyclic aminoketone that resembles amphetamine and the diet drug diethylpropion (Tenuate) in its molecular structure (Figure 9–1).

PHARMACOLOGICAL ACTIONS

Bupropion is well absorbed from the gastrointestinal (GI) tract. Peak plasma concentrations of bupropion are usually reached within 2 hours of oral administration, and peak levels of the sustained-release version are seen after 3 hours. The mean half-life of the compound is 12 hours, ranging from 8 to 40 hours.

The mechanism of action for the antidepressant effects of bupropion is poorly understood. It was initially thought that bupropion acts through the blockade of dopamine reuptake. However, central nervous system (CNS) concentrations of bupropion are probably not sufficient to result in significant dopamine reuptake inhibition. Nonetheless, some data indicate that bupropion exerts its antidepressant effects by increasing the functional efficiency of noradrenergic systems. Regarding the effects of bupropion on smoking cessation, it is a noncompetitive inhibitor of nicotinic acetylcholine receptors and thus may interfere with the addictive actions of nicotine.

THERAPEUTIC INDICATIONS

Depression

The therapeutic efficacy of bupropion in depression is well established in both outpatient and inpatient settings. Improvement in sleep early in the course of treatment is seen less often with bupropion than with some other antidepressants, because

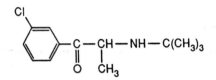

Figure 9-1.   Molecular structure of bupropion.

of its lack of sedation; however, it does not disrupt sleep architecture as much as the SSRIs. It is also of use in hypoactive sexual desire that may accompany depression.

Bipolar Disorders

Bupropion may be less likely than tricyclics to precipitate mania in persons with bipolar I disorder, although it is not free of this risk. It may be less likely than other antidepressants to exacerbate or induce rapid-cycling bipolar II disorder.

Attention-Deficit/Hyperactivity Disorder

Bupropion is a major second-line agent, after the sympathomimetics, for treatment of attention-deficit/hyperactivity disorder (ADHD). It can be nearly as efficacious as methylphenidate (Ritalin) for childhood and adult ADHD. Bupropion is an appropriate choice for persons with comorbid ADHD and depression or persons with comorbid ADHD, conduct disorder, or substance abuse.

Cocaine Detoxification

Some clinicians have reported that bupropion can be used to reduce the cravings for cocaine in persons who have withdrawn from the substance.

Smoking Cessation

Bupropion is indicated for use in combination with behavioral modification programs for smoking cessation. Success of smoking cessation efforts is best associated with a high degree of motivation and structured behavioral support. Bupropion and nicotine substitutes (Nicoderm, Nicotrol) individually increase the success rate, and they act synergistically in combination.

PRECAUTIONS AND ADVERSE REACTIONS

The most common adverse effects associated with use of bupropion are headache, insomnia, upper respiratory complaints, and nausea. Restlessness, agitation, and irritability may also occur. Most likely because of its potentiating effects on dopaminergic neurotransmission, bupropion has rarely been associated with psychotic symptoms, including hallucinations, delusions, and catatonia, as well as delirium. Most notable about bupropion is the absence of significant drug-induced orthostatic hypotension, weight gain, daytime drowsiness, and anticholinergic effects. Some persons, however, may experience dry mouth or constipation, and weight loss may occur in about 25 percent of persons. Bupropion causes no significant cardiovascular or clinical laboratory changes.

A major advantage of bupropion over SSRIs is that bupropion is virtually devoid of any adverse effects on sexual functioning, whereas the SSRIs are associated with such effects in up to 80 percent of all persons. Some people taking bupropion experience increased sexual responsiveness and even spontaneous orgasm.

At dosages of 300 mg a day or less of the sustained-release preparation, the incidence of seizures is 0.05 percent, which is no worse than the incidence of seizures with other antidepressants. The risk of seizures increases to about 0.1 percent 400 mg a day. Risk factors for seizures, such as past history of seizures, use of alcohol, recent benzodiazepine withdrawal, organic brain disease, head trauma, or epileptiform discharges on electroencephalogram (EEG), warrant critical examination of the decision to use bupropion.

Because high dosages (more than 400 mg a day) of bupropion may be associated with a euphoric feeling, bupropion may be relatively contraindicated in persons with histories of substance abuse. The use of bupropion by pregnant women has not been studied and is not recommended. Because bupropion is secreted in breast milk, the use of bupropion in nursing women is not recommended.

Overdoses with bupropion are associated with a generally favorable outcome, except in the cases of huge doses and mixed-drug overdoses. Seizures occur in about a third of all overdoses, and fatalities can involve uncontrollable seizures, bradycardia, and cardiac arrest. In general, however, bupropion is safer in overdose cases than are other antidepressants, except perhaps the SSRIs.

DRUG INTERACTIONS

Bupropion should not be used concurrently with monoamine oxidase inhibitors (MAOIs) because of the possibility of inducing a hypertensive crisis, and at least 14 days should pass after the discontinuation of an MAOI before initiating treatment with bupropion. Addition of bupropion may permit persons taking antiparkinsonian medications to lower the doses of their dopaminergic drugs. However, delirium, psychotic symptoms, and dyskinetic movements may be associated with the coadministration of bupropion and dopaminergic agents such as levodopa (Larodopa), pergolide (Permax), ropinirol (Requip), pramipexole (Mirapex), amantadine (Symmetrel), and bromocriptine (Parlodel).

Bupropion in combination with lithium (Eskalith) is effective and well tolerated in some persons with refractory depression, but this combination may rarely cause CNS toxicity, including seizures.

The combination of bupropion and fluoxetine (Prozac) is one of the most effective and well-tolerated treatments for all types of depression, but a few case reports indicate that panic, delirium, or seizures may be associated with this combination. Patients with panic disorder are sensitive to the activating effects of bupropion and may have an exacerbation of their anxiety.

Carbamazepine (Tegretol) may decrease plasma concentrations of bupropion, and bupropion may increase plasma concentrations of valproic acid (Depakene).

LABORATORY INTERFERENCES

A report has appeared indicating that bupropion may give a false positive result on urinary amphetamine screens. No other reports have appeared of laboratory interferences clearly associated with bupropion treatment. Clinically nonsignificant changes in the ECG (premature beats and nonspecific ST-T changes) and decreases in the white blood cell count (by about 10 percent) have been reported in a small number of persons.

DOSAGE AND CLINICAL GUIDELINES

Bupropion is available in 75- and 100-mg tablets, and sustained-release bupropion is available in 100- and 150-mg tablets. Initiation of treatment in the average adult person should be at 100 mg orally twice a day or 150 mg of the sustained-release version once a day. On the fourth day of treatment, the dosage can be raised to 100 mg three times a day or 300 mg a day of the sustained-release formulation taken in the morning or in two divided doses. As 300 mg is the recommended dosage, the person should be maintained on this dosage for several weeks before increasing the dosage further. Because of the risk of seizures, increases in dosage should never exceed 100 mg in a 3-day period; a single dose of bupropion should never exceed 150 mg, and a single dose of sustained-release bupropion should never exceed 300 mg. The total daily dosage should not exceed 450 mg of the immediate-release formulation or 400 mg of the sustained-release version.

For smoking cessation, the patient should start taking 150 mg a day of sustained-release bupropion 10 to 14 days before quitting smoking. On the fourth day, the dosage should be increased to 150 mg twice daily. Treatment generally lasts 7 to 12 weeks.

For a more detailed discussion of this topic, see Golden RN, Nicholas LM: Bupropion, Sec 31.11, p 2324, in CTP/VII.

10

Buspirone

Buspirone (BuSpar) is indicated for the treatment of anxiety disorders. Unlike the benzodiazepines and the barbiturates, buspirone does not have sedative, hypnotic, muscle-relaxant, or anticonvulsant effects; carries a low potential for abuse; and is not associated with withdrawal phenomena or cognitive impairment.

CHEMISTRY

The molecular structure of buspirone is chemically distinct from currently available benzodiazepines, barbiturates, and antidepressants (Figure 10–1).

PHARMACOLOGICAL ACTIONS

Buspirone is well absorbed from the gastrointestinal (GI) tract and is unaffected by food intake. The drug reaches peak plasma levels in 60 to 90 minutes after oral administration. The short half-life (2 to 11 hours) necessitates dosing three times daily.

In contrast to benzodiazepines and barbiturates, which act on the γ-aminobutyric acid (GABA)-associated chloride ion channel, buspirone has no effect on that receptor mechanism. Rather, buspirone acts as an agonist or partial agonist on serotonin 5-HT_{1A}-receptors. Buspirone also has activity at 5-HT_2 and dopamine D_2 receptors, although the significance of the effects at these receptors is unknown. At D_2 receptors, it has properties of both an agonist and an antagonist. The fact that buspirone takes 2 to 3 weeks to exert its therapeutic effects implies that whatever its initial effects, the therapeutic effects may involve the modulation of several neurotransmitters and intraneuronal mechanisms.

THERAPEUTIC INDICATIONS

Generalized Anxiety Disorder

Buspirone is safe and effective for treatment of generalized anxiety disorder. Compared with benzodiazepines, buspirone is generally more effective for symptoms of anger and hostility, equally effective for psychic symptoms of anxiety, and less effective for somatic symptoms of anxiety. The full benefit of buspirone is evident only at dosages above 30 mg a day. Buspirone offers several advantages over the benzodiazepines in long-term use, including lack of development of withdrawal symptoms upon discontinuation and less need to return to benzodiazepines once the initial course of drug treatment is terminated (Table 10–1). Buspirone is not associ-

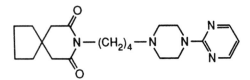

Figure 10-1. Molecular structure of buspirone.

ated with any abuse potential, even in groups of persons who are at high risk for addictive behavior.

Compared with the benzodiazepines, buspirone has a delayed onset of action and lacks any euphoric effect. Unlike benzodiazepines, buspirone has no immediate effects, and the patient should be told that a full clinical response may take 2 to 4 weeks. If an immediate response is needed, the patient can be started on a benzodiazepine and then withdrawn from the drug after buspirone's effects begin. Sometimes the sedative effects of benzodiazepines, which are not found with buspirone, are desirable; however, these sedative effects may cause impaired motor performance and cognitive deficits.

Other Disorders

Buspirone is not effective in the treatment of panic disorder or social phobia; however, buspirone may reduce the increased arousal and flashbacks associated with posttraumatic stress disorder. Evidence of the efficacy of high-dosage buspirone (30 to 90 mg a day) for depressive disorders is mixed. It is sometimes used to augment serotonergic antidepressant drugs for major depressive and obsessive-compulsive disorders.

Because buspirone does not act on the GABA-chloride ion channel complex, the drug is not recommended for the treatment of withdrawal from benzodiazepines, alcohol, or sedative-hypnotic drugs, except as treatment of comorbid anxiety symptoms.

Buspirone can effectively reduce aggression and anxiety in persons with organic brain disease or traumatic brain injury. It may also reduce comorbid oppositional-

TABLE 10-1
COMPARISON OF BENZODIAZEPINES AND BUSPIRONE

	Benzodiazepine	Buspirone
Effect of single dose	Yes	No
Full therapeutic action	Days	Weeks
Sedating	Yes	No
Dependence liability	Yes	No
Impair performance	Yes	No
Suppress sedative withdrawal symptoms	Yes	No
History of previous benzodiazepine response	Good response	Poor response
Side effects	Sedation, memory impairment	Restlessness, nervousness

From Silver JM, Yudofsky SC, Hurowitz G. Psychopharmacology and electroconvulsive therapy. In: *The American Psychiatric Press Textbook of Psychiatry.* 2nd edition (American Psychiatric Press, Washington, DC, 1994), with permission.

defiant symptoms, aggressive behavior, hyperactivity, impulsivity, inattention, and mood in children with attention-deficit/hyperactivity disorder (ADHD). Buspirone may also reduce hyperactivity associated with autistic spectrum disorders.

Buspirone may be beneficial for treatment of the physical and psychic symptoms of premenstrual dysphoric disorder. At higher dosages, buspirone may ameliorate the sexual inhibition of the selective serotonin reuptake inhibitors (SSRIs). It is also used to treat SSRI-induced bruxism.

PRECAUTIONS AND ADVERSE REACTIONS

The most common adverse effects of buspirone are headache, nausea, dizziness, and, rarely, insomnia. No sedation is associated with buspirone. Some persons may report a minor feeling of restlessness, although that symptom may reflect an incompletely treated anxiety disorder. No deaths have been reported from overdoses of buspirone, and the median lethal dose (LD_{50}) is estimated to be 160 to 550 times the recommended daily dose. Buspirone should be used with caution by persons with hepatic and renal impairment, pregnant women, and nursing mothers. Buspirone can be used safely by the elderly.

DRUG INTERACTIONS

The coadministration of buspirone and haloperidol (Haldol) results in increased blood concentrations of haloperidol. Buspirone should not be used with monoamine oxidase inhibitors (MAOIs) to avoid hypertensive episodes, and a 2-week washout period should pass between the discontinuation of MAOI use and the initiation of treatment with buspirone. Erythromycin (E-mycin), itraconazole (Sporonox), nefazodone (Serzone), and grapefruit juice may raise plasma concentrations of buspirone.

LABORATORY INTERFERENCES

Single doses of buspirone can cause transient elevations in growth hormone, prolactin, and cortisol concentrations, although the effects are not clinically significant.

DOSAGE AND CLINICAL GUIDELINES

Buspirone is available in single-scored 5- and 10-mg tablets and triple-scored 15-30-mg tablets; treatment is usually initiated with either 5 mg orally three times daily or 7.5 mg orally twice daily. The dosage can be raised 5 mg every 2 to 4 days to the usual dosage range of 15 to 60 mg a day.

Switching from a Benzodiazepine to Buspirone

Buspirone is as effective as the benzodiazepines in the treatment of anxiety in persons who have not received benzodiazepines in the past; however, buspirone does not achieve the same response in patients who have received benzodiazepines in the past. The reason is probably the absence of the immediate mildly euphoric and sedative effects of the benzodiazepines. The most common clinical problem, therefore, is how to initiate buspirone therapy in a person who is currently taking benzodiazepines. There are two alternatives. First, the clinician can start buspirone treatment gradually while the benzodiazepine is being withdrawn. Second, the clinician can start buspirone treatment and bring the person up to a therapeutic dosage for 2 to 3 weeks while the person is still receiving the regular dosage of the benzodiazepine, and then slowly taper the benzodiazepine dosage. The coadministration of buspirone and benzodiazepines may be effective in the treatment of anxiety disorders that have not responded to treatment with either drug alone.

For a more detailed discussion of this topic, see Brawman-Mintzer O, Lydiard RB, Ballenger JC: Buspirone, Sec 31.12, p 2329, in CTP/VII.

11

Calcium Channel Inhibitors

Calcium channel inhibitors are used in psychiatry as antimanic agents for persons who do not respond well to first-line agents such as lithium (Eskalith), valproic acid (Depakene), carbamazepine (Tegretol), or other anticonvulsants. Calcium channel inhibitors include nifedipine (Procardia, Adalat), nimodipine (Nimotop), isradipine (DynaCirc), amlodipine (Norvasc, Lotrel), nicardipine (Cardene), nisoldipine (Sular), nitrendipine, and verapamil (Calan). They are used for control of mania and ultradian bipolar disorder (mood cycling in less than 24 hours).

CHEMISTRY

The molecular structures of the calcium channel inhibitors that are most relevant to psychiatry are shown in Figure 11–1.

PHARMACOLOGICAL ACTIONS

The calcium channel inhibitors are well absorbed from the gastrointestinal (GI) tract, with significant first-pass hepatic metabolism. Considerable intraindividual and interindividual variations are seen in the plasma concentrations of the drugs after a single dose. The half-life of verapamil after the first dose is 2 to 8 hours; the half-life increases to 5 to 12 hours after the first few days of therapy. The half-lives of the other calcium channel blockers range from 1 to 2 hours for nimodipine and isradipine, to 30 to 50 hours for amlodipine (Table 11–1).

The calcium channel inhibitors discussed in this section inhibit the influx of calcium into neurons through L-type (long-acting) voltage-dependent calcium channels.

THERAPEUTIC INDICATIONS

Bipolar Disorder

There are mixed reports about the efficacy of verapamil for both short-term and maintenance treatment of bipolar disorders, to be used following trials of lithium, carbamazepine, and valproate. The other drugs, such as nimodipine, isradipine, and amlodipine, may be particularly effective in the treatment of manic episodes and of rapid-cycling or ultrarapid cycling bipolar disorders. The clinician should begin treatment with a short-acting drug such as nimodipine or isradipine, beginning with a low dosage and increasing the dosage every 4 to 5 days until a clinical response is seen or adverse effects appear. Once symptoms are controlled, a longer-acting drug,

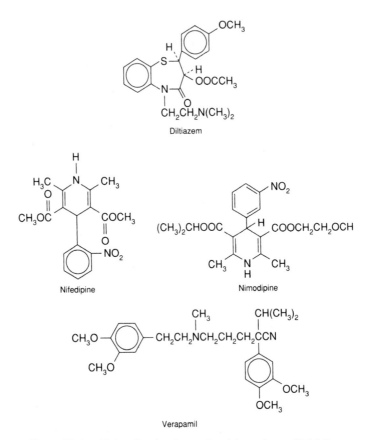

Figure 11-1.   Molecular structures of calcium channel inhibitors.

such as amlodipine, can be substituted as maintenance therapy. Failure to respond to verapamil does not exclude a favorable response to one of the other drugs.

Recurrent Brief Depressive Disorder

This disorder, characterized by brief (1- to 3-day) but possibly severe depressive episodes, may not be affected by standard antidepressants or lithium. Early experience shows that the calcium channel inhibitors may be effective for persons with recurrent brief depressive disorder; however, more trials are needed.

Other Psychiatric Indications

Calcium channel inhibitors may be beneficial in Tourette's disorder, Huntington's disease, Alzheimer's disease, panic disorder, premenstrual dysphoric disorder, and intermittent explosive disorder. Well-controlled studies have found a lack of ef-

TABLE 11–1
HALF-LIVES, DOSAGES, AND EFFECTIVENESS OF SELECTED CALCIUM CHANNEL INHIBITORS IN PSYCHIATRIC DISORDERS

	Verapamil (Calan, Isoptin)	Nimodipine (Nimotop)	Iaradipine (DynaCirc)	Amlodipine (Norvasc)
Half-life	Short (5–12 h)	Short (1–2 h)	Short ($1\frac{1}{2}$–2 h)	Long (30–50 h)
Starting dosage	30 mg ti.d.	30 mg t.i.d.	2.5 mg b.i.d.	5 mg h.s.
Peak daily dosage	480 mg	240–450 mg	15 mg	10–15 mg
Antimanic	++	++	(++)	a
Antidepressant	±	+	(+)	a
Antiultradian[b]	±	++	(++)	a

[a] No systematic studies, only case reports.
[b] Rapid-cycling bipolar disorder.
Table adapted from Robert M. Post, M.D.

ficacy for calcium channel inhibitors in schizophrenia, tardive dyskinesia, and major depression.

PRECAUTIONS AND ADVERSE REACTIONS

The most common adverse effects associated with calcium channel inhibitors are those due to vasodilation: dizziness, headache, tachycardia, nausea, dysesthesias, and peripheral edema. Verapamil and diltiazem (Cardizem) in particular can cause hypotension, bradycardia, and AV heart block, which necessitates close monitoring and sometimes discontinuation of the drugs. In all patients with cardiovascular disease, the drugs should be used with caution. Other common adverse effects include constipation, fatigue, rash, coughing, and wheezing. Adverse effects noted with diltiazem include hyperactivity, akathisia, and parkinsonism; with verapamil, delirium, hyperprolactinemia, and galactorrhea; with nimodipine, subjective sense of chest tightness and skin flushing; and with nifedipine, depression. The drugs have not been evaluated for safety in pregnant women and are best avoided. Because the drugs are secreted in breast milk, nursing mothers should also avoid the drugs.

DRUG INTERACTIONS

Calcium channel inhibitors should not be used by persons taking β-adrenergic receptor antagonists, hypotensives (e.g., diuretics, vasodilators, and angiotensin-converting enzyme inhibitors), or antiarrhythmic drugs (e.g., quinidine and digoxin) without consultation with an internist or cardiologist. Verapamil and diltiazem but not nifedipine have been reported to precipitate carbamazepine-induced neurotoxicity. Cimetidine (Tagamet) has been reported to increase plasma concentrations of nifedipine and diltiazem. Some patients who are treated with lithium and calcium channel inhibitors concurrently may be at increased risk for the signs and symptoms of neurotoxicity, and deaths have occurred.

LABORATORY INTERFERENCES

No known laboratory interferences are associated with the use of calcium channel inhibitors.

DOSAGE AND CLINICAL GUIDELINES

Verapamil is available in 40-, 80-, and 120-mg tablets; 120-, 180- and 240-mg sustained-release tablets; and 100-, 120-, 180-, 200-, 240-, 300-, and 360-mg sustained-release capsules. The starting dosage is 40 mg orally three times a day and can be raised in increments every 4 to 5 days up to 80 to 120 mg three times a day. The patient's blood pressure, pulse, and electrocardiogram (ECG) (in patients more than 40 years old or with a history of cardiac illness) should be routinely monitored.

Nifedipine is available in 10- and 20-mg capsules and 30-, 60-, and 90-mg extended-release tablets. Administration should be started at 10 mg orally three or four times a day and can be increased up to a maximum dosage of 120 mg a day.

Nimodipine is available in 30-mg capsules. It has been used at 60 mg every 4 hours for ultra-rapid-cycling bipolar disorder, and sometimes briefly at up to 630 mg per day.

Isradipine is available in 2.5- and 5-mg capsules and 5- or 10-mg controlled-release tablets. Administration should be started at 2.5 mg a day and can be increased up to a maximum of 15 mg a day in divided doses.

Amlodipine is available in 2.5-, 5-, and 10-mg tablets. Administration should start at 5 mg once at night and can be increased to a maximum dosage of 10 to 15 mg a day.

Diltiazem is available in 30-, 60-, 90-, and 120-mg tablets; 60-, 90-, 120-, 180-, 240-, 300-, and 360-mg extended-release capsules; and 60-, 90-, 120-, 180-, 240-, 300-, and 360-mg extended-release tablets. Administration should start with 30 mg orally four times a day and can be increased up to a maximum of 360 mg a day.

Elderly persons are more sensitive to the calcium channel inhibitors than are younger adults. No specific information is available regarding the use of the agents for children.

For a more detailed discussion of this topic, see Post RM: Calcium Channel Inhibitors, Sec 31.13, p 2334, in CTP/VII.

12

Carbamazepine

Carbamazepine (Tegretol) is effective for the treatment of acute mania and for the prophylactic treatment of bipolar I disorder. It is a first-line agent along with lithium (Eskalith) and valproic acid (Depakene). Carbamazepine is also used to treat partial and generalized-onset epilepsy and trigeminal neuralgia. A cogener, oxycarbazepine (Trilepetal) is also available but its use in psychiatry is limited at this time.

CHEMISTRY

The molecular structure of carbamazepine (Figure 12–1) is similar to the tricyclic structure of imipramine (Tofranil).

PHARMACOLOGICAL ACTIONS

Carbamazepine is absorbed slowly and erratically from the gastrointestinal (GI) tract, and absorption is enhanced when the drug is taken with meals. Peak plasma concentrations are reached 2 to 8 hours after a single dose, and steady-state levels are reached after 2 to 4 days on a steady dosage. The suspension formulation is absorbed somewhat faster, and the extended-release formulation somewhat slower, than the standard formulation. The half-life of carbamazepine at the initiation of treatment has a wide range; during long-term administration the half-life decreases to a range of 12 to 17 hours because of the induction of hepatic enzymes, which reaches its maximum level after about 1 month of therapy. The extended-release formulation permits achievement of smooth steady-state concentrations with twice-daily dosing. Carbamazepine is metabolized in the liver, and the 10,11-epoxide metabolite is active as an anticonvulsant; its activity in the treatment of bipolar disorders is unknown.

The anticonvulsant effects of carbamazepine are thought to be mediated mainly by binding to voltage-dependent sodium channels in the inactive state and prolonging their inactivation. This secondarily reduces voltage-dependent calcium channel activation and, therefore, synaptic transmission. Additional effects include reduction of currents through N-methyl-D-aspartate (NMDA) glutamate-receptor channels, competitive antagonism of adenosine A_1 receptors, and potentiation of central nervous system (CNS) catecholamine neurotransmission. Whether any or all of these mechanisms also result in mood stabilization is not known.

THERAPEUTIC INDICATIONS

Bipolar Disorder

Manic Episodes. Carbamazepine is effective in the treatment of acute mania, with efficacy comparable to that of lithium and antipsychotics. Carbamazepine is

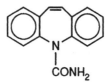

Figure 12-1. Molecular structure of carbamazepine.

also effective as a second-line agent in the prophylaxis of both manic and depressive episodes in bipolar disorders, after lithium and valproic acid. Carbamazepine is an effective antimanic agent in 50 to 70 percent of all persons within 2 to 3 weeks of initiation, and it may be effective in some persons who are not responsive to lithium, such as persons with dysphoric mania, rapid cycling, or a negative family history of mood disorders. The antimanic effects of carbamazepine can be augmented by concomitant administration of lithium, valproic acid, thyroid hormones, dopamine receptor antagonists, or serotonin-dopamine antagonists. Some persons may respond to carbamazepine but not lithium or valproic acid, and vice versa. Tolerance for the antimanic effects of carbamazepine can develop in some persons.

Depressive Episodes. The available data indicate that carbamazepine is an effective treatment for depression in some persons. About 25 to 33 percent of depressed persons respond to carbamazepine. That percentage is significantly smaller than the 60 to 70 percent response rate for standard antidepressants. Nevertheless, carbamazepine is an alternative drug for depressed persons who have not responded to conventional treatments, including electroconvulsive therapy (ECT), or who have a marked or rapid periodicity in their depressive episodes.

Schizophrenia and Schizoaffective Disorder

Carbamazepine is effective in the treatment of schizophrenia and schizoaffective disorder. Persons with prominent positive symptoms (e.g., hallucinations) may be likely to respond, as are persons who display impulsive aggressive outbursts.

Impulse-Control Disorders

Several studies have reported that carbamazepine is effective in controlling impulsive, aggressive behavior in nonpsychotic persons of all ages, including children and the elderly. Other drugs for impulse-control disorders, particularly intermittent explosive disorder, include lithium, propranolol (Inderal), and antipsychotics. Because of the risk of serious adverse effects with carbamazepine, treatment with other agents is warranted before initiating a trial with carbamazepine.

Carbamazepine is also effective in controlling nonacute agitation and aggressive behavior in schizophrenic persons. Diagnoses to be ruled out before treatment with carbamazepine is begun include akathisia and neuroleptic malignant syndrome. Lorazepam (Ativan) is more effective than carbamazepine for the control of acute agitation.

Posttraumatic Stress Disorder

Carbamazepine has been suggested, along with antidepressants, benzodiazepines, lithium, β-adrenergic receptor antagonists, and α_2-adrenergic receptor agonists, as a treatment for posttraumatic stress disorder (PTSD). Carbamazepine is particularly useful for management of agitation and aggression in PTSD.

Alcohol and Benzodiazepine Withdrawal

According to several studies, carbamazepine is as effective as the benzodiazepines in the control of symptoms associated with alcohol withdrawal. It may also assist in withdrawal from chronic alcohol or benzodiazepine use, especially in seizure-prone persons. However, the lack of any advantage of carbamazepine over the benzodiazepines for alcohol withdrawal and the potential risk of adverse effects with carbamazepine limit the clinical usefulness of this application.

PRECAUTIONS AND ADVERSE REACTIONS

Although the drug's hematological effects are not dose related, most of the adverse effects of carbamazepine are correlated with plasma concentrations above 9 μg/mL. The rarest but most serious adverse effects of carbamazepine are blood dyscrasias, hepatitis, and exfoliative dermatitis (Table 12–1). Otherwise, carbamazepine is relatively well tolerated by persons except for mild GI and CNS effects that can be significantly reduced if the dosage is increased slowly and minimal effective plasma concentrations are maintained.

Blood Dyscrasias

Severe blood dyscrasias (aplastic anemia, agranulocytosis) occur in about 1 in 125,000 persons treated with carbamazepine. There does not appear to be a correlation between the degree of benign white blood cell suppression (leukopenia), which is seen in 1 to 2 percent of persons, and the emergence of life-threatening blood dyscrasias. Persons should be warned that the emergence of such symptoms as fever, sore throat, rash, petechiae, bruising, and easy bleeding can potentially herald a serious dyscrasia and should cause the person to seek medical evaluation immediately. Routine hematological monitoring in carbamazepine-treated persons is recom-

TABLE 12–1
ADVERSE EVENTS ASSOCIATED WITH CARBAMAZEPINE

Dosage-Related Adverse Effects	Idiosyncratic Adverse Effects
Double or blurred vision	Agranulocytosis
Vertigo	Stevens-Johnson syndrome
Gastrointestinal disturbances	Aplastic anemia
Task performance impairment	Hepatic failure
Hematological effects	Rash
	Pancreatitis

mended at 3, 6, 9 and 12 months. If there is no significant evidence of bone marrow suppression by that time, many experts would reduce the interval of monitoring. However, even assiduous monitoring may fail to detect severe blood dyscrasias before they cause symptoms.

Hepatitis

Within the first few weeks of therapy, carbamazepine can cause both a hepatitis associated with increases in liver enzymes, particularly transaminases, and a cholestasis associated with elevated bilirubin and alkaline phosphatase. Mild transaminase elevations warrant observation only, but persistent elevations more than three times the upper limit of normal indicate discontinuation of carbamazepine. Hepatitis can recur if the drug is reintroduced to the person and can result in death.

Exfoliative Dermatitis

A benign pruritic rash occurs in 10 to 15 percent of persons treated with carbamazepine, usually occurring within the first few weeks of treatment. Approximately three persons per million per week may experience life-threatening dermatological syndromes, including exfoliative dermatitis, erythema multiforme, Stevens-Johnson syndrome, and toxic epidermal necrolysis. The possible emergence of these serious dermatological problems causes most clinicians to discontinue carbamazepine use in a person who develops any type of rash. If carbamazepine seems to be the only effective drug for a person who has a benign rash with carbamazepine treatment, a retrial of the drug can be undertaken with pretreatment of the person with prednisone (40 mg a day) in an attempt to treat the rash, although other symptoms of an allergic reaction (e.g., fever and pneumonitis) may develop, even with steroid pretreatment. The risk of drug rash is about equal between valproic acid and carbamazepine in the first 2 months of use but is subsequently much higher for carbamazepine.

Gastrointestinal Effects

The most common adverse effects of carbamazepine are nausea, vomiting, gastric distress, constipation, diarrhea, and anorexia. The severity of the adverse effects is reduced if the dosage of carbamazepine is increased slowly and kept at the minimal effective plasma concentration. Unlike lithium and valproate, carbamazepine does not appear to cause weight gain.

Central Nervous System Effects

Acute confusional states can occur with carbamazepine alone but occur most often in combination with lithium or antipsychotic drugs. Elderly persons and persons with cognitive disorders are at increased risk for CNS toxicity from carbamazepine.

The symptoms of CNS toxicity include dizziness, ataxia, clumsiness, sedation, diplopia, hyperreflexia, clonus, and tremor. These symptoms can be reduced by a slow upward titration of the dosage. The incidence of cognitive disturbances is about equal to carbamazepine, lithium, and valproic acid.

Other Adverse Effects

Carbamazepine decreases cardiac conduction (although less than the tricyclic drugs do) and can thus exacerbate preexisting cardiac disease. Carbamazepine should be used with caution in persons with glaucoma, prostatic hypertrophy, diabetes, or a history of alcohol abuse. Carbamazepine occasionally activates vasopressin-receptor function, which results in a condition resembling the syndrome of secretion of inappropriate antidiuretic hormone (SIADH), characterized by hyponatremia and, rarely, water intoxication. This is the opposite of the renal effects of lithium, i.e., nephrogenic diabetes insipidus. Augmentation of lithium with carbamazepine does not reverse the lithium effect, however. Emergence of confusion, severe weakness, or headache in a person taking carbamazepine should prompt measurement of serum electrolytes.

Carbamazepine use rarely elicits an immune hypersensitivity response consisting of fever, rash, eosinophilia, and possibly fatal myocarditis.

Some evidence indicates that minor cranial facial abnormalities, fingernail hypoplasia, and spina bifida in infants may be associated with the maternal use of carbamazepine during pregnancy. Therefore, pregnant women should not use carbamazepine unless absolutely necessary. The risk of neural tube defects can be reduced by maternal intake of folic acid 1 to 4 mg daily for at least 3 months prior to conception. Carbamazepine is secreted in breast milk, but its use during breast-feeding is considered safe by the American Academy of Pediatrics.

DRUG INTERACTIONS

Principally because it induces several hepatic enzymes, carbamazepine may interact with many drugs (Table 12–2). For the most part, addition of carbamazepine lowers the plasma concentrations of affected drugs, and monitoring for a decrease in clinical effects is frequently indicated. Coadministration with lithium, antipsychotic drugs, verapamil (Calan), or nifedipine (Procardia) can precipitate carbamazepine-induced CNS adverse effects. Carbamazepine can decrease the blood concentrations of oral contraceptives, resulting in breakthrough bleeding and uncertain prophylaxis against pregnancy. Carbamazepine should not be administered with monoamine oxidase inhibitors (MAOIs), which should be discontinued at least 2 weeks before initiating treatment with carbamazepine. Carbamazepine may significantly induce the metabolism of bupropion (Wellbutrin).

LABORATORY INTERFERENCES

Carbamazepine treatment is associated with a transient decrease in thyroid hormones (thyroxine [T_4] and triiodothyronine [T_3]) without an associated increase in

TABLE 12-2
CARBAMAZEPINE-DRUG INTERACTIONS

Effect of Carbamazepine on Plasma Concentrations of Concomitant Agents	Agents That May Affect Carbamazepine Plasma Concentrations
Carbamazepine may decrease drug plasma concentration of	*Agents that may increase carbamazepine plasma concentration*
Acetaminophen	Allopurinol
Alprazolam	Cimetidine
Amitriptyline	Clarithromycin
Bupropion	Danazol
Clomipramine	Diltiazem
Clonazepam	Erythromycin
Clozapine	Fluoxetine
Cyclosporine	Fluvoxamine
Desipramine	Gemfibrozil
Dicumarol	Itraconazole
Doxepine	Ketoconazole
Doxycycline	Isoniazid[a]
Ethosuximide	Itraconazole
Felbamate	Lamotrigine
Fentanyl	Lorantadine
Fluphenazine	Macrolides
Haloperidol	Nefazadone
Hormonal contraceptives	Nicotinamide
Imipramine	Propoxyphene
Lamotrigine	Terfenadine
Methadone	Troleandromycin
Methsuximide	Valproate[a]
Methylprednisolone	Verapamil
Nimodipine	Viloxazine
Pancuronium	
Phensuximide	*Drugs that may decrease carbamazepine plasma concentrations*
Phenytoin	Carbamazepine (autoinduction)
Primidone	Cisplatin
Theophylline	Doxorubicin HCl
Valproate	Felbamate
Warfarin	Phenobarbital
Carbamazepine may increase drug plasma concentrations of	Phenytoin
Clomipramine	Primidone
Phenytoin	Rifampin[b]
Primidone	Theophylline
	Valproate

[a] Increased concentrations of the active 10, 11-epoxide.
[b] Decreased concentrations of carbamazepine and increased concentrations of the 10, 11-epoxide.
Table by Carlos A. Zarate, Jr., M.D., and Mauricio Tohen, M.D.

thyroid-stimulating hormone (TSH). Carbamazepine is also associated with an increase in total serum cholesterol, primarily by increasing high-density lipoproteins. The thyroid and cholesterol effects are not clinically significant. Carbamazepine may interfere with the dexamethasone suppression test and may also cause false-positive pregnancy test results.

DOSAGE AND CLINICAL GUIDELINES

Carbamazepine can be used alone or with an antipsychotic drug for the treatment of manic episodes, although carbamazepine-induced CNS adverse effects (drowsiness, dizziness, ataxia) are likely to occur with this combination of drugs. Persons who do not respond to lithium alone may respond when carbamazepine is added to the lithium treatment. If a person then responds, an attempt should be made to withdraw the lithium to assess whether the person can be treated successfully with carbamazepine alone. When lithium and carbamazepine are used together, the clinician should minimize or discontinue any antipsychotics, sedatives, or anticholinergic drugs the person may be taking, to reduce the risks for adverse effects associated with taking multiple drugs. The combination of lithium and carbamazepine must be monitored closely for CNS toxicity, which may be fatal if not properly treated. The lithium and the carbamazepine should both be used at standard therapeutic plasma concentrations before a trial of combined therapy is considered to have been a therapeutic failure. A 3-week trial of carbamazepine at therapeutic plasma concentrations usually suffices to determine whether the drug will be effective in the treatment of acute mania; a longer trial is necessary to assess efficacy in the treatment of depression. Carbamazepine is also used in combination with valproic acid (Depakene), another anticonvulsant that is effective in bipolar disorders. When carbamazepine and valproate are used in combination, the dosage of carbamazepine should be decreased, because valproate displaces carbamazepine binding on proteins, and the dosage of valproate may need to be increased.

Pretreatment Medical Evaluation

The person's medical history should include information about preexisting hematological, hepatic, and cardiac diseases, because all three can be relative contraindications for carbamazepine treatment. Persons with hepatic disease require only one third to one half the usual dosage; the clinician should be cautious about raising the dosage in such persons and should do so only slowly and gradually. The laboratory examination should include a complete blood count with platelet count, liver function tests, serum electrolytes, and an electrocardiogram in persons more than 40 years of age or with a preexisting cardiac disease. An electroencephalogram (EEG) is not necessary before the initiation of treatment, but it may be helpful in some cases for the documentation of objective changes correlated with clinical improvement.

Initiation of Treatment

Carbamazepine is available in 100- and 200-mg tablets and as a 100 mg/5 mL suspension. The usual starting dosage is 200 mg orally two times a day; however, with titration, three-times-a-day dosing is optimal. An extended-release version suitable for twice-a-day maintenance dosing is available in 100-, 200-, and 400-mg tablets. Carbamazepine should be taken with meals, and the drug should be stored in a cool, dry place. Carbamazepine can lose one third of its potency when stored in a humid environment, such as a bathroom. In a hospital setting with seriously ill persons, the dosage can be raised by not more than 200 mg a day until a dosage of 600 to 1200 mg a day is reached. This relatively rapid titration, however, is often associated with adverse effects and may adversely affect compliance with the drug. In less ill persons and in outpatients, the dosage should be raised no more quickly than 200 mg every 2 to 7 days to minimize the occurrence of minor adverse effects such as nausea, vomiting, drowsiness, and dizziness. When discontinuing treatment with carbamazepine, the clinician generally should taper the dosage, although the drug can safely be stopped abruptly in most persons.

Blood Concentrations

The anticonvulsant blood concentration range for carbamazepine is 4 to 12 $\mu g/$ mL, and this range should be reached before determining that carbamazepine is not effective in the treatment of a mood disorder. It is clinically prudent to come up to that range gradually, since the person is likely to tolerate a gradual increase of carbamazepine better than a rapid increase. The clinician should titrate carbamazepine up to the highest well-tolerated dosage before deciding that the drug is ineffective. Plasma concentrations should be determined when a person has been receiving a steady dosage for at least 5 days. Blood for the determination of plasma levels is drawn in the morning before the first daily dose of carbamazepine is taken. The total daily dosage necessary to achieve plasma concentrations in the usual therapeutic range varies from 400 to 1600 mg a day, with a mean around 1000 mg a day.

Routine Laboratory Monitoring

The most serious potential effects of carbamazepine are agranulocytosis and aplastic anemia. Although it has been suggested that complete laboratory blood assessments be performed every 2 weeks for the first 2 months of treatment and quarterly thereafter, this conservative approach may not be justified by a cost-benefit analysis and may not detect a serious blood dyscrasia before it occurs. The Food and Drug Administration (FDA) has revised the package insert for carbamazepine to suggest that blood monitoring be performed at the discretion of the physician. Education about the signs and the symptoms of a developing hematological problem is probably more effective than is frequent blood monitoring in protecting against blood dyscrasias. It has also been suggested that liver and renal function tests be conducted quarterly, although the benefit of conducting tests this frequently has been questioned. It seems reasonable, however, to assess hematological status, along with liver and renal functions, whenever a routine examination of the person is being conducted. A monitoring protocol is listed in Table 12–3.

TABLE 12–3
LABORATORY MONITORING OF CARBAMAZEPINE FOR ADULT PSYCHIATRIC DISORDERS

	Baseline	Weekly to Stability	Monthly for 6 Mo	6–12 Mo
CBC[a]	+	+	+	+
Bilirubin	+		+	+
Alanine aminotransferase	+		+	+
Aspartate aminotransferase	+		+	+
Alkaline phosphatase	+		+	+
Carbamazepine level		+		+

[a] Complete blood count.

The following laboratory values should prompt the physician to discontinue carbamazepine treatment and to consult a hematologist: total white blood cell count below 3000/mm^3, erythrocytes below 4.0×10^6 per mm^3, neutrophils below 1500/mm^3, hematocrit less than 32 percent, hemoglobin less than 11 grams per 100 mL, platelet count below 100,000/mm^3, reticulocyte count below 0.3 percent, and a serum iron concentration below 150 mg per 100 mL.

For a more detailed discussion of this topic, see Zarate CA, Tohen M: Carbamazepine, Sec 31.7a, p 2282, in CTP/VII.

13

Chloral Hydrate

Chloral hydrate is a hypnotic agent rarely used in psychiatry because there are numerous safer options, such as the benzodiazepines. It is most frequently used as a sedative for pediatric procedures.

CHEMISTRY

The molecular structure of chloral hydrate is shown in Figure 13–1.

PHARMACOLOGICAL ACTIONS

Chloral hydrate is well absorbed from the gastrointestinal (GI) tract. The parent compound is metabolized within minutes by the liver to the active metabolite trichloroethanol, which has a half-life of 8 to 11 hours. A dose of chloral hydrate induces sleep in about 30 to 60 minutes and maintains sleep for 4 to 8 hours. It probably potentiates γ-aminobutyric (GABAergic) neurotransmission, which suppresses neuronal excitability.

THERAPEUTIC INDICATIONS

The major indication for chloral hydrate is for induction of sleep. It should be used no more than 2 or 3 days, because longer-term treatment is associated with an increased incidence and severity of adverse effects. Tolerance develops to the hypnotic effects of chloral hydrate after 2 weeks of treatment. The benzodiazepines are superior to chloral hydrate for all psychiatric uses.

PRECAUTIONS AND ADVERSE REACTIONS

Chloral hydrate has adverse effects on the central nervous system (CNS), gastrointestinal (GI) system, and skin. The sedation may extend into the next day and is associated with impaired motor coordination. Chloral hydrate has no analgesic properties and may cause excitement or agitation in the presence of pain. High doses (over 4 grams) may be associated with stupor, confusion, ataxia, falls, or coma. The GI effects include nonspecific irritation, nausea, vomiting, flatulence, and an unpleasant taste. With long-term use and overdose, gastritis and gastric ulceration can develop. The drug may aggravate GI inflammatory conditions. The dermatological effects, although not common, include rashes, urticaria, purpura, eczema, and erythema multiforme. The dermatological lesions are sometimes accompanied by fever.

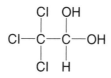

Figure 13-1. Molecular structure of chloral hydrate.

Chloral hydrate should be avoided in persons with severe renal, cardiac, or hepatic disease or with porphyria. Chloral hydrate is secreted in breast milk and should not be used during pregnancy or by nursing women.

In addition to the development of tolerance, dependence on chloral hydrate can occur, with symptoms similar to those of alcohol dependence. The symptoms of intoxication include confusion, ataxia, dysarthria, bradycardia, arrhythmia, and severe drowsiness. The lethal dose of chloral hydrate is between 5,000 and 10,000 mg, thus making chloral hydrate a particularly poor choice for potentially suicidal persons. The lethality of the drug is potentiated by other CNS depressants, including alcohol. Hepatic and renal damage can follow overdose attempts, resulting in jaundice and albuminuria.

DRUG INTERACTIONS

Chloral hydrate sedation occurs in addition to sedation due to other centrally acting agents. Because of metabolic interference, chloral hydrate should be strictly avoided with alcohol, a notorious concoction known as a "Mickey Finn." Use of chloral hydrate less than 24 hours before receiving intravenous furosemide (Lasix) can cause diaphoresis, flushes, and an unsteady blood pressure. Chloral hydrate may displace warfarin (Coumadin) from plasma proteins and enhance anticoagulant activity; this combination should be avoided.

LABORATORY INTERFERENCES

Chloral hydrate administration can lead to false-positive results for urine glucose determinations that use cupric sulfate (e.g., Clinitest) but not in tests that use glucose oxidase (e.g., Clinistix and Tes-Tape). Chloral hydrate may also interfere with the determination of urinary catecholamines and 17-hydroxycorticosteroids.

DOSAGE AND CLINICAL GUIDELINES

Chloral hydrate is available in 500-mg capsules, 500 mg/5 mL solution, and 324-, 500-, and 648-mg rectal suppositories. The standard dose of chloral hydrate is 500 to 2000 mg at bedtime. Because the drug is a GI irritant, it should be administered with excess water, milk, other liquids, or antacids to decrease gastric irritation.

For a more detailed discussion of this topic, see Labbate LA, Arana GW, Ballenger JC: Chloral Hydrate, Sec 31.14, p 2343, in CTP/VII.

14

Cholinesterase Inhibitors

Donepezil (Aricept), rivastigmine (Exelon), and tacrine (Cognex) are cholinesterase inhibitors used for the treatment of mild-to-moderate cognitive impairment in dementia of the Alzheimer's type. They reduce the inactivation of the neurotransmitter acetylcholine and thus potentiate cholinergic neurotransmission, which in turn produces a modest improvement in memory and goal-directed thought. These drugs are most useful for persons with mild- to-moderate memory loss who have enough preservation of their basal forebrain cholinergic neurons to benefit from augmentation of cholinergic neurotransmission.

Donepezil is well tolerated and widely used. Tacrine is rarely used, because of its potential for hepatotoxicity. There are fewer clinical data available for rivastigmine, which appears more likely to cause gastrointestinal (GI) and neuropsychiatric adverse effects than is donepezil.

CHEMISTRY

The molecular structures of donepezil, rivastigmine, tacrine, and galanthamine are shown in Figure 14–1.

PHARMACOLOGICAL ACTIONS

Donepezil is absorbed completely from the GI tract. Peak plasma concentrations are reached about 3 to 4 hours after oral dosing. The half-life of donepezil is 70 hours in the elderly, and it is taken only once daily. Steady-state levels are achieved within about 2 weeks. Presence of stable alcoholic cirrhosis reduces clearance of donepezil by 20 percent. Rivastigmine is rapidly and completely absorbed from the GI tract and reaches peak plasma concentrations in 1 hour, but this is delayed by up to 90 minutes if rivastigmine is taken with food. The half-life of rivastigmine is 1 hour, but because it remains bound to cholinesterases, a single dose is therapeutically active for 10 hours, and it is taken twice daily.

Tacrine is absorbed rapidly from the GI tract. Peak plasma concentrations are reached about 90 minutes after oral dosing. The half-life of tacrine is about 2 to 4 hours, thereby necessitating four-times-daily dosing.

The primary mechanism of action of cholinesterase inhibitors is reversible, nonacylating inhibition of acetylcholinesterase and butyrylcholinesterase, the enzymes that catabolize acetylcholine in the central nervous system (CNS). The enzyme inhibition increases synaptic concentrations of acetylcholine, especially in hippocampus and cerebral cortex. Unlike tacrine, which is nonselective for all forms of acetylcholinesterase, donepezil appears to be selectively active within the CNS and to have little activity in the periphery. Donepezil's favorable side effect profile appears to correlate with its lack of inhibition of cholinesterases in the GI tract. Rivastigmine

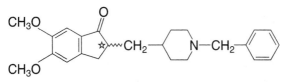

Donepezil

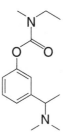

Rivastigmine

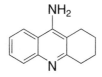

Tacrine

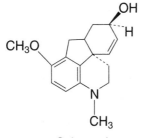

Galantamine

Figure 14-1. Molecular structures of cholinesterase inhibitors.

appears to have somewhat more peripheral activity than donepezil and is thus more likely to cause GI adverse effects than is donepezil.

THERAPEUTIC INDICATIONS

Donepezil, rivastigmine, and tacrine are effective for the treatment of cognitive impairment in dementia of the Alzheimer's type. Based on numerous well-controlled studies, the cholinesterase inhibitors in long-term use slow the progression of memory loss and diminish apathy, depression, hallucinations, anxiety, euphoria, and purposeless motor behaviors. Functional autonomy is less well preserved. Some persons note immediate improvement in memory, mood, psychotic symptoms, and interpersonal skills. Others note little initial benefit, but are able to retain their cognitive and adaptive faculties at a relatively stable level for many months. Use of cholinesterase inhibitors may delay or reduce the need for nursing home placement.

Donepezil may be beneficial for the treatment of dementia due to diffuse Lewy body disease and for treatment of cognitive deficits due to traumatic brain injury. Donepezil is under study for treatment of mild cognitive impairment less severe than that due to Alzheimer's disease. People with multi-infarction and other types of dementia may not respond to acetylcholinesterase inhibitors. Occasionally, cholinesterase inhibitors elicit an idiosyncratic catastrophic reaction, with signs of grief and agitation, that is self-limited once the drug is discontinued. Use of cholinesterase inhibitors to improve cognition by nondemented individuals should be discouraged.

PRECAUTIONS AND ADVERSE REACTIONS

Donepezil

Donepezil is generally well tolerated at recommended dosages. Less than 3 percent of persons taking donepezil experience nausea, diarrhea, and vomiting. These mild symptoms are more common with a 10-mg dose than with a 5-mg dose, and when present, they tend to resolve after 3 weeks of continued use. Donepezil may cause weight loss. Donepezil treatment has been infrequently associated with bradyarrhythmias, especially in persons with underlying cardiac disease. A small number of persons experience syncope.

Rivastigmine

Rivastigmine is generally well tolerated, but recommended dosages may need to be scaled back in the initial period of treatment to limit GI and CNS adverse effects. These mild symptoms are more common at dosages above 6 mg a day, and when present, they tend to resolve once the dosage is lowered. The most common adverse effects associated with rivastigmine are nausea, vomiting, dizziness, headache, diarrhea, abdominal pain, anorexia, fatigue, and somnolence. Rivastigmine may cause weight loss, but it does not appear to cause hepatic, renal, hematological, or electrolyte abnormalities.

Tacrine

Tacrine is cumbersome to titrate and use, and it poses the risk of potentially significant elevations in hepatic transaminase levels in 25 to 30 percent of persons, nausea and vomiting in about 20 percent of persons, and diarrhea and other cholinergic symptoms in about 11 percent of persons. Aside from elevated transaminase levels, the most common specific adverse effects associated with tacrine treatment are nausea, vomiting, myalgia, anorexia, and rash, but only nausea, vomiting, and anorexia have been found to have a clear relation to the dosage. Transaminase elevations characteristically develop during the first 6 to 12 weeks of treatment, and cholinergically mediated events are dosage related.

Hepatotoxicity.   Tacrine is associated with increases in the plasma activities of alanine aminotransferase (ALT) and aspartate aminotransferase (AST). The ALT measurement is the more sensitive indicator of the hepatic effects of tacrine. About 95 percent of patients who develop elevated ALT serum levels do so in the first 18 weeks of treatment. The average length of time for elevated ALT concentrations to return to normal after stopping tacrine treatment is 4 weeks.

For routine monitoring of hepatic enzymes, AST and ALT activities should be measured weekly for the first 18 weeks, every month for the second 4 months, and every 3 months thereafter. Weekly assessments of AST and ALT should be performed for at least 6 weeks after any increase in dosage. Patients with mildly elevated ALT activity should be monitored weekly, and not be rechallenged with tacrine until the ALT activity returns to the normal range. For any patient with elevated ALT activity and jaundice, tacrine treatment should be stopped, and the patient should not be given the drug again.

DRUG INTERACTIONS

The metabolism of donepezil may be increased by phenytoin (Dilantin), carbamazepine (Tegretol), dexamethasone (Decadron), rifampin (Rifadin), or phenobarbital (Solfoton). All cholinesterase inhibitors should be used cautiously with drugs that also possess cholinomimetic activity, such as succinylcholine (Anectine) or bethanechol (Urecholine). The coadministration of cholinesterase inhibitors and drugs that have cholinergic antagonist activity (e.g., tricyclic drugs) is probably counterproductive. Donepezil is highly protein bound, but it does not displace other protein-bound drugs, such as furosemide (Lasix), digoxin (Lanoxin), or warfarin (Coumadin). Rivastigmine circulates mostly unbound to serum proteins and has no significant known drug interactions.

LABORATORY INTERFERENCES

No laboratory interferences have been associated with donepezil, rivastigmine, or tacrine.

DOSAGE AND CLINICAL GUIDELINES

Before the initiation of treatment with cholinesterase inhibitors, potentially treatable causes of dementia should be ruled out and the diagnosis of dementia of the Alzheimer's type should be established with a thorough neurological evaluation. Detailed neuropsychological testing can detect early signs of Alzheimer's disease. Psychiatric evaluation also should focus on depression, anxiety, and psychosis.

Donepezil is available in 5- and 10-mg tablets. Treatment should be initiated at 5-mg each night. If well tolerated and of some discernible benefit after 4 weeks, the dosage should be increased to a maintenance dosage of 10-mg each night. Donepezil absorption is unaffected by meals.

Rivastigmine is available in 1.5-, 3-, 4.5-, and 6-mg capsules. The recommended initial dosage is 1.5 mg twice daily for a minimum of 2 weeks, after which increases of 1.5 mg a day can be made at intervals of at least 2 weeks to a target dosage of 6 mg a day, taken in two equal dosages. If tolerated, the dosage may be further titrated upward to a maximum of 6 mg twice daily. The risk of adverse GI events can be reduced by administration of rivastigmine with food.

Tacrine is available in 10-, 20-, 30-, and 40-mg capsules. Before the initiation of tacrine treatment, a complete physical and laboratory examination should be conducted, with special attention to liver function tests and baseline hematological indexes. Treatment should be initiated at 10 mg four times a day and then raised by increments of 10 mg a dose every 6 weeks up to 160 mg a day; the person's tolerance of each dosage is indicated by the absence of unacceptable side effects and lack of elevation of ALT activity. Tacrine should be given four times daily—ideally 1 hour before meals, since the absorption of tacrine is reduced by about 25 percent when it is taken during the first 2 hours after meals. If tacrine is used, the specific guidelines for tacrine-induced ALT listed above should be followed.

GALANTAMINE

Galantamine is a tertiary amine of the phenthrene group that competitively inhibits acetylcholinesterase but not butyrylcholinesterase. The compound is plant derived, naturally occurring, and is an agonist at nicotinic sites without producing desensitization, as well as a cholinesterase inhibitor. This ability to enhance the sensitivity of the acetylcholine receptor is possessed only by galantamine and physostigmine. The mechanism of action is analogous to that of benzodiazepines at the γ-aminobutyric acid (GABA) A site. Consequently, the drug has an in vivo cholinomimetic activity that is even stronger than its acetylcholinesterase inhibitory properties alone would predict. Galantamine's properties are interesting because in animals the combination of agonist and cholinesterase inhibitor may have an additive effect with fewer adverse events. Placebo-controlled clinical trials have demonstrated improved scores on the Alzheimer's Disease Assessment Scale (ADAS) and activities-of-daily-living measures. The usual effective daily dosage of galantamine is 20 to 40 mg in divided doses. The drug has been approved in Austria, and multicenter clinical trials are under way in Europe and the United States.

For a more detailed discussion of this topic, see SC Samuels, KL Davis: Cholinesterase Inhibitors, Sec 31.15, p 2346 in CTP/VII.

15

Dantrolene

Dantrolene (Dantrium) is a direct-acting skeletal muscle relaxant, which is used in treatment of neuroleptic malignant syndrome.

CHEMISTRY

The molecular structure of dantrolene is shown in Fig. 15–1.

PHARMACOLOGICAL ACTIONS

About one third of orally administered dantrolene is slowly absorbed from the gastrointestinal (GI) tract. Peak plasma concentrations are seen about 5 hours after oral administration, and the elimination half-life of dantrolene is about 9 hours. Dantrolene is metabolized by the liver and excreted in the urine.

Dantrolene produces skeletal muscle relaxation by directly affecting the contractile response of the muscles at a site inside the skeletal muscle cell. The skeletal muscle relaxant effect is the basis of its efficacy in reducing the muscle destruction and hyperthermia associated with neuroleptic malignant syndrome.

THERAPEUTIC INDICATIONS

Intravenous (i.v.) dantrolene reduces muscle spasm in about 80 percent of persons with neuroleptic malignant syndrome. Dantrolene is almost always used in conjunction with appropriate supportive measures and a dopamine receptor agonist. Muscle relaxation and a general and dramatic improvement in symptoms can appear within minutes of administration, although in most cases the beneficial effects can take several hours to appear. Some evidence indicates that dantrolene treatment must be continued for some time, perhaps days to a week or more, to minimize the risk of the recurrence of symptoms. Dantrolene has been used in efforts to treat other psychiatric conditions characterized by life-threatening muscle rigidity, such as catatonia and serotonin syndrome.

PRECAUTIONS AND ADVERSE REACTIONS

The most common adverse effects of dantrolene include muscle weakness, drowsiness, dizziness, light-headedness, nausea, diarrhea, malaise, and fatigue. These effects are generally transient. The central nervous system (CNS) effects of dantrolene include slurred speech, headache, visual disturbances, alteration of taste, depression, confusion, hallucinations, nervousness, and insomnia. More-serious ad-

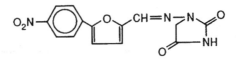

Figure 15-1.   Molecular structure of dantrolene.

verse effects, which appear only with long-term use, include hepatitis, seizures, and pleural effusion with pericarditis. Dantrolene should be used with caution by patients with hepatic, renal, or chronic lung disease.

Dantrolene can cross the placenta and is, thus, contraindicated for pregnant women and should not be used by nursing mothers except in emergency situations, such as neuroleptic malignant syndrome. No data are available regarding the use of dantrolene by the elderly, and no unique problems have been associated with its use by children.

DRUG INTERACTIONS

The risk of liver toxicity may be increased in patients who are also taking estrogens. Dantrolene should be used with caution by patients who are using other drugs that produce drowsiness, most notably the benzodiazepines. In the case of neuroleptic malignant syndrome, however, the general guidelines regarding dantrolene must be weighed against the severity of the syndrome. Dantrolene should not be given i.v. in combination with calcium channel blockers.

LABORATORY INTERFERENCES

No known laboratory interferences are associated with dantrolene, although experience with its use in patients with neuroleptic malignant syndrome is still limited.

DOSAGE AND CLINICAL GUIDELINES

In addition to the immediate discontinuation of antipsychotic drugs, medical support to cool the patient, and the monitoring of vital signs and renal output, dantrolene in dosages of 1 mg per kg can be given orally four times daily, or 1 to 5 mg per kg can be given i.v. to reduce muscle spasms in patients with neuroleptic malignant syndrome. Although some clinicians have recommended low dosages (2.5 mg per kg per day) because of the adverse effects, other clinicians indicate that daily dosages of 10 mg per kg are most likely to be effective. Dantrolene is supplied as 25-, 50-, and 100-mg capsules and in a 20-mg parenteral preparation for reconstitution with 60 mL of sterile water.

For a more detailed discussion of this topic, see DeBattista C, Schatzberg AF: Other Pharmacological and Biological Therapies, Sec 31.33, p 2521, in CTP/VII.

16

Disulfiram

Disulfiram (Antabuse) is used in the treatment of alcohol dependence. Its main effect is to produce a rapid and violently unpleasant reaction in a person who ingests even a small amount of alcohol. Because of the risk of severe and even fatal disulfiram-alcohol reactions, disulfiram therapy is used less often today than previously.

CHEMISTRY

The structural formula of disulfiram is shown in Figure 16–1.

PHARMACOLOGICAL ACTIONS

Disulfiram is almost completely absorbed from the gastrointestinal (GI) tract after oral administration. Its half-life is estimated to be 60 to 120 hours. Therefore, 1 or 2 weeks may be needed before disulfiram is totally eliminated from the body after the last dose has been taken.

The metabolism of ethanol proceeds through oxidation via alcohol dehydrogenase to the formation of acetaldehyde, which is further metabolized to acetyl-coenzyme A (acetyl-CoA) by aldehyde dehydrogenase. Disulfiram is an aldehyde dehydrogenase inhibitor that interferes with the metabolism of alcohol by producing a marked increase in blood acetaldehyde concentration. The accumulation of acetaldehyde (to a level up to 10 times higher than occurs in the normal metabolism of alcohol) produces a wide array of unpleasant reactions, called the *disulfiram-alcohol reaction*, characterized by nausea, throbbing headache, vomiting, hypertension, flushing, sweating, thirst, dyspnea, tachycardia, chest pain, vertigo, and blurred vision. The reaction occurs almost immediately after the ingestion of one alcoholic drink and may last up to 30 minutes.

THERAPEUTIC INDICATIONS

The primary indication for disulfiram use is as an aversive conditioning treatment for alcohol dependence. Either the fear of having a disulfiram-alcohol reaction or the memory of having had one is meant to condition the person not to use alcohol. Usually, describing the severity and the unpleasantness of the disulfiram-alcohol reaction graphically enough discourages the person from imbibing alcohol. Disulfiram treatment should be combined with such treatments as psychotherapy, group therapy, and support groups like Alcoholics Anonymous (AA). Treatment with disulfiram requires careful monitoring, since a person can simply decide not to take the medication.

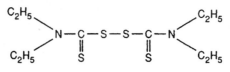

Figure 16-1.   Molecular formula of disulfiram.

PRECAUTIONS AND ADVERSE REACTIONS

With Alcohol Consumption

The intensity of the disulfiram-alcohol reaction varies with each person. In extreme cases it is marked by respiratory depression, cardiovascular collapse, myocardial infarction, convulsions, and death. Therefore, disulfiram is contraindicated for a person with significant pulmonary or cardiovascular disease. In addition, disulfiram should be used with caution, if at all, by a person with nephritis, brain damage, hypothyroidism, diabetes, hepatic disease, seizures, polydrug dependence, or an abnormal electroencephalogram (EEG). Most fatal reactions occur in persons who are taking more than 500 mg a day of disulfiram and who consume more than 3 ounces of alcohol. The treatment of a severe disulfiram-alcohol reaction is primarily supportive to prevent shock.

Without Alcohol Consumption

The adverse effects of disulfiram in the absence of alcohol consumption include fatigue, dermatitis, impotence, optic neuritis, a variety of mental changes, and hepatic damage. A metabolite of disulfiram inhibits dopamine-β-hydroxylase, the enzyme that metabolizes dopamine into norepinephrine and epinephrine, and thus may exacerbate psychosis in persons with psychotic disorders.

DRUG INTERACTIONS

Disulfiram increases the blood concentration of diazepam (Valium), paraldehyde, phenytoin (Dilantin), caffeine, tetrahydrocannabinol (the active ingredient in marijuana), barbiturates, anticoagulants, isoniazid (Nydrazid), and tricyclic drugs. Disulfiram should not be administered concomitantly with paraldehyde, because paraldehyde is metabolized to acetaldehyde in the liver.

LABORATORY INTERFERENCES

In rare instances, disulfiram has been reported to interfere with the incorporation of iodine-131 into protein-bound iodine. Disulfiram may reduce urinary concentrations of homovanillic acid, the major metabolite of dopamine, because of its inhibition of dopamine hydroxylase.

DOSAGE AND CLINICAL GUIDELINES

Disulfiram is supplied in 250- and 500-mg tablets. The usual initial dosage is 500 mg a day taken by mouth for the first 1 or 2 weeks, followed by a maintenance dosage of 250 mg a day. The dosage should not exceed 500 mg a day. The maintenance dosage range is 125 to 500 mg a day.

The person taking disulfiram must be instructed that the ingestion of even the smallest amount of alcohol will bring on a disulfiram-alcohol reaction, with all its unpleasant effects. In addition, the person should be warned against ingesting any alcohol-containing preparations, such as cough drops, tonics of any kind, and alcohol-containing foods and sauces. Some reactions have occurred in patients who used alcohol-based after shave lotions, toilet water, colognes, or perfumes and inhaled the fumes; therefore, precautions must be explicit and should include any topically applied preparations containing alcohol, such as perfume.

Disulfiram should not be administered until the person has abstained from alcohol for at least 12 hours. Persons should be warned that the disulfiram-alcohol reaction may occur as long as 1 or 2 weeks after the last dose of disulfiram. Persons taking disulfiram should carry identification cards describing the disulfiram-alcohol reaction and listing the name and the telephone number of the physician to be called.

For a more detailed discussion of this topic, see DeBattista C, Schatzberg AF: Other Pharmacological and Biological Therapies, Sec 31.33, p 2521, in CTP/VII.

17

Dopamine Receptor Agonists and Precursors: Apomorphine, Bromocriptine, Levodopa, Pergolide, Pramipexole, and Ropinirole

Dopamine receptor agonists and precursors increase the amount of dopamine in the brain. They are used by psychiatrists to treat various adverse effects of antipsychotic drugs, including (1) parkinsonism, (2) extrapyramidal symptoms, (3) akinesia, (4) focal perioral tremors, (5) hyperprolactinemia, (6) galactorrhea, and (7) and neuroleptic malignant syndrome. The drugs in this class most commonly prescribed are bromocriptine (Parlodel), levodopa (Larodopa), and carbidopa-levodopa (Sinemet). New dopamine receptor agonists include ropinirole (Requip), pramipexole (Mirapex), and pergolide (Permax), which are better tolerated than bromocriptine. Apomorphine (Uprima) is under investigation for approval by the Food and Drug Administration for treatment of erectile dysfunction.

CHEMISTRY

Levodopa is the natural precursor of dopamine. The formulation of levodopa combined with carbidopa reduces the incidence of non-central nervous system (CNS) adverse effects experienced with use of levodopa alone. Bromocriptine and pergolide are ergotamine derivatives. Apomorphine is structurally related to morphine and other opioids. The molecular structures of dopamine receptor agonists and carbidopa (Lodosyn) are shown in Figure 17–1.

PHARMACOLOGICAL ACTIONS

Levodopa, or L-dopa, is rapidly absorbed after oral administration, and peak plasma levels are reached after 30 to 120 minutes. The half-life of levodopa is 90 minutes. Absorption of levodopa can be significantly reduced by changes in gastric pH and by ingestion with meals. Bromocriptine, pergolide, and ropinirole are rapidly absorbed but undergo first-pass metabolism such that only about 30 to 55 percent of the dosage is bioavailable. Peak concentrations are achieved 1½ to 3 hours after oral administration. Pergolide has a half-life of about 27 hours, and a single dose has 5 to 6 hours of clinical activity. The half-life of ropinirole is 6 hours. Pramipexole is rapidly absorbed with little first-pass metabolism and reaches peak concentrations in 2 hours. Its half-life is 8 hours.

Apomorphine can be administered subcutaneously, sublingually, intravenously, intranasally, orally, and rectally. Enteral administration is contraindicated because

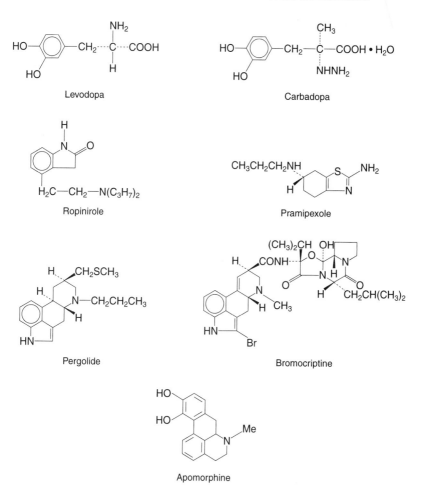

Figure 17-1. Molecular structures of dopamine receptor agonists and carbadopa.

of extensive first-pass metabolism and excessive nausea, vomiting, and azotemia. As formulated for treatment of erectile dysfunction, in a controlled-release sublingual tablet, onset of action occurs within about 15 minutes of administration, coincident with achievement of peak cerebrospinal fluid concentrations. Absorption is unaffected by food. Duration of action is 1 to 2 hours.

Once levodopa enters the dopaminergic neurons of the CNS, it is converted by dopa decarboxylase into the neurotransmitter dopamine. Apomorphine, bromocriptine, pergolide, ropinirole, and pramipexole act directly on dopamine receptors. Dopamine, pramipexole, and ropinirole bind about 20 times more selectively to dopamine D_3 than D_2 receptors; the corresponding ratio for pergolide is 5, and for bromocriptine is less than 2. Apomorphine binds selectively to D_1 and D_2 receptors, with little affinity for D_3 and D_4 receptors. Levodopa, pramipexole, and ropinirole have no significant activity at nondopaminergic receptors, but pergolide and bromocriptine bind to serotonin 5-HT$_1$ and 5-HT$_2$, and α_1, α_2, and β-adrenergic receptors.

THERAPEUTIC INDICATIONS

Medication-Induced Movement Disorders

In present day clinical psychiatry, dopamine receptor agonists are used for the treatment of medication-induced parkinsonism, extrapyramidal symptoms, akinesia, and focal perioral tremors. Their use has diminished sharply, however, because the incidence of medication-induced movement disorders is much lower with the use of the newer, atypical antipsychotics (serotonin-dopamine antagonists [SDAs]).

For the treatment of medication-induced movement disorders, most clinicians rely on anticholinergics, amantadine (Symmetrel), and antihistamines because they are equally effective and have few adverse effects. Bromocriptine remains in use in the treatment of neuroleptic malignant syndrome; however, the incidence of this disorder is diminishing with the decreasing use of dopamine receptor antagonists.

Dopamine receptor agonists are also used to counteract the hyperprolactinemic effects of dopamine receptor antagonists, which result in the side effects of amenorrhea and galactorrhea. Dopamine receptor agonists may reduce the pharmacological effects of cocaine but are not effective in reducing the craving for cocaine associated with withdrawal.

Sexual Dysfunction

All dopamine receptor agonists can improve erectile dysfunction. However, they are rarely used because therapeutic dosages frequently cause intolerable adverse effects and sildenafil (Viagra) is better tolerated and more effective. A sublingual formulation of apomorphine that controls the rate of transmucosal absorption facilitated intercourse in 47 percent of men at the 2 mg dose and 56 percent of men at the 4 mg dose. Higher doses were not tolerated, mainly due to nausea. Placebo response under the same conditions was 33 percent.

Sublingual apomorphine may find a therapeutic niche in treatment of erectile dysfunction in men in whom sildenafil is contraindicated due to use of nitrate-containing medications. However, the safety of coadministration of apomorphine and nitrates has not yet been determined.

PRECAUTIONS AND ADVERSE REACTIONS

Adverse effects are common with dopamine receptor agonists, thus limiting the usefulness of these drugs. Adverse effects are dosage dependent and include nausea, vomiting, orthostatic hypotension, headache, dizziness, and cardiac arrhythmias. To reduce the risk of orthostatic hypotension, the initial dosage of all dopamine receptor agonists should be quite low, with incremental increases in dosage at intervals of at least 1 week. These drugs should be used with caution in persons with hypertension, cardiovascular disease, and hepatic disease. After long-term use, persons, particularly elderly persons, may experience choreiform and dystonic movements and psychiatric disturbances, including hallucinations, delusions, confusion, depression, and mania and other behavioral changes.

Long-term use of bromocriptine and pergolide can produce retroperitoneal and pulmonary fibrosis, pleural effusions, and pleural thickening.

In general, ropinirole and pramipexole have a similar but much milder adverse effect profile than levodopa, bromocriptine, and pergolide. Pramipexole and ropinirole may cause irresistible sleep attacks that occur suddenly, without warning and have caused motor vehicle accidents.

The most common adverse effects of apomorphine are nausea, orthostatic hypotension, sedation, bradycardia, syncope, perspiration, and vomiting. Apomorphine's sedative effects are exacerbated with concurrent use of alcohol or other CNS depressants.

Dopamine receptor agonists are contraindicated during pregnancy and for nursing mothers especially, because they inhibit lactation.

DRUG INTERACTIONS

Dopamine receptor antagonists are capable of reversing the effects of dopamine receptor agonists, but this is not usually clinically significant. The concurrent use of tricyclic drugs and dopamine receptor agonists has been reported to cause symptoms of neurotoxicity, such as rigidity, agitation, and tremor. They may also potentiate the hypotensive effects of diuretics and other antihypertensive medications. Dopamine receptor agonists should not be used in conjunction with monoamine oxidase inhibitors (MAOIs), including selegiline (Eldepryl), and MAOIs should be discontinued at least 2 weeks before the initiation of dopamine receptor agonist therapy.

Benzodiazepines, phenytoin (Dilantin), and pyridoxine may interfere with the therapeutic effects of dopamine receptor agonists. Ergot alkaloids and bromocriptine should not be used concurrently, as they may cause hypertension and myocardial infarction. Progestins, estrogens, and oral contraceptives may interfere with the effects of bromocriptine and may raise plasma concentrations of ropinirole. Ciprofloxacin (Cipro) can raise plasma concentrations of ropinirole, and cimetidine (Tagamet) can raise plasma concentrations of pramipexole.

LABORATORY INTERFERENCES

Levodopa administration has been associated with false reports of elevated serum and urinary uric acid concentrations, urinary glucose test results, urinary ketone test results, and urinary catecholamine concentrations. No laboratory interferences have been associated with the administration of the other dopamine receptor agonists.

DOSAGE AND CLINICAL GUIDELINES

Table 17–1 lists the various dopamine receptor agonists and their formulations. For the treatment of antipsychotic-induced parkinsonism the clinician should start

TABLE 17–1
AVAILABLE PREPARATIONS OF DOPAMINE RECEPTOR AGONISTS AND CARBIDOPA

Generic Name	Trade Name	Preparations
Bromocriptine	Parlodel	2.5 mg, 5 mg tablets
Carbidopa	Lodosyn	25 mg[a]
Levodopa	Larodopa	100, 250, 500 mg tablets
Levodopa-carbidopa (cocareldopa)	Sinemet, Atamet	100/10 mg, 100/25 mg, 250/25 mg tablets; 100/25, 200/50 extended-release tablets
Pergolide	Permax	0.05, 0.25, and 1 mg tablets
Pramipexole	Mirapex	0.125, 0.25, 0.5, 1, 1.5 mg tablets
Ropinirole	Requip	0.25, 0.5, 1, 2, 5 mg tablets

[a]Drug only available directly through the manufacturer.

with a 100 mg dose of levodopa three times a day, which may be increased until the person is functionally improved. The maximum dosage of levodopa is 2000 mg a day, but most persons respond to dosages below 1000 mg per day. The dosage of the carbidopa component of the levodopa-carbidopa formulation should total at least 75 mg a day.

The dosage of bromocriptine for mental disorders is uncertain, although it seems prudent to begin with low dosages (1.25 mg twice daily) and to increase the dosage gradually. Bromocriptine is usually taken with meals to help reduce the likelihood of nausea.

The starting dosage of pergolide is 0.05 mg daily, which can be increased by 0.1 to 0.15 mg a day every 3 days for four increments, then by 0.25 mg per day every 3 days divided into three equal daily dosages, until therapeutic benefit or adverse effects emerge. The average dosage for treatment of idiopathic Parkinson's disease is 3 mg per day, and the maximum dosage is 5 mg per day.

The starting dosage of pramipexole is 0.125 mg three times daily, which is increased to 0.25 mg three times daily in the second week and is increased by 0.25 mg per dose each week until therapeutic benefit or adverse effects emerge. Persons with idiopathic Parkinson's disease usually experience benefit at total daily doses of 1.5 mg, and the maximum daily dose is 4.5 mg.

For ropinirole, the starting dosage is 0.25 mg three times daily and is increased by 0.25 mg per dose each week to a total daily dose of 3 mg, then by 0.5 mg per dosage each week to a total daily dose of 9 mg, then by 1 mg per dose each week to a maximum dosage of 24 mg a day, until therapeutic benefit or adverse effects emerge. The average daily dose for persons with idiopathic Parkinson's disease is about 16 mg.

Sublingual apomorphine for treatment of erectile dysfunction has been tested in 2- and 4-mg formulations. It is taken at least 15 minutes before initiation of sexual intercourse. Clinical guidelines regarding the minimum time interval between doses are not yet available.

For a more detailed discussion of this topic, see DeBattista C, Schatzber AF: Other Pharmacological and Biological Therapies, Sec 31.33, p 2521, in CTP/VII.

18

Dopamine Receptor Antagonists: Typical Antipsychotics

The dopamine receptor antagonists are so named because they are high-affinity antagonists of dopamine receptors. Other terms used to refer to these drugs are *typical, traditional,* or *conventional* antipsychotics. They are used in the treatment of schizophrenia and other psychotic disorders. The dopamine receptor antagonists include chlorpromazine (Thorazine), thioridazine (Mellaril), fluphenazine (Prolixin), and haloperidol (Haldol) among others (Table 18–1).

A new class of antipsychotic agents, the serotonin-dopamine antagonists (SDAs), also called *newer, novel,* or *atypical* antipsychotics, has appeared, which has fewer neurological adverse effects than the dopamine receptor antagonists and is effective against a broader range of psychotic symptoms. Differentiating the two classes of antipsychotics—dopamine receptor antagonists and SDAs—is increasingly important since they have different mechanisms of action and different clinical effects.

CHEMISTRY

The molecular structures of the dopamine receptor antagonists are shown in Figure 18–1.

PHARMACOLOGICAL ACTIONS

Most dopamine receptor antagonists are incompletely absorbed after oral administration, although liquid preparations are absorbed more efficiently than are other formulations. The half-lives of the these drugs range from 10 to 20 hours, and all can be given in one daily oral dose once the person is in a stable condition and has adjusted to any adverse effects. Many drugs are also available in parenteral forms that can be given intramuscularly in emergency situations, resulting in more rapid and more reliable attainment of therapeutic plasma concentrations than is possible with oral administration. Peak plasma concentrations are usually reached 1 to 4 hours after oral administration and 30 to 60 minutes after parenteral administration.

In the United States, two antipsychotics, haloperidol and fluphenazine, are available in long-acting depot parenteral formulations for administration once every 1 to 4 weeks, depending on the dose and the person. It can take up to 6 months of treatment with depot formulations to reach steady-state plasma levels, indicating that oral therapy should perhaps be continued during the first month or so of depot antipsychotic treatment. The long half-life of the depot formulation also means that detectable concentrations of the antipsychotic are present long after the last administration of the drug.

TABLE 18-1
DOPAMINE RECEPTOR ANTAGONIST DRUGS, TRADE NAMES, POTENCIES, AND DOSAGES

Generic Name	Trade Name	Potency[a] (mg of drug equivalent to 100 mg chlorpromazine)	Usual Adult Dosage Range (mg a day)	Usual Single i.m. Dosage (mg)
Phenothiazines				
Aliphatic				
Chlorpromazine	Thorazine	100—low	300–800	25–50
Triflupromazine	Vesprin	25–50—low	100–150	20–60
Promazine	Sparine	40—low	40–800	50–150
Piperazine				
Prochlorperazine	Compazine	15—medium	40–150	10–20
Perphenazine	Trilafon	10—medium	8–40	5–10
Trifluoperazine	Stelazine	3–5—high	6–20	1–2
Fluphenazine	Proixin, Permitil	1.5–3—high	1–20	2–5
Acetophenazine	Tindal (no longer manufactured)	25—medium	60–120	—
Butaperazine	Repoise (not sold in U.S.)	10—medium	—	—
Carphenazine	Proketazine (not sold in U.S.)	25—medium	—	—
Piperidine				
Thioridazine[c]	Mellaril	100—low	200–700[b]	—
Mesoridazine	Serentil	50—low	75–300	25
Piperacetazine	Quide (not sold in U.S.)	10—medium	—	—
Thioxanthenes				
Chlorprothixene	Taractan (no longer manufactured)	50—low	50–400	25–50
Thiothixene	Navane	2–5—high	6–30	2–4
Dibenzoxazepine				
Loxapine	Loxitane	10–15—medium	60–100	12.5–50
Dihydroindole				
Molindone	Moban	6–10—medium	50–100	—
Butyrophenones				
Haloperidol	Haldol	2–5—high	6–20	2–6
Droperidol	Inapsine	10—medium	—	—
Diphenylbutylpiperidine				
Pimozide[c]	Orap	1—high	1–10	—

[a] Recommended adult dosages are 200 to 400 mg a day of chlorpromazine or an equivalent amount of another drug.
[b] Maximum 800 mg.
[c] Second-line drug because of cardiotoxicity.

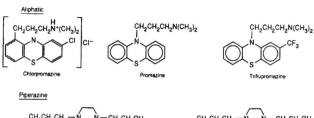

Phenothiazines

Aliphatic

Chlorpromazine   Promazine   Triflupromazine

Piperazine

Fluphenazine   Perphenazine

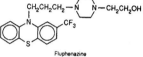

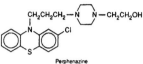

Prochlorperazine   Trifluoperazine

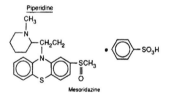

Piperidine

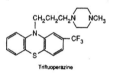

Mesoridazine   Thoridazine

Thioxanthene

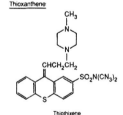

A   Thiothixene

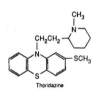

Figure 18-1. Molecular structures of dopamine receptor antagonists and reserpine.

The typical antipsychotic drugs appear to reduce psychotic symptoms through inhibition of dopamine binding to dopamine D_2 receptors. The antipsychotic effects appear to derive from inhibition of dopaminergic neurotransmission in the mesocortical dopamine projection, while the parkinsonian adverse effects are the consequence of blockade of the nigrostriatal pathway. Inhibition of the tuberoinfundibular tract is responsible for the endocrine effects of the drugs. The drugs reduce

Dibenzoxazepine

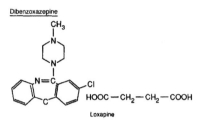

Loxapine

Dihydroindole

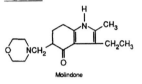

Molindone

Butyrophenones

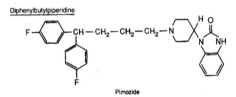

Droperidol

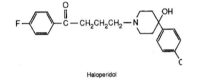

Haloperidol

Diphenylbutylpiperidine

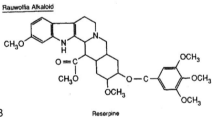

Pimozide

Rauwolfia Alkaloid

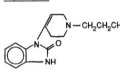

B   Reserpine

Figure 18-1. *Continued*

psychotic symptoms due to either a primary psychiatric disorder, such as schizophrenia, or another medical condition.

Most of the neurological and endocrinological adverse effects can be explained by their blockade of dopamine receptors. In addition, various antipsychotics also block noradrenergic, cholinergic, and histaminergic receptors, thus accounting for the variation in adverse-effect profiles seen among the drugs. The drugs fall on a spectrum of potency, which ranges from high-potency drugs, which are more likely to cause parkinsonian adverse effects, to low potency drugs, which are more likely to interact with nondopaminergic receptors and thus have cardiotoxic, epileptogenic, and anticholinergic adverse effects.

THERAPEUTIC INDICATIONS

Primary Psychotic Disorders

Dopamine receptor antagonists are effective in both the short-term and the long-term management of schizophrenia, schizophreniform disorder, schizoaffective disorder, delusional disorder, brief psychotic disorder, manic episodes, and major depressive disorder with psychotic features. They both reduce acute symptoms and prevent future exacerbations.

Schizophrenia. About 75 percent of all persons with schizophrenia relapse over the course of 1 year if treated with a placebo, compared with only 15 to 25 percent who relapse after taking dopamine receptor antagonists. Furthermore, the symptoms during the relapses are less severe in the persons receiving maintenance treatment than in those not receiving antipsychotic treatment.

In general, the dopamine receptor antagonists are thought to be more effective in the treatment of the positive symptoms of schizophrenia (e.g., hallucinations, delusions, and agitation) than in the treatment of the negative symptoms (e.g., emotional withdrawal and ambivalence) or the cognitive dissociations. The dopamine receptor antagonists themselves may also contribute to the negative symptoms. It is also generally believed that paranoid symptoms are more effectively treated than are nonparanoid symptoms and that women are more responsive than men are. Some persons do not respond to any of the dopamine receptor antagonists but may show improvement with the SDAs. The latter drugs also have been demonstrated to improve negative and cognitive as well as positive symptoms.

Bipolar Disorders. Antipsychotics are often used in combination with antimanic drugs to treat psychosis or manic excitement in bipolar I disorder. The standard drugs for treatment of bipolar disorder, lithium (Eskalith), carbamazepine (Tegretol), and valproate (Depakene), generally have a slower onset of action than do antipsychotics in the treatment of the acute symptoms. The general practice is to use combination therapy at the initiation of treatment and then gradually withdraw the antipsychotics.

Combination treatment with an antipsychotic and an antidepressant is one of the treatments of choice for major depressive disorder with psychotic features; the other is electroconvulsive therapy (ECT).

Persons with schizoaffective disorder and delusional disorder often respond favorably to treatment with these drugs. Some persons with borderline personality disorder who have marked psychotic symptoms as part of their disorder are also at least partially responsive to antipsychotic drugs, although these persons in particular also require psychotherapeutic treatment.

Secondary Psychoses

Secondary psychoses are psychotic syndromes that are associated with an identified organic cause, such as a brain tumor, a dementing disorder (e.g., dementia of the Alzheimer's type), or substance abuse. The dopamine receptor antagonists are generally effective in the treatment of psychotic symptoms associated with these syndromes. The high-potency dopamine receptor antagonists are usually safer than the low-potency dopamine receptor antagonists in such persons because the high-potency drugs have lower cardiotoxic, epileptogenic, and anticholinergic activities. Dopamine receptor antagonists should not be used to treat withdrawal symptoms associated with ethanol or barbiturate intoxication because of the risk that such treatment will cause withdrawal seizures. The drug of choice in such patients is usually a benzodiazepine. Agitation and psychosis associated with such neurological conditions as dementia of the Alzheimer's type also respond to antipsychotic treatment. High-potency drugs and low dosages are generally preferable; however, even with high-potency drugs, as many as 25 percent of elderly persons may experience episodes of hypotension. Low dosages of high-potency drugs, such as 0.5 to 5 mg a day of haloperidol, usually suffice for the treatment of these persons, although thioridazine 10 to 50 mg a day is also used because of its particularly potent sedative properties.

Severe Agitation and Violent Behavior

Dopamine receptor antagonists are used to treat persons who are severely agitated and violent, although other drugs such as benzodiazepines are also effective for the immediate control of such behavior. Symptoms such as extreme irritability, lack of impulse control, severe hostility, gross hyperactivity, and agitation respond to short-term treatment with dopamine receptor antagonists. Mentally handicapped children, especially those with profound mental retardation and autistic disorder, often have associated episodes of violence, aggression, and agitation that respond to treatment with antipsychotic drugs; however, the repeated administration of antipsychotics to control disruptive behavior in children is controversial. If dopamine receptor antagonists are used, the high-potency drugs, which cause little sedation, (e.g., 0.5 to 1 mg a day of haloperidol) are preferred to the more sedating, low-potency drugs.

Tourette's Disorder

Dopamine receptor antagonists are used to treat Tourette's disorder. Haloperidol and pimozide (Orap) are the most frequently used drugs in this class. Many clinicians prefer to use clonidine (Catapres) for this indication because of the lower risk of neurological side effects.

Other Psychiatric and Nonpsychiatric Indications

Some clinicians use low dosages of typical antipsychotic drugs (0.5 mg of haloperidol daily) to treat severe anxiety. The risk of inducing neurological

TABLE 18–2
POTENCIES AND ADVERSE EFFECT PROFILES OF DOPAMINE RECEPTOR ANTAGONISTS

Drug	Potency	Sedative Effect	Hypotensive Effect	Anticholinergic Effect	Extrapyramidal Effect
Phenothiazines					
Aliphatic					
Chlorpromazine (Thorazine)	Low	High	High	Medium	Low
Piperidines					
Mesoridazine (Serentil)	Low	Medium	Medium	Medium	Medium
Thioridazine (Mellaril)	Low	High	High	High	Low
Piperazines					
Fluphenazine (Prolixin, Permitil)	High	Medium	Low	Low	High
Perphenazine (Trilafon)	Medium	Low	Low	Low	High
Trifluoperazine (Stelazine)	High	Medium	Low	Low	High
Thioxanthene					
Thiothixene (Navane)	High	Low	Low	Low	High
Dibenzodiazepines					
Loxapine (Loxitane)	Medium	Medium	Medium	Medium	High
Butyrophenones					
Droperidol (Inapsine— injection only)	Medium	Low	Low	Low	High
Haloperidol (Haldol)	High	Low	Low	Low	High
Indolone					
Molindone (Moban)	Medium	Medium	Low	Medium	High
Diphenylbutylpiperidine					
Pimozide (Orap)	High	Low	Low	Low	High

From Hyman SE, Arana GW, Rosenbaum JF. *Handbook of Psychiatric Drug Therapy*, 3rd edition. Little, Brown, Boston, Massachusetts, 1996, with permission.

side effects must be carefully weighed against the potential therapeutic benefits in such cases. Other miscellaneous indications for the use of dopamine receptor antagonists include the treatment of nausea, emesis, intractable hiccups, and pruritus. The rare neurological disorders ballismus and hemiballismus (which affects only one side of the body), characterized by propulsive movements of the limbs away from the body, also respond to treatment with antipsychotic agents.

PRECAUTIONS AND ADVERSE REACTIONS

One generalization about the adverse effects of typical antipsychotics is that low-potency drugs cause most nonneurological adverse effects and high-potency drugs cause most neurological adverse events (Table 18–2).

Nonneurological Adverse Effects

Cardiac Effects. Low-potency dopamine receptor antagonists are more cardiotoxic than are high-potency drugs. Chlorpromazine causes prolongation of the QT and PR intervals, blunting of the T waves, and depression of the ST segment. Thioridazine, in particular, has marked effects on the T wave and is associated with malignant arrhythmias at high doses.

Sudden Death. The cardiac effects of dopamine receptor antagonists have been hypothesized to be related to sudden death in persons treated with the drugs, but this is a controversial area. Some studies show no change in the incidence of sudden death with the introduction of antipsychotics. In addition, both low- and high-potency drugs were involved in the reported cases. Furthermore, many reports were of persons with other medical problems who were also treated with several other drugs.

Orthostatic (Postural) Hypotension. Orthostatic (postural) hypotension is mediated by adrenergic blockade and is most common with low-potency drugs, particularly chlorpromazine, thioridazine, and chlorprothixene. It occurs most frequently during the first few days of treatment, and tolerance develops rapidly for the adverse effects. The chief dangers of orthostatic hypotension are that persons may faint, fall, and injure themselves, although such occurrences are not common.

When using intramuscular (i.m.) low-potency dopamine receptor antagonists, the clinician should measure the person's blood pressure (lying and standing) before and after the first dose and during the first few days of treatment. When appropriate, persons should be warned of the possibility of fainting and should be given the usual instructions to rise from bed gradually, sit at first with their legs dangling, wait for a minute, and sit or lie down if they feel faint. Patients should avoid all caffeine and alcohol, should drink at least 2 liters of fluid a day, and if not under treatment for hypertension should add liberal amounts of salt to their diet. Support hose may help some persons.

If hypotension does occur in persons receiving the medications, the symptoms can usually be managed by having them lie down with the feet higher than the head, then pump their legs as if bicycling. On rare occasions, volume expansion or vasopressor agents, such as norepinephrine (Levophed), may be indicated. Because hypotension is produced by α-adrenergic blockade, the drugs also block the α-adrenergic stimulating properties of epinephrine, leaving the β-adrenergic stimulating effects untouched. Therefore, the administration of epinephrine results in a paradoxical worsening of hypotension and is contraindicated in cases of antipsychotic-induced hypotension. Pure α-adrenergic pressor agents, such as metaraminol (Aramine) and norepinephrine, are the drugs of choice in the treatment of the disorder.

Hematological Effects. An often transient leukopenia with a white blood cell (WBC) count of about 3500 is a common but not serious problem. Agranulocytosis, a life-threatening hematological problem, occurs most often with chlorpromazine and thioridazine but is seen with almost all dopamine receptor antagonists. Agranulocytosis occurs most frequently during the first 3 months of treatment, with an incidence of about 5 in 10,000 persons treated with dopamine receptor antagonists. Routine complete blood counts (CBCs) are not indicated; however, if a person reports a sore throat and fever, a CBC should be done immediately to check for the possibility. If the blood indexes are low, administration of dopamine receptor antagonists should be stopped, and the person should be transferred to a medical facility. The mortality rate for the complication may be as high as 30 percent. Thrombocytopenic or nonthrombocytopenic purpura, hemolytic anemias, and pancytopenia may occur rarely in persons treated with dopamine receptor antagonists.

Peripheral Anticholinergic Effects. Peripheral anticholinergic effects, consisting of dry mouth and nose, blurred vision, constipation, urinary retention, and mydriasis, are common, especially with low-potency dopamine receptor antagonists, for example, chlorpromazine, thioridazine, mesoridazine (Serentil), and trifluoperazine (Stelazine). Some persons also have nausea and vomiting.

Dry mouth can be a troubling symptom for some persons and can endanger continued compliance. Persons can be advised to rinse out their mouths frequently with water and not to chew gum or candy containing sugar, as this can result in fungal infections of the mouth or an increased incidence of dental caries. Constipation should be treated with the usual laxative preparations, but the condition can still progress to paralytic ileus in some persons. A decrease in the dopamine receptor antagonist dosage or a change to a less anticholinergic drug is warranted in such cases. Pilocarpine (Salagen) may be used to treat paralytic ileus, although the relief is only transitory. Bethanechol (Urecholine) (20 to 40 mg a day) may be useful in some persons with urinary retention.

Endocrine Effects. Blockade of the dopamine receptors in the tuberoinfundibular tract results in the increased secretion of prolactin, which can result in breast enlargement, galactorrhea, impotence in men, and amenorrhea and inhibited orgasm in women. The newer antipsychotics olanzapine (Zyprexa), quetiapine (Seroquel), and clozapine (Clozaril), in contrast, are not particularly associated with an increase in prolactin levels and may be the drugs of choice for persons experiencing disturbing side effects from increased prolactin release.

Sexual Adverse Effects. The incidence of the disturbing sexual effects of dopamine receptor antagonists may be underestimated. As many as 50 percent of men taking antipsychotics report ejaculatory and erectile disturbances. Sildenafil (Viagra) or alprostadil (Muse, Caverject, Edex) may be effective treatments for this erectile disorder. Although bromocriptine (Parlodel) and yohimbine (Yocon) can be successful in some persons, they increase the risk of exacerbating the underlying psychosis. Both men and women taking dopamine receptor antagonists can experience anorgasmia and decreased libido. Thioridazine is particularly associated with decreased libido and retrograde ejaculation in men. Priapism and reports of painful orgasms have also been described, both possibly resulting from α_1-adrenergic antagonist activity.

Weight Gain. Weight gain, which can be significant in some cases, is a common adverse effect of treatment with typical antipsychotics. Molindone (Moban) and, perhaps, loxapine (Loxitane) are not associated with the symptom and may be indicated in persons for whom weight gain is a serious health hazard or a reason for noncompliance.

Dermatological Effects.   Allergic dermatitis and photosensitivity occur in a small percentage of persons, most commonly those taking low-potency drugs, particularly chlorpromazine. A variety of skin eruptions—urticarial, maculopapular, petechial, and edematous eruptions—have been reported. The eruptions occur early in treatment, generally in the first few weeks, and remit spontaneously. A photosensitivity reaction that resembles a severe sunburn also occurs in some persons taking chlorpromazine. Persons should be warned of this adverse effect, should spend no more that 30 to 60 minutes in the sun, and should use sunscreens. Chlorpromazine is also associated with some cases of a blue-gray discoloration of skin areas exposed to sunlight. The skin changes often begin with a tan or golden brown color and progress to such colors as slate gray, metallic blue, and purple.

Ophthalmological Effects.   Thioridazine is associated with irreversible pigmentation of the retina when given in dosages above 800 mg a day. An early symptom of the side effect can sometimes be nocturnal confusion related to difficulty with night vision. The pigmentation is similar to that seen in retinitis pigmentosa, and it can progress even after thioridazine administration is stopped, finally resulting in blindness.

In contrast, chlorpromazine is associated with a relatively benign pigmentation of the eyes, characterized by whitish brown granular deposits concentrated in the anterior lens and posterior cornea and visible only by slit-lens examination. The deposits can progress to opaque white and yellow-brown granules, often stellate. Occasionally, the conjunctiva is discolored by a brown pigment. No retinal damage is seen, and vision is almost never impaired. The deposits usually appear only in persons who have ingested 1 to 3 kg of chlorpromazine throughout their lives.

Jaundice.   Obstructive or cholestatic jaundice is rare with typical antipsychotic treatment. It usually occurs in the first month and begins with symptoms of upper abdominal pain, nausea and vomiting, a flu-like syndrome, fever, rash, eosinophilia, bilirubin in the urine, and increases in serum bilirubin, alkaline phosphatase, and hepatic transaminases. If jaundice occurs, the medication should be discontinued.

Overdoses.   The symptoms of overdose include extrapyramidal symptoms, mydriasis, decreased deep tendon reflexes, tachycardia, and hypotension. With the exception of overdoses of thioridazine and mesoridazine, the outcome of overdose is generally favorable unless the person has also ingested other central nervous system (CNS) depressants, such as alcohol and benzodiazepines. The severe symptoms of overdose include delirium, coma, respiratory depression, and seizures. Haloperidol may be among the safest typical antipsychotics in overdose. After an overdose, the electroencephalogram (EEG) shows diffuse slowing and low voltage. Thioridazine overdose can lead to heart block and ventricular fibrillation, resulting in death.

The treatment should include the use of activated charcoal, if possible, and gastric lavage. The use of emetics is not indicated, since the antiemetic actions of the dopamine receptor antagonists inhibit their efficacy. Seizures can be treated with intravenous (i.v.) diazepam (Valium) or phenytoin (Dilantin). Hypotension can be treated with either norepinephrine or dopamine (Dopastat) but not epinephrine (Adrenalin).

Neurological Adverse Effects

Neuroleptic-Induced Parkinsonism. Parkinsonian adverse effects occur in approximately 15 percent of patients, usually within 5 to 90 days of the treatment's initiation. Symptoms include muscle stiffness, cogwheel rigidity, shuffling gait, stooped posture, and drooling. The pill-rolling tremor of idiopathic parkinsonism is rare, but a regular, coarse tremor similar to essential tremor may be present. Rabbit syndrome is a focal, perioral tremor that resembles the other parkinsonian effects of antipsychotics but can occur late in treatment. The mask-like facies, bradykinesia, and akinesia of the parkinsonian syndrome are often misdiagnosed as being part of the negative symptom picture of schizophrenia.

Women are affected about twice as often as men, and the syndrome can occur at all ages, although it is most frequent after age 40. All antipsychotics can cause the symptoms, especially high-potency drugs with low anticholinergic activity. Chlorpromazine and thioridazine are less likely to be involved. The incidence of parkinsonism is markedly lower with clozapine, olanzapine, quetiapine, and risperidone (Risperdal), although the risk of parkinsonian symptoms increases modestly with risperidone as the dose is increased above 6 mg a day. The blockade of dopaminergic transmission in the nigrostriatal tract is the cause of neuroleptic-induced parkinsonism. The differential diagnosis should also include other causes of idiopathic parkinsonism, other organic causes of parkinsonism, and depression. The syndrome can be treated with anticholinergic agents, amantadine (Symadine, Symmetrel), or diphenhydramine (Benadryl). Although amantadine may have fewer side effects, it may be less effective at reducing muscular rigidity. Levodopa (Larodopa) does not work in these patients, and it may exacerbate the psychosis. Anticholinergics should be withdrawn after 4 to 6 weeks to assess whether the patient has a tolerance to the parkinsonian effects; approximately 50 percent of patients need continued treatment. Even after the antipsychotics are withdrawn, parkinsonian symptoms may last for up to 2 weeks and even up to 3 months in elderly patients. In such patients it is reasonable to continue administering the anticholinergic drug after stopping antipsychotic use.

Neuroleptic-Induced Acute Dystonia. About 10 percent of all persons experience dystonia as an adverse effect of typical antipsychotics, usually in the first few hours or days of treatment. Dystonic movements result from a slow, sustained muscular contraction or spasm that can result in an involuntary movement. Dystonia can involve the neck (spasmodic torticollis or retrocollis), the jaw (forced opening resulting in a dislocation of the jaw or trismus), the tongue (protrusions, twisting), and the entire body (opisthotonos). Involvement of the eyes can result in an oculogyric crisis, characterized by upward and lateral movement of the eyes. Unlike other types of dystonia, an oculogyric crisis may also occur late in treatment. Other dystonias include blepharospasm and glossopharyngeal dystonia, resulting in dysarthria, dysphagia, and even trouble breathing, which can cause cyanosis. Children are particularly likely to evidence opisthotonos, scoliosis, lordosis, and writhing movements. Dystonia can be painful and frightening and often results in noncompliance with the dopamine receptor antagonist treatment regimen.

Dystonia is most common in young men (less than 40 years old) but can occur at any age in either sex. Although it is most common with i.m. doses of high-potency dopamine receptor antagonists, dystonia can occur with any dopamine receptor antagonist. The mechanism of action is thought to be the dopaminergic hyperactivity in the basal ganglia that occurs when the CNS levels of the dopamine receptor antagonist drug begin to fall between doses. Dystonia can fluctuate spontaneously, responding to reassurance and resulting in the clinician's false impression that the movement is hysterical or completely under conscious control. The differential diagnosis of a dystonic movement should include seizures and tardive dyskinesia.

Prophylaxis with anticholinergics or related drugs (see Table 42–3 in Chapter 42) usually prevents the development of dystonia, although the risks of prophylactic treatment weigh against the benefit. Treatment with i.m. anticholinergics or i.v. or i.m. diphenhydramine (50 mg) almost always relieves the symptoms. Diazepam (10 mg i.m.), amobarbital (Amytal), caffeine, sodium benzoate, and hypnosis have also been reported to be effective. Although tolerance for the adverse effect usually develops, it is sometimes prudent to change the antipsychotic (e.g., from typical to atypical) if the person is particularly concerned about recurrence of the reaction.

Neuroleptic-Induced Acute Akathisia. Akathisia is a subjective feeling of muscular discomfort that can cause a person to be agitated, pace relentlessly, alternately sit and stand in rapid succession, and feel generally dysphoric. The symptoms are primarily motor and cannot be controlled by the person's will. Akathisia can appear at any time during treatment. The disorder is probably underdiagnosed because the symptoms are mistakenly attributed to psychosis, agitation, or lack of cooperation.

Once akathisia is recognized and diagnosed, the antipsychotic dosage should be reduced to the minimal effective level or another drug should be substituted, such as one of the newer antipsychotics. Treatment can also be attempted with anticholinergics or amantadine, although those drugs are not particularly effective for akathisia. Drugs that may be more effective include propranolol (Inderal) (30 to 120 mg a day), benzodiazepines, and clonidine. In some cases of akathisia, no treatment seems to be effective.

Neuroleptic-Induced Tardive Dyskinesia. The word "tardive," like "tardy," refers to "late." Tardive dyskinesia is a delayed effect of antipsychotics; it rarely occurs until after 6 months of treatment. The disorder consists of abnormal, involuntary, irregular choreoathetoid movements of the muscles of the head, the limbs, and the trunk. The severity of the movements ranges from minimal—often missed by persons and their families—to grossly incapacitating. Perioral movements are the most common and include darting, twisting, and protruding movements of the tongue; chewing and lateral jaw movements; lip puckering; and facial grimacing. Finger movements and hand clenching are also common. Torticollis, retrocollis, trunk twisting, and pelvic thrusting are seen in severe cases. Respiratory dyskinesia has also been reported. Dyskinesia is exacerbated by stress and disappears during sleep. Other late-appearing movement disorders have been noted and have been referred to, depending on the symptoms, as tardive dystonia, tardive parkinsonism, and tardive Tourette's disorder.

All of the dopamine receptor antagonists have been associated with tardive dyskinesia. Some data indicate that thioridazine is less associated with tardive dyskinesia than the other drugs. The longer persons take typical antipsychotics, the more likely they are to experience tardive dyskinesia. About 10 to 20 percent of persons who are treated for more than a year and about 15 to 20 percent of long-term hospital patients have tardive dyskinesia. Women are more likely to be affected than are men, and persons over 50 years of age, persons with brain damage, children, and persons with mood disorders are also at high risk. Before the introduction of antipsy-chotics in the early 1950s, 1 to 5 percent of schizophrenic persons had similar ab-normal movements, indicating that the pattern of movement disorders is related to the underlying pathophysiology of schizophrenia itself.

The three basic approaches to tardive dyskinesia are prevention, diagnosis, and management. Prevention is best achieved by using these drugs only when clearly in-dicated and in the lowest effective dosages. Persons should be examined regularly for the appearance of abnormal movements, preferably by using a standardized rat-ing scale (see Table 42–2 in Chapter 42). When abnormal movements are detected, a differential diagnosis should be considered (Table 18–3).

Once a diagnosis of tardive dyskinesia is made, the clinician must regularly con-duct objective ratings of the movement disorder. Although tardive dyskinesia often emerges while the person is taking a steady dosage of medication, it is even more likely to emerge when the dosage is reduced. Once tardive dyskinesia is recognized, the clinician should consider reducing the dosage of the drug or even stopping the medication altogether. The newer SDAs should be considered for the treatment of tardive dyskinesias, because they reduce the abnormal movements and have the low-est risk of exacerbating the condition.

When tardive dyskinesia was first recognized, the movement disorder was be-lieved to be chronic and progressive; however, tardive dyskinesia develops rapidly, stabilizes, and often remits, sometimes even when the person continues the same drug treatment. Between 5 and 40 percent of all cases of tardive dyskinesia eventu-ally remit, and between 50 and 90 percent of all mild cases remit. However, tardive dyskinesia is less likely to remit in elderly persons than in young persons.

Tardive dyskinesia has no single effective treatment. Lowering the dosage of the drug or switching to another drug (e.g., clozapine, olanzapine, or quetiapine) are the

TABLE 18–3
DIFFERENTIAL DIAGNOSIS FOR TARDIVE DYSKINESIA-LIKE MOVEMENTS

Common—Schizophrenic mannerisms and stereotypies
    Dental problems (e.g., ill-fitting dentures)
    Maige's syndrome and other senile dyskinesias
Drug induced—Antidepressants
    Antihistamines
    Antimalarials
    Antipsychotics
    Heavy metals
    Levodopa
    Phenytoin
    Sympathomimetics
CNS—Anoxia induced
    Hepatic failure
    Huntington's disease
    Parathyroid hypoactivity
    Postencephalitic
    Pregnancy (chorea gravidarum)
    Renal failure
    Sydenham's chorea
    Systemic lupus erythematosus
    Thyroid hyperactivity
    Torsion dystonia
    Tumors
    Wilson's disease

primary treatment strategies. In persons who cannot continue taking any antipsychotic medication, lithium, carbamazepine, or benzodiazepines may be effective in reducing both the movement disorder symptoms and the psychotic symptoms. Vitamin E has also shown some benefit in tardive dyskinesia in high dosages.

Neuroleptic Malignant Syndrome. Neuroleptic malignant syndrome is a life-threatening complication that can occur at any time during the course of dopamine receptor antagonist treatment. The motor and behavioral symptoms include muscular rigidity and dystonia, akinesia, mutism, obtundation, and agitation. The autonomic symptoms include hyperpyrexia (up to 107°F), sweating, and increased pulse rate and blood pressure. Laboratory findings include increased WBC, creatinine phosphokinase, liver enzymes, plasma myoglobin, and myoglobinuria, occasionally associated with renal failure. The symptoms usually evolve over 24 to 72 hours, and the untreated syndrome lasts 10 to 14 days. The diagnosis is often missed in the early stages, and the withdrawal or agitation may mistakenly be considered to reflect increased psychosis. Men are affected more frequently than are women, and young persons are affected more commonly than elderly persons. The mortality rate can reach 20 to 30 percent or even higher when depot medications are involved.

The first step in treatment is the immediate discontinuation of dopamine receptor antagonist drugs; medical support to cool the person; monitoring of vital signs, electrolytes, fluid balance, and renal output; and symptomatic treatment of fever. Antiparkinsonian medications may reduce some of the muscle rigidity. Dantrolene (Dantrium), a skeletal muscle relaxant (0.8 to 2.5 mg per kg every 6 hours, up to a total dosage of 10 mg a day), may be useful in the treatment of this disorder. Once the person can take oral medications, dantrolene can be given in doses of 100 to 200 mg a day. Bromocriptine (20 to 30 mg a day in four divided doses) or perhaps amantadine can be added to the regimen. Treatment should usually be continued for 5 to 10 days. When drug treatment is restarted, the clinician should consider switching to a low-potency drug or one of the newer antipsychotic drugs (Chapter 29).

Epileptogenic Effects. Dopamine receptor antagonist administration is associated with slowing and increased synchronization of the EEG. This effect may be the mechanism by which some antipsychotics decrease the seizure threshold. Chlorpromazine, thioridazine, and other low-potency drugs are thought to be more epileptogenic than are high-potency drugs. Molindone may be the least epileptogenic of the dopamine receptor antagonist drugs. The risk of inducing a seizure by drug administration warrants consideration when the person already has a seizure disorder or an organic brain lesion.

Sedation. Sedation is primarily a result of the blockade of histamine H_1 receptors. Chlorpromazine is the most sedating typical antipsychotic; thioridazine, chlorprothixene, and loxapine are also sedating; and the high-potency antipsychotics are much less sedating (Table 18–2). Patients taking antipsychotics should be warned about driving and operating machinery. Giving the entire daily dose at bedtime usually eliminates any problems from sedation, and tolerance for this adverse effect often develops.

Central Anticholinergic Effects. The symptoms of central anticholinergic activity include severe agitation; disorientation to time, person, and place; hallucinations; seizures; high fever; and dilated pupils. Stupor and coma may ensue. The treatment of anticholinergic toxicity consists of discontinuing the causal agent or agents, close medical supervision, and physostigmine (Antilirium, Eserine), 2 mg by slow i.v. infusion, repeated within 1 hour as necessary. Too much physostigmine is dangerous, and symptoms of physostigmine toxicity include hypersalivation and sweating. Atropine sulfate (0.5 mg) can reverse the effects of physostigmine toxicity.

Prevention and Treatment of Some Neuroleptic-Induced Movement Disorders. A variety of drugs may be used to prevent and treat medication-induced movement disorders, particularly neuroleptic-induced parkinsonism and neuroleptic-induced acute dystonia. The drugs include anticholinergics, amantadine, antihistamines, benzodiazepines, β-receptor antagonists, and clonidine. Most acute dystonia and parkinsonism symptoms are effectively treated by these drugs, and acute akathisia may also respond in some cases.

Whether prophylactic treatment with these drugs is warranted when starting to administer a dopamine receptor antagonist to a person remains controversial. The proponents of prophylactic treatment argue that the increased likelihood of avoiding adverse neurological effects is humane and increases the possibility of future compliance. The opponents of the practice argue that a large proportion (30 to 50 percent) of persons do not need antiparkinsonian drugs, and that their use may increase the likelihood of tardive dyskinesia, autonomic side effects, cognitive impairment, hyperthermia, and anticholinergic toxicity. Many of the drugs used to treat parkinsonian symptoms also have some abuse liability and may be associated with changes in the plasma concentrations of the antipsychotics. A reasonable compromise is to use the drugs prophylactically in persons under the age of 45 who are at risk for adverse effects, particularly dystonia, and not to use the drugs prophylactically in persons over 45 who are at increased risk for anticholinergic toxicity.

Once patients start taking drugs to treat a movement disorder, they should be treated for 4 to 6 weeks. Then the clinician should attempt to taper and stop the medication over a 1-month period. Many patients become tolerant for the neurological adverse effects and no longer require treatment for the neuroleptic-induced movement disorder.

Most clinicians use one of the anticholinergic drugs (such as benztropine [Cogentin]) or diphenhydramine for prophylaxis or treatment of neurological adverse effects. Of these drugs, diphenhydramine is the most sedating, biperiden (Akineton) is neither sedating nor stimulating, and trihexyphenidyl (Artane) may be slightly stimulating. Amantadine is most often used when one of the anticholinergic drugs is ineffective. Although amantadine does not typically exacerbate the psychosis of schizophrenia, some persons become tolerant for its antiparkinsonian effects. Amantadine is also sedating for some persons.

Pregnancy and Lactation

If possible, antipsychotics should be avoided during pregnancy, particularly in the first trimester, unless the benefit outweighs the risk. In fact, however, there is a low correlation between the presence of congenital malformations in the infant and the use of antipsychotics during pregnancy, except perhaps for chlorpromazine. Antipsychotic use in the second and third trimesters is probably relatively safe. High-potency drugs are preferable to low-potency drugs, since the low-potency drugs are associated with hypotension.

All dopamine receptor antagonists probably do pass into breast milk. Women who are taking dopamine receptor antagonists should not breast-feed their infants, since available data do not prove that the practice is safe.

DRUG INTERACTIONS

Because of their many receptor effects and because of the metabolism of most of the dopamine receptor antagonists in the liver, many pharmacokinetic and pharmacodynamic drug interactions are associated with these drugs (Table 18–4).

Antacids

Antacids and cimetidine (Tagamet) taken within 2 hours of antipsychotic administration can reduce the absorption of these drugs.

Anticholinergics

Anticholinergics may decrease the absorption of dopamine receptor antagonists. The additive anticholinergic activity of dopamine receptor antagonists, anticholinergics, and tricyclic drugs may result in anticholinergic toxicity.

Anticonvulsants

Phenothiazines, especially thioridazine, may decrease the metabolism of and cause toxic concentrations of phenytoin. Barbiturates may increase the metabolism of dopamine receptor antagonists, and these drugs may lower the person's seizure threshold.

Antidepressants

Tricyclic drugs and dopamine receptor antagonists may decrease each other's metabolism, resulting in increased plasma concentrations of both drugs. The anticholinergic, sedative, and hypotensive effects of the drugs may also be additive.

Antihypertensives

Typical antipsychotics may inhibit the hypotensive effects of α-methyldopa (Aldomet). Conversely, typical antipsychotics may have an additive effect on some hypotensive drugs. Antipsychotic drugs have a variable effect on the hypotensive effects of clonidine. Propranolol coadministration increases the blood concentrations of both drugs.

CNS Depressants

Dopamine receptor antagonists potentiate the CNS-depressant effects of sedatives, antihistamines, opiates, opioids, and alcohol, particularly in persons with impaired respiratory status. When these agents are taken with alcohol, the risk for heat stroke may be increased.

TABLE 18–4
ANTIPSYCHOTIC DRUG INTERACTIONS

Interacting Medication	Mechanism	Clinical Effect
Drug interactions assessed to have major severity		
β-Adrenergic receptor antagonists	Synergistic pharmacologic-effect; antipsychotic inhibits metabolism of propranolol; antipsychotic increases plasma concentrations	Severe hypotension
Anticholinergics	Pharmacodynamic effects	Decreased antipsychotic effect
	Additive anticholinergic effect	Anticholinergic toxicity
Barbiturates	Phenobarbital induces antipsychotic metabolism	Decreased antipsychotic concentrations
Carbamazepine	Induces antipsychotic metabolism	Up to 50% reduction in antipsychotic concentrations
Charcoal	Reduces GI absorption of antipsychotic and adsorbs drug during enterohepatic circulation	May reduce antipsychotic effect or cause toxicity when during overdose or for GI disturbances
Cigarette smoking	Induction of microsomal enzymes	Reduced plasma concentrations of antipsychotic agents
Epinephrine, norepinephrine	Antipsychotic antagonizes pressor effect	Hypotension
Ethanol	Additive CNS depression	Impaired psychomotor skills
Fluvoxamine	Fluvoxamine inhibits metabolism of haloperidol and clozapine	Increased concentrations of haloperidol and clozapine
Guanethidine	Antipsychotic antagonizes guanethidine reuptake	Impaired antihypertensive effect
Lithium	Unknown	Rare reports of neurotoxicity
Meperidine	Additive CNS depression	Hypotension and sedation
Drug interactions assessed to have minor or moderate severity		
Amphetamines, anorexiants	Decreased pharmacological effect of amphetamine; drug-disease state interaction	Diminished weight loss effect; amphetamines may exacerbate psychosis; treatment-refractory schizophrenics may improve
Angiotensin-converting enzyme inhibitors	Additive hypotensive crisis	Hypotension, postural intolerance
Antacids containing aluminum	Insoluble complex formed in GI tract	Possible reduced antipsychotic effect
Antidepressants (AD) nonspecific	Decreased metabolism of AD through competitive inhibition	Increased AD concentration
Benzodiazepines	Increased pharmacological effect of the benzodiazepine	Respiratory depression, stupor, hypotension
Bromocriptine	Antipsychotic antagonizes dopamine receptor stimulation	Increased prolactin
Caffeinated beverages	Form precipitate with antipsychotic solutions	Possible diminished antipsychotic effect
Cimetidine	Reduced antipsychotic absorption and clearance	Decreased antipsychotic effect
Clonidine	Antipsychotic potentiates α-adrenergic hypotensive effect	Hypotension or hypertension
Disulfiram	Impairs antipsychotic metabolism	Increased antipsychotic concentrations
Methyldopa	Unknown	Blood pressure elevations
Phenytoin	Induction of antipsychotic metabolism; decreased phenytoin metabolism	Decreased antipsychotic concentrations; increased phenytoin levels
Serotonin-specific reuptake inhibitors	Impair antipsychotic metabolism; pharmacodynamic interaction	Sudden onset of extrapyramidal symptoms
Valproic acid	Antipsychotic inhibits valproic acid metabolism	Increased valproic acid half-life and levels

From Ereshosky L, Overman GP, Karp JK. Current psychotropic dosing and monitoring guidelines. *Prim Psychiatry* 1996;3:21, with permission.

Other Substances

Cigarette smoking may decrease the plasma levels of typical antipsychotic drugs. Epinephrine has a paradoxical hypotensive effect in persons taking typical antipsychotics. These drugs may decrease the blood concentration of warfarin (Coumadin), resulting in decreased bleeding time. Phenothiazines, thioridazine, and pimozide should not be coadministered with other agents that prolong the QT interval. Thioridazine is contraindicated in patients taking drugs that inhibit the cytochrome P450 (CYP) 2D6 isoenzyme or in patients with reduced levels of CYP 2D6.

LABORATORY INTERFERENCES

Dopamine receptor antagonist drugs have been reported to interfere with some laboratory tests. Chlorpromazine and perphenazine (Trilafon) have been reported to cause both false-positive and false-negative results in immunological pregnancy tests and falsely elevated bilirubin (with reagent test strips) and urobilinogen (with Ehrlich's reagent test) values. These drugs have also been associated with an abnormal shift in results of glucose tolerance test, although that shift may reflect the effects of the drugs on the glucose-regulating system. Phenothiazines have been reported to interfere with the measurement of 17-ketosteroids and 17-hydroxycorticosteroids.

DOSAGE AND CLINICAL GUIDELINES

Dopamine receptor antagonist drugs are remarkably safe in short-term use. Some contraindications exist however. These include (1) a history of a serious allergic response, (2) the possible ingestion of a substance that will interact with the antipsychotic to induce CNS depression (e.g., alcohol, opioids, barbiturates, and benzodiazepines) or anticholinergic delirium (e.g., scopolamine and possibly phencyclidine [PCP]), (3) the presence of a severe cardiac abnormality, (4) a high risk for seizures from organic and idiopathic causes, (5) the presence of narrow-angle glaucoma or prostatic hypertrophy if a drug with high anticholinergic activity is to be used, and (6) the presence or a history of tardive dyskinesia. Antipsychotics should be administered with caution in persons with hepatic disease, since impaired hepatic metabolism may result in high plasma concentrations. The usual assessment should include a CBC with WBC indexes, liver function tests, and an electrocardiogram, especially in women over 40 and men over 30. The elderly and children are more sensitive to side effects than are young adults, so the dosage of the drug should be adjusted accordingly.

Choice of Drug

The general guidelines for choosing a particular psychotherapeutic drug should be followed (Chapter 1). If no other rationale prevails, the choice should be based on adverse-effect profiles and the psychiatrist's preference. Although high-potency antipsychotics are associated with more neurological adverse effects, current clinical practice greatly favors using them because of the higher incidence of other adverse effects (e.g., cardiac, hypotensive, epileptogenic, sexual, and allergic) with the low-potency drugs. There is a myth in psychiatry that hyperexcitable patients respond best to chlorpromazine because it is more sedating, whereas withdrawn patients respond best to high-potency antipsychotics, such as fluphenazine. That hypothesis has never been proved; if sedation is a desired goal, either the antipsychotic can be given in divided doses or a sedative drug, such as a benzodiazepine, can also be administered.

Some research supports the clinical observation that an unpleasant reaction by the patient to the first dose of an antipsychotic correlates highly with future poor response and noncompliance. Such experiences include a subjective negative feeling, oversedation, and acute dystonia. If a patient reports such a reaction, the clinician may be well advised to switch the patient to a different antipsychotic.

Dosage and Schedule

Various patients may respond to widely different dosages of antipsychotics; therefore, there is no set dosage for any given antipsychotic drug. It is reasonable clinical practice to begin at a low dosage and increase it as necessary. It is important to remember that the maximal effects of a particular dosage may not be evident for 4 to 6 weeks. Available preparations of dopamine receptor antagonists are given in Table 18–5.

Short-Term Treatment.   The equivalent of 5 to 10 mg of haloperidol is a reasonable dose for an adult person in an acute state. A geriatric person may benefit from as little as 1 mg of haloperidol. The administration of more than 50 mg of chlorpromazine in one injection may result in serious hypotension. Administration of the antipsychotic i.m. results in peak plasma levels in about 30 minutes, versus 90 minutes using the oral route. Doses of drugs for i.m. administration are about half those given by the oral route. In a short-term treatment setting, the person should be observed for 1 hour after the first dose of medication. After that time, most clinicians administer a second dose or a sedative agent (e.g., a benzodiazepine) to achieve effective behavioral control. Possible sedatives include lorazepam (Ativan) (2 mg i.m.) and amobarbital (50 to 250 mg i.m.).

Rapid Neuroleptization.   Rapid neuroleptization (also called psychotolysis) is the practice of administering hourly i.m. doses of antipsychotic medications until marked sedation of the person is achieved. However, several research studies have shown that merely waiting several more hours after one dose yields the same clinical improvement as is seen with repeated doses. Nevertheless, clinicians must be careful to keep persons from becoming violent while they are psychotic. Clinicians can help prevent violent episodes by the use of adjuvant sedatives or by temporarily using physical restraints until the persons can control their behavior.

Early Treatment.   Agitation and excitement are usually the first symptoms to improve with antipsychotic treatment. About 75 percent of persons with a short history of illness show significant improvement in their psychosis. In persons with a long history of illness, a full 6 weeks may be necessary to evaluate the extent of the improvement in psychotic symptoms. Psychotic symptoms, both positive and negative, usually continue to improve 3 to 12 months after the initiation of treatment.

TABLE 18–5
DOPAMINE RECEPTOR ANTAGONIST PREPARATIONS

	Tablets	Capsules	Solution	Parenteral	Rectal Suppositories
Acetophenazine	20 mg	—	—	—	—
Chlorpromazine	10, 25, 50, 100, 200 mg	30, 75, 150, 200, 300 mg	10 mg/5 mL, 30 mg/mL, 100 mg/mL	25, mg/mL	25, 100 mg
Droperidol	—	—	—	2.5 mg/mL	—
Fluphenazine	1, 2.5, 5, 10 mg	—	2.5 mg/5 mL, 5L, 5mg/mL	2.5 mg/mL (i.m. only)	—
Fluphenazine decanoate	—	—	—	25 mg/mL	—
Fluphenazine enanthate	—	—	—	25 mg/mL	—
Haloperidol	0.5, 1, 2, 10, 20 mg	—	2 mg/mL	5 mg/mL (i.m. only)	—
Haloperidol decanoate	—	—	—	50 mg/mL, 100 mg/mL (i.m. only)	—
Loxapine	—	5, 10, 25, 50 mg	25 mg/mL	50 mg/mL	—
Mesoridazine	10, 25, 50, 100 mg	—	25 mg/mL	25 mg/mL	—
Molindone	5, 10, 25, 50, 100 mg	—	20 mg/mL	—	—
Perphenazine	2, 4, 8, 16 mg	—	16 mg/5 mL	5 mg/mL	—
Pimozide	2 mg	—	—	—	—
Prochlorperazine	5, 10, 25 mg	10, 15, 30 mg (SR)	5 mg/5 mL	5 mg/mL	2.5, 5, 25 mg
Promazine	25, 50, 100 mg	—	—	25 mg/mL, 50 mg/mL	—
Thioridazine	10, 15, 25, 50, 100, 150, 200 mg	—	25 mg/5 mL, 100 mg/5 mL, 30 mg/mL, 100 mg/mL	—	—
Thiothixene	—	1, 2, 5, 10, 20 mg	5 mg/mL	10 mg (i.m. only), 2 mg/mL (i.m. only)	—
Trifluoperazine	1, 2, 5, 10 mg	—	10 mg/mL	2 mg/mL	—
Triflupromazine	—	—	—	10 mg/mL 20 mg/mL	—

The equivalent of 10 to 20 mg of haloperidol or 400 mg of chlorpromazine a day is adequate treatment for most persons with schizophrenia. Some research studies indicate that 5 mg of haloperidol or 200 mg of chlorpromazine may, in fact, be just as effective as higher doses. It is a reasonable practice to give antipsychotic drugs in divided doses when initiating treatment, to minimize the peak plasma levels and reduce the incidence of side effects. The total daily dose can be consolidated into a single daily dose after the first week or two of treatment. The single daily dose is usually given at bedtime to help induce sleep and to reduce the incidence of adverse effects. However, bedtime dosing for elderly persons may increase their risk of falling if they get out of bed during the night. The sedative effects of typical antipsychotics last only a few hours, in contrast to the antipsychotic effects, which last for 1 to 3 days.

Intermittent Medications.   It is common clinical practice to order medications to be given intermittently as needed (p.r.n.). Although this practice may be reasonable during the first few days that a person is hospitalized, the amount of time the person takes antipsychotic drugs, rather than an increase in dosage, is what produces therapeutic improvement. Clinicians on in-patient service, may feel pressured by staff members to write as-needed antipsychotic orders; such orders should include specific symptoms, how often the drugs should be given, and how many doses can be given each day. Clinicians may choose to use small doses for the as-needed doses (e.g., 2 mg haloperidol) or use a benzodiazepine instead (e.g., 2 mg lorazepam i.m.). If as-needed doses of an antipsychotic are necessary after the first week of treatment, the clinician may want to consider increasing the standing daily dosage of the drug.

Maintenance Treatment.   The first 3 to 6 months after a psychotic episode is usually considered a period of stabilization. After that time, the dosage of the antipsychotic can be decreased about 20 percent every 6 months until the minimum effective dosage is found. A person is usually maintained on antipsychotic medications for 1 to 2 years after the first psychotic episode. Antipsychotic treatment is often continued for 5 years after a second psychotic episode, and lifetime maintenance is considered after the third psychotic episode, although attempts to reduce the daily dosage can be made every 6 to 12 months.

Antipsychotic drugs are effective in controlling psychotic symptoms, but persons may report that they prefer being off the drugs, because they feel better without them. This problem is less common with the newer antipsychotic SDAs. The clinician must discuss maintenance medication with patients and take into account their wishes, the severity of their illnesses, and the quality of their support systems. It is essential for the clinician to know enough about the patient's life to try to predict upcoming stressors that might require increasing the dosage or closely monitoring compliance.

Long-Acting Depot Medications.   Because some persons with schizophrenia do not comply with oral antipsychotic regimens, long-acting depot preparations may be needed (Table 18–6). A clinician usually administers the i.m. preparations once every 1 to 4 weeks. Depot medications may be associated with increased adverse effects, including tardive dyskinesia.

Two depot preparations, a decanoate and an enanthate, of fluphenazine and a decanoate preparation of haloperidol are available in the United States. The preparations are injected i.m. into an area of large muscle tissue, from which they are absorbed slowly into the blood. Decanoate preparations can be given less frequently

TABLE 18–6
USE OF LONG-ACTING DOPAMINE RECEPTOR ANTAGONISTS

Dosage
  a. Stabilize patient on lowest effective dose of oral preparation.
  b. Usual dosage conversion:
    10 mg/day oral fluphenazine = 12.5–25 mg/2 weeks fluphenazine decanoate
    10 mg/day oral haloperidol = 100–200 mg/4 weeks haloperidol decanoate
  c. As with all other antipsychotic medications, the lowest effective dose should be used. Note that patients with chronic schizophrenia have been adequately maintained or doses of fluphenazine deconoate as low as 5 mg/2 weeks.
  d. Supplementation with oral medication may be necessary for the first several months until the optimum dosage regimen has been determined.
Techniques of injection
  a. Using a 2-inch needle, inject no more than 3 mL of medication per injection into upper quadrant of buttock (to inject more than 3 mL, use alternate buttocks and vary injection sites).
  b. After drawing up medication, draw a small air bubble of 0.1 mL into syringe and change needle for injection.
  c. Wipe injection site with alcohol swab and allow to dry before giving injection, otherwise alcohol may infiltrate subcutaneous tissue and cause local irritation.
  d. Stretch the skin over the injection site to one side and hold firmly.
  e. Inject medication slowly, including air bubble, which forces last drop from needle into the muscle and prevents any medication from being deposited in subcutaneous tissue as needle is withdrawn.
  f. Wait about 10 seconds before withdrawing needle, then do so quickly and release skin.
  g. Do not massage injection site, as this may force medication to ooze from muscle and infiltrate subcutaneous tissue.
  h. Precautions should also be taken with glass ampules to avoid injection of glass particles.

Technique for injecting long-acting neuroleptics. *Br J Psychiatry* 1982;144:316, with permission.

than enanthate preparations because they are absorbed more slowly. Although stabilizing a person on the oral preparation of the specific drugs is not necessary before initiating the depot form, it is good practice to give at least one oral dose of the drug to assess the possibility of an adverse effect, such as severe extrapyramidal symptoms or an allergic reaction.

The correct dosage and frequency of administration are difficult to predict for depot preparations. It is reasonable to begin with either 12.5 mg (0.5 mL) of fluphenazine preparation or 25 mg (0.5 mL) of haloperidol decanoate. If symptoms emerge in the next 2 to 4 weeks, the person can be treated temporarily with additional oral medications or with additional small depot injections. After 3 to 4 weeks the depot injection can be increased to a single dose equal to the total of the doses given during the initial period.

A good reason to initiate depot treatment with low doses is that the absorption of the preparations may be faster than usual at the onset of treatment, resulting in frightening episodes of dystonia that eventually discourage compliance with the medication. Some clinicians keep persons drug free for 3 to 7 days before initiating depot treatment and give small doses of the depot preparations (3.125 mg fluphenazine or 6.25 mg haloperidol) every few days to avoid those initial problems. Because the major indication for depot medication is poor compliance with oral forms, the clinician should go slowly with what is practically the last method of achieving compliance.

Plasma Concentrations. Interindividual variation in the metabolism of the antipsychotics is significant, resulting in part from genetic differences among persons and from pharmacokinetic interactions with other drugs. If a person has not improved after 4 to 6 weeks of treatment, the plasma concentration of the drug should be determined if such a test is available. Other possible indications for determining the plasma concentration are questions regarding compliance, concern regarding pharmacokinetic interactions, and the development of significant akathisia or akinesia.

The blood sample must be obtained after the person has been taking a particular dosage for at least five times the half-life of the drug, to approach steady-state concentrations. It is also standard practice to obtain plasma samples at trough levels— just before the daily dose is given, usually at least 12 hours after the previous dose and most commonly 20 to 24 hours after the previous dose. The quality of the laboratories that perform the analyses varies significantly; therefore, the clinician must obtain the normal ranges for a particular laboratory and must test the laboratory with multiple plasma samples from well-controlled persons. Having taken all these precautions, the clinician is still left with the reality that most antipsychotics have no well-defined dose-response curve. The best-studied drug is haloperidol, which may have a therapeutic window ranging from 2 to 15 ng/mL. Other therapeutic ranges that have been reasonably well documented are 30 to 100 ng/mL for chlorpromazine and 0.8 to 2.4 ng/mL for perphenazine.

Treatment-Resistant Persons.   Various studies indicate that 10 to 35 percent of persons with schizophrenia fail to obtain significant benefit from the antipsychotic drugs. Persons are often defined as being treatment-resistant if they have failed at least two adequate trials of antipsychotics from two pharmacological classes. Adequate trials are usually defined at least 6 weeks of daily doses equivalent to 20 mg of haloperidol or 1000 mg of chlorpromazine. It is useful to determine plasma concentrations for such persons, since one possibility is that they are slow metabolizers and are grossly overmedicated with a particular drug. More likely, however, they simply do not respond to the antipsychotic drugs. Studies have shown that up to two thirds of nonresponders to typical antipsychotic drugs may respond to SDAs.

Adjuvant Treatments.   Medications that have been reported to be useful as adjuvants to antipsychotics include lithium, carbamazepine, β-adrenergic receptor antagonists, antidepressants, and benzodiazepines. Of these medications, the most robust data support the use of lithium as an adjuvant medication. When using the combination of lithium and antipsychotics, the clinician should use slightly lower dosages of each initially to avoid the development of delirium or neurotoxicity. The use of carbamazepine has also been reported to be an effective addition to antipsychotic drug treatment, although the coadministration of carbamazepine can lower the plasma concentrations of the antipsychotic as much as 50 percent because of the induction of hepatic enzymes. Benzodiazepines have been reported to be effective as an adjuvant treatment; however their withdrawal must be monitored carefully to avoid significant worsening of symptoms. An increasing body of data supports the use of antidepressants in schizophrenic persons who have significant depressive symptoms.

For a more detailed discussion of this topic, see Marder SR, van Kammen DP: Dopamine Receptor Antagonists (Typical Antipsychotics), Sec 31.17, p 2356 in CTP/VII.

19

Lithium

Lithium (Eskalith, Lithobid, Lithonate) is the most commonly used short-term, long-term, and prophylactic treatment for bipolar I disorder. It is also used as an adjunctive medication in the treatment of major depressive disorder, schizoaffective disorder, therapy-resistant schizophrenia, anorexia nervosa, and bulimia nervosa and for control of chronic aggression in both children and adults.

CHEMISTRY

Lithium (Li), a monovalent ion, is the third lightest element and the lightest of the alkali metals (group IA of the periodic table), a group that also includes sodium, potassium, rubidium, cesium, and francium. No other element of group IA has antimanic properties. Lithium exists in nature as both ^{6}Li (7.42 percent) and ^{7}Li (92.58 percent). The latter isotope allows the imaging of lithium by magnetic resonance spectroscopy. Some 300 mg of lithium is contained in 1597 mg of lithium carbonate (Li_2CO_3).

PHARMACOLOGICAL ACTIONS

After ingestion, lithium is completely absorbed by the gastrointestinal (GI) tract. Serum concentrations peak in 1 to 1½ hours for standard preparations and in 4 to 4½ hours for controlled-released preparations. Lithium does not bind to plasma proteins, is not metabolized, and is excreted through the kidneys. The plasma half-life is initially 1.3 days and is 2.4 days after administration for more than 1 year. The blood–brain barrier permits only slow passage of lithium, which is why a single overdose does not necessarily cause toxicity and why long-term lithium intoxication is slow to resolve. The half-life of lithium is about 20 hours, and equilibrium is reached after 5 to 7 days of regular intake. Renal clearance of lithium is decreased with renal insufficiency (common in the elderly) and is increased in adolescents, which may necessitate twice or thrice daily dosing. The excretion of lithium is complex during pregnancy; excretion increases during pregnancy but decreases after delivery. Lithium is excreted in breast milk and in insignificant amounts in the feces and sweat.

The molecular mechanism of the mood-stabilizing effects of lithium is not known. Speculation has touched on several known cellular pathways, but no consistent associations have been found.

THERAPEUTIC INDICATIONS

Bipolar I Disorder

Manic Episodes. Lithium controls acute mania and prevents relapse in about 80 percent of persons with bipolar I disorder and in a somewhat smaller percentage of persons with mixed (mania and depression) episodes, rapid-cycling bipolar disorder, or mood changes in encephalopathy. Lithium alone at therapeutic concentrations exerts its antimanic effects in 1 to 3 weeks. To control mania initially, a benzodiazepine, such as clonazepam (Klonopin) or lorazepam (Ativan), or a dopamine receptor antagonist, such as haloperidol (Haldol) or chlorpromazine (Thorazine), should also be administered for the first few weeks.

Lithium is effective as long-term prophylaxis of both manic and depressive episodes in about 70 to 80 percent of persons with bipolar I disorder.

Depressive Episodes.   Lithium is effective in the treatment of major depressive disorder and depression associated with bipolar I disorder. Because antidepressants can trigger mania in persons with bipolar disorders, lithium monotherapy is an ideal treatment for both mania and depression in persons with bipolar disorder. Lithium may also be prescribed with an antidepressant for long-term maintenance of persons with bipolar disorder. Tricyclic and tetracyclic drugs are considered more likely to trigger severe mania than are bupropion (Wellbutrin) or selective serotonin reuptake inhibitors (SSRIs). Augmentation of lithium therapy with valproate (Depakene) or carbamazepine (Tegretol) is usually well tolerated, with little risk of precipitation of mania.

When a depressive episode occurs in a person taking maintenance lithium, the differential diagnosis should include lithium-induced hypothyroidism, substance abuse, and lack of compliance with the lithium therapy. Possible treatment approaches include increasing the lithium concentration (up to 1 to 1.2 mEq/L), adding supplemental thyroid hormone (e.g., 25 μg a day liothyronine [Cytomel]) even in the presence of normal findings on thyroid function tests, augmentation with valproate or carbamazepine, the judicious use of antidepressants, electroconvulsive therapy (ECT), and psychotherapy. Once the acute depressive episode resolves, other therapies should be tapered off in favor of lithium monotherapy, if clinically tolerated.

Maintenance.   Maintenance treatment with lithium markedly decreases the frequency, the severity, and the duration of manic and depressive episodes in persons with bipolar I disorder. Lithium provides relatively more effective prophylaxis for mania than for depression, and supplemental antidepressant strategies may be necessary either intermittently or continuously. Lithium maintenance is almost always indicated after the second episode of bipolar I disorder depression or mania and should be considered after the first episode for adolescents or for persons who have a family history of bipolar I disorder. Others who benefit from lithium maintenance are those who have poor support systems, had no precipitating factors for the first episode, have a high suicide risk, had a sudden onset of the first episode, or had a first episode of mania. Clinical studies have shown that lithium reduces the incidence of suicide in bipolar I disorder patients sixfold or sevenfold. Lithium is also effective treatment for persons with severe cyclothymic disorder.

Initiating maintenance therapy after the first manic episode is considered a wise approach based on several observations. First, each episode of mania increases the risk of subsequent episodes. Second, among people responsive to lithium, relapses are 28 times more likely after lithium use is discontinued. Third, case reports describe persons who initially responded to lithium, discontinued taking it, and then had a relapse but no longer responded to lithium in subsequent episodes. Continued maintenance treatment with lithium is often associated with increasing efficacy and reduced mortality. Therefore, an episode of depression or mania that occurs after a relatively short time of lithium maintenance does not necessarily represent treatment failure. However, lithium treatment alone may begin to lose its effectiveness after several years of successful use. If this occurs, then supplemental treatment with carbamazepine or valproate may be useful.

Maintenance lithium dosages often can be adjusted to achieve plasma concentration somewhat lower than that needed for treatment of acute mania. If lithium use is to be discontinued, then the dosage should be slowly tapered. Abrupt discontinuation of lithium therapy is associated with increased risk of recurrence of manic and depressive episodes.

Major Depressive Disorder

The primary indication for lithium in major depressive disorder is as an adjuvant to antidepressant use in persons who have failed to respond to the antidepressants alone. About 50 percent of antidepressant nonresponders do respond when lithium 300 mg, three times daily, is added to the antidepressant regimen. Some persons respond rapidly, in days; for most persons, several weeks are required to assess the efficacy of the regimen. Lithium alone may effectively treat depressed persons who actually have bipolar I disorder but have not yet had their first manic episode. Moreover, lithium has been reported to be effective in persons with major depressive disorder whose disorder has a particularly marked cyclicity.

Schizoaffective Disorder and Schizophrenia

Among persons with schizoaffective disorder, those with predominant mood symptoms—either bipolar type or depressive type—are more likely to respond to lithium than are those with predominant psychotic symptoms. Serotonin-dopamine antagonists (SDAs) and dopamine receptor antagonists are the treatments of choice for persons with schizoaffective disorder, whereas lithium is a useful augmentation agent, particularly for persons whose symptoms are resistant to treatment with SDAs and dopamine receptor antagonists. Lithium augmentation of an SDA or dopamine receptor antagonist treatment, however, may be an effective treatment for persons with schizoaffective disorder even in the absence of a prominent mood disorder component. Some persons with schizophrenia who cannot take antipsychotic drugs may benefit from lithium treatment alone. The intermittent aggressive outbursts of some persons with schizophrenia may also be reduced by lithium treatment.

Aggression

Lithium has been used to treat aggressive outbursts in persons with schizophrenia, prison inmates, those with intermittent explosive disorder, and children with conduct disorder and to treat aggression and self-mutilation in persons with mental retardation. Treatment response is more likely in the presence of a more "affective" (explosive) subtype of aggression and less likely if aggression is "predatory" (planned). Less success has been reported in the treatment of aggressiveness associated with head trauma and epilepsy.

PRECAUTIONS AND ADVERSE EFFECTS

The most common adverse effects from lithium treatment are increased thirst, polyuria, gastric distress, weight gain, tremor, fatigue, and mild cognitive impairment (Table 19–1). Gastric distress may include nausea, vomiting, and diarrhea and can often be reduced by further dividing the dosage, administering the lithium with food, or switching among the various lithium preparations. Weight gain and edema can be impossible to treat other than by encouraging the patient to eat less and to exercise moderately. The tremor affects mostly the fingers and sometimes can be worse at peak levels of the drug. It can be reduced by further dividing the dosage. Propranolol (Inderal) (30 to 160 mg a day in divided doses) reduces the tremor significantly in most patients. The fatigue and mild cognitive impairment may decrease with time. Rare neurological adverse effects include symptoms of mild parkinsonism, ataxia, and dysarthria. Patients with brain impairment are at risk of neurotoxicity. Lithium may exacerbate Parkinson's disease. Lithium should be used with caution in diabetic patients, as it may induce seizures or exacerbate a seizure disorder. Dehydrated, debilitated, and medically ill patients are susceptible to side effects and toxicity. Leukocytosis is a common benign effect of lithium treatment.

Gastrointestinal Effects

GI symptoms can include nausea, decreased appetite, vomiting, and diarrhea and can be diminished by dividing the dosage, administering the lithium with food, or switching to another lithium preparation. The lithium preparation least likely to cause diarrhea is lithium citrate. Some lithium preparations contain lactose, which can cause diarrhea in lactose-intolerant persons. Persons taking slow-release formulations of lithium who experience diarrhea due to unabsorbed medication in the lower part of the GI tract may experience less diarrhea with standard-release preparations. Diarrhea may also respond to antidiarrheal preparations such as loperamide (Imodium, Kaopectate), bismuth subsalicylate (Pepto-Bismol), or diphenoxylate with at-

TABLE 19–1
ADVERSE EFFECTS OF LITHIUM

Neurological
  Benign, nontoxic: dysphoria, lack of spontaneity, slowed reaction time, memory difficulties
  Tremor: postural, occasional extrapyramidal
  Toxic: coarse tremor, dysarthria, ataxia, neuromuscular irritability, seizures, coma, death
  Miscellaneous: peripheral neuropathy, benign intracranial hypertension, myasthenia gravis–like syndrome, altered creativity, lowered seizure threshold
Endocrine
  Thyroid: goiter, hypothyroidism, exophthalmos, hyperthyroidism (rare)
  Parathyroid: hyperparathyroidism, adenoma
Cardiovascular
  Benign T-wave changes, sinus node dysfunction
Renal
  Concentrating defect, morphological changes, polyuria (nephrogenic diabetes insipidus), reduced GFR, nephrotic syndrome, renal tubular acidosis
Dermatological
  Acne, hair loss, psoriasis, rash
Gastrointestinal
  Appetite loss, nausea, vomiting, diarrhea
Miscellaneous
  Altered carbohydrate metabolism, weight gain, fluid retention

ropine (Lomotil).Weight gain results from a poorly understood effect of lithium on carbohydrate metabolism. Weight gain can also result from lithium-induced edema.

Neurological Effects

Tremor. A lithium-induced postural tremor may occur that is usually 8 to 12 Hz and is most notable in outstretched hands, especially in the fingers, and during tasks involving fine manipulations. The tremor can be reduced by dividing the daily dosage, using a sustained-release formulation, reducing caffeine intake, reassessing the concomitant use of other medicines, and treating comorbid anxiety. β-Adrenergic receptor antagonists, such as propranolol, 30 to 120 mg a day in divided doses, and primidone (Mysoline), 50 to 250 mg a day, are usually effective in reducing the tremor. In persons with hypokalemia, potassium supplementation may improve the tremor. When a person taking lithium has a severe tremor, the possibility of lithium toxicity should be suspected and evaluated.

Cognitive Effects. Lithium use has been associated with dysphoria, lack of spontaneity, slowed reaction times, and impaired memory. The presence of these symptoms should be noted carefully, because they are a frequent cause of noncompliance. The differential diagnosis for such symptoms should include depressive disorders, hypothyroidism, hypercalcemia, other illnesses, and other drugs. Some, but not all, persons have reported that fatigue and mild cognitive impairment decrease with time.

Other Neurological Effects. Uncommon neurological adverse effects include symptoms of mild parkinsonism, ataxia, and dysarthria, although the last two symptoms may also be due to lithium intoxication. Lithium is rarely associated with development of peripheral neuropathy, benign intracranial hypertension (pseudotumor cerebri), findings resembling myasthenia gravis, and increased risk of seizures.

Renal Effects

The most common adverse renal effect of lithium is polyuria with secondary polydipsia. The symptom is particularly a problem in 25 to 35 percent of persons taking lithium, who may have a urine output of more than 3 liters a day (normal, 1 to 2 liters a day). The polyuria primarily results from lithium antagonism to the effects of antidiuretic hormone, which thus causes diuresis. When polyuria is a significant problem, the person's renal function should be evaluated and followed up with 24-hour urine collections for creatinine clearance determinations. Treatment consists of fluid replacement, the use of the lowest effective dosage of lithium, and single daily dosing of lithium. Treatment can also involve the use of a thiazide or potassium-sparing diuretic—for example, amiloride (Midamor), spironolactone (Aldactone), triamterene (Dyrenium), or amiloride-hydrochlorothiazide (Moduretic). If treatment with a diuretic is initiated, the lithium dosage should be halved, and the diuretic should not be started for 5 days, because the diuretic is likely to increase lithium retention.

The most serious renal adverse effects, which are rare and associated with continuous lithium administration for 10 years or more, involve appearance of nonspecific interstitial fibrosis, associated with gradual decreases in glomerular filtration rate and increases in serum creatinine concentrations, and rarely with renal failure. Lithium occasionally is associated with nephrotic syndrome and features of distal renal tubular acidosis. It is prudent for persons taking lithium to check their serum creatinine concentration, urine chemistries, and 24-hour urine volume at yearly intervals.

Thyroid Effects

Lithium affects thyroid function, causing a generally benign and often transient diminution in the concentrations of circulating thyroid hormones. Reports have attributed goiter (5 percent of persons), benign reversible exophthalmos, hyperthyroidism, and hypothyroidism (7 to 10 percent of persons) to lithium treatment. Lithium-induced hypothyroidism is more common in women (14 percent) than in men (4.5 percent). Women are at highest risk during the first two years of treatment. Persons taking lithium to treat bipolar disorder are twice as likely to develop hypothyroidism if they develop rapid cycling. About 50 percent of persons receiving long-term lithium treatment have laboratory abnormalities, such as an abnormal thyrotropin-releasing hormone (TRH) response, and about 30 percent have elevated concentrations of thyroid-stimulating hormone (TSH). If symptoms of hypothyroidism are present, replacement with levothyroxine (Synthroid) is indicated. Even in the absence of hypothyroid symptoms, some clinicians treat persons with significantly elevated TSH concentrations with levothyroxine. In lithium-treated persons, TSH concentrations should be measured every 6 to 12 months. Lithium-induced hypothyroidism should be considered when evaluating depressive episodes that emerge during lithium therapy.

Cardiac Effects

The cardiac effects of lithium, which resemble those of hypokalemia on the electrocardiogram (ECG), are caused by the displacement of intracellular potassium by the lithium ion. The most common changes on the ECG are T wave flattening or inversion. The changes are benign and disappear after the lithium is excreted from the body. Nevertheless, baseline ECGs are essential and should be repeated annually.

Because lithium also depresses the pacemaking activity of the sinus node, lithium treatment can result in sinus dysrhythmias, heart block, and episodes of syncope. Lithium treatment, therefore, is contraindicated in persons with sick sinus syndrome. In rare cases, ventricular arrhythmias and congestive heart failure have been associated with lithium therapy. Lithium cardiotoxicity is more prevalent in persons on a low-salt diet, those taking certain diuretics or angiotensin-converting enzyme inhibitors, and those with fluid-electrolyte imbalances or any renal insufficiency.

Dermatological Effects

Several cutaneous adverse effects, which may be dose dependent, have been associated with lithium treatment. The most prevalent effects include acneiform, follicular, and maculopapular eruptions; pretibial ulcerations; and worsening of psoriasis. Alopecia has also been reported. Many of those conditions respond favorably to changing to another lithium preparation and the usual dermatological measures. Lithium concentrations should be monitored if tetracycline is used for the treatment of acne, because it can increase the retention of lithium. Occasionally, aggravated psoriasis or acneiform eruptions may force the discontinuation of lithium treatment.

Lithium Toxicity and Overdoses

The early signs and symptoms of lithium toxicity include neurological symptoms, such as coarse tremor, dysarthria, and ataxia; GI symptoms; cardiovascular changes; and renal dysfunction. The later signs and symptoms include impaired consciousness, muscular fasciculations, myoclonus, seizures, and coma (Table 19–2). Risk factors include exceeding the recommended dosage; reduced excretion due to renal impairment, low-sodium diet, or drug interaction; and dehydration. Elderly persons are more vulnerable to the effects of increased serum lithium concentrations. The higher the lithium concentration and the longer the lithium concentration has been high, the worse are the symptoms of lithium toxicity. Lithium toxicity is a medical emergency, since it can result in permanent neuronal damage and death.

The treatment of lithium toxicity (Table 19–3) involves discontinuing the lithium and treating the dehydration. Unabsorbed lithium can be removed from the GI tract by ingestion of polystyrene sulfonate (Kayexalate) or polyethylene glycol solution (GoLYTELY) but not activated charcoal. Ingestion of a single large dose may create clumps of medication in the stomach, which can be removed by gastric lavage

TABLE 19–2
SIGNS AND SYMPTOMS OF LITHIUM TOXICITY

Mild-to-moderate intoxication (lithium level = 1.5–2.0 mEq/L)	
Gastrointestinal	Vomiting
	Abdominal pain
	Dryness of mouth
Neurological	Ataxia
	Dizziness
	Slurred speech
	Nystagmus
	Lethargy or excitement
	Muscle weakness
Moderate-to-severe intoxication (lithium level = 2.0–2.5 mEq/L)	
Gastrointestinal	Anorexia
	Persistent nausea and vomiting
Neurological	Blurred vision
	Muscle fasciculations
	Clonic limb movements
	Hyperactive deep tendon reflexes
	Choreoathetoid movements
	Convulsions
	Delirium
	Syncope
	Electroencephalographic changes
	Stupor
	Coma
	Circulatory failure (lowered blood pressure, cardiac arrhythmias, and conduction abnormalities)
Severe lithium intoxication (lithium level >2.5 mEq/L) Generalized convulsions Oliguria and renal failure Death	

From Marangell LB, Silver JM, Yudofsky SC: Psychopharmacology and electroconvulsive therapy. In: *The American Psychiatric Press Textbook of Psychiatry*, ed 3. American Psychiatric Press, Washington, DC, 1999, with permission.

TABLE 19-3
MANAGEMENT OF LITHIUM TOXICITY

1. The patient should immediately contact his or her personal physician or go to a hospital emergency room.
2. Lithium should be discontinued and the patient instructed to ingest fluids, if possible.
3. Physical examination should be completed, including vital signs and a neurological examination with complete formal mental status examination.
4. Lithium level, serum electrolytes, renal function tests, and electrocardiogram should be obtained as soon as possible.
5. For significant acute ingestion, residual gastric contents should be removed by induction of emesis, gastric lavage, and absorption with activated charcoal.
6. Vigorous hydration and maintenance of electrolyte balance are essential.
7. For any patient with a serum lithium level greater than 4.0 mEq/L or with serious manifestations of lithium toxicity, hemodialysis should be initiated.
8. Repeat dialysis may be required every 6–10 hours, until the lithium level is within nontoxic range and the patient has no signs or symptoms of lithium toxicity.

From Marangell LB, Silver JM, Yudofsky SC: Psychopharmacology and electroconvulsive therapy. In: *The American Psychiatric Press Textbook of Psychiatry*, ed 3. American Psychiatric Press, Washington, DC, 1999, with permission.

with a wide-bore tube. The value of forced diuresis is still debated. In the most serious cases, hemodialysis is the most effective means of rapid removal of excessive amounts of serum lithium. Postdialysis serum lithium concentrations may rise as lithium is redistributed from tissues to blood, and repeat dialysis may be needed. Neurological improvement may lag behind clearance of serum lithium by several days, because lithium crosses the blood–brain barrier slowly.

Adolescents

The serum lithium concentrations for adolescents is similar to that for adults. Although the side-effect profile is similar in adolescents and adults, weight gain and acne associated with lithium use can be particularly troublesome to an adolescent.

Elderly Persons

Lithium is a safe and effective drug for the elderly. However, the treatment of elderly persons taking lithium may be complicated by the presence of other medical illnesses, decreased renal function, special diets that affect lithium clearance, and generally increased sensitivity to lithium. Elderly persons should initially be given low dosages, their dosages should be switched less frequently than are those of younger persons, and a longer time must be allowed for renal excretion to equilibrate with absorption before lithium can be assumed to have reached its steady-state concentrations.

Pregnant Women

Lithium should not be administered to pregnant women in the first trimester because of the risk of birth defects. The most common malformations involve the cardiovascular system, most commonly Ebstein's anomaly of the tricuspid valves. The risk of Ebstein's malformation in lithium-exposed fetuses is 1 in 1000, which is 20 times the risk in the general population. The possibility of fetal cardiac anomalies can be evaluated with fetal echocardiography. The teratogenic risk of lithium (4 to

12 percent) is higher than that for the general population (2 to 3 percent) but appears to be lower than that associated with use of valproate or carbamazepine. A woman who continues to take lithium during pregnancy should use the lowest effective dosage. The maternal lithium concentration must be monitored closely during pregnancy and especially after pregnancy, because of the significant decrease in renal lithium excretion as renal function returns to normal in the first few days after delivery. Adequate hydration can reduce the risk of lithium toxicity during labor. Lithium prophylaxis is recommended for all women with bipolar disorder as they enter the postpartum period. Lithium is excreted into breast milk and should be taken by a nursing mother only after careful evaluation of potential risks and benefits. Signs of lithium toxicity in infants include lethargy, cyanosis, abnormal reflexes, and sometimes hepatomegaly.

Miscellaneous Effects

Lithium should be used with caution in diabetic persons, who should monitor their blood glucose concentrations carefully to avoid diabetic ketoacidosis. Benign, reversible leukocytosis is commonly associated with lithium treatment. Dehydrated, debilitated, and medically ill persons are most susceptible to adverse effects and toxicity.

DRUG INTERACTIONS

Lithium drug interactions are summarized in Table 19–4.

Lithium has been used successfully with dopamine receptor antagonists for many years. However, coadministration of higher dosages of dopamine receptor antagonists and lithium may result in a synergistic increase in the symptoms of lithium-induced neurological adverse effects. This interaction may occur with use of any dopamine receptor antagonist.

The coadministration of lithium and anticonvulsants—including carbamazepine, valproate, and clonazepam—may increase lithium concentrations and aggravate lithium-induced neurological adverse effects. Used wisely, however, the coadministration of lithium and anticonvulsants can be therapeutically beneficial to some persons. Treatment with the combination should be initiated at slightly lower dosages than usual, and the dosages should be increased gradually. Changes from one to another treatment for mania should be made carefully, with as little temporal overlap between the drugs as possible.

Most diuretics (e.g., thiazide and potassium sparing) can increase lithium concentrations; when treatment with such a diuretic is stopped, the clinician may need to increase the person's daily lithium dosage. Osmotic and loop diuretics, carbonic anhydrase inhibitors, and xanthines (including caffeine) may reduce lithium concentrations to below therapeutic concentrations. Angiotensin-converting enzyme inhibitors may cause an increase in lithium concentrations, whereas the AT_1 angiotensin II receptor inhibitors losartan (Cozaar) and irbesartan (Avapro) do not alter lithium concentrations. A wide range of nonsteroidal anti-inflammatory drugs can decrease lithium clearance, thereby increasing lithium concentrations. These drugs include indomethacin (Indocin), phenylbutazone (Azolid), diclofenac (Voltaren),

TABLE 19–4
DRUG INTERACTIONS WITH LITHIUM

Drug Class	Reaction
Antipsychotics	Case reports of encephalopathy, worsening of extrapyramidal adverse effects, and neuroleptic malignant syndrome. Inconsistent reports of altered red blood cell and plasma concentrations of lithium, antipsychotic drug, or both
Antidepressants	Occasional reports of a serotonin-like syndrome with potent serotonin reuptake inhibitors
Anticonvulsants	No significant pharmacokinetic interactions with carbamazepine or valproate; reports of neurotoxicity with carbamazepine; combinations helpful for treatment resistance
Nonsteroidal anti-inflammatory drugs	May reduce renal lithium clearance and increase serum concentration; toxicity reported (exception is aspirin)
Diuretics	
Thiazides	Well-documented reduced renal lithium clearance and increased serum concentration; toxicity reported
Potassium sparing	Limited data, may increase lithium concentration
Loop	Lithium clearance unchanged (some case reports of increased lithium concentration)
Osmotic (mannitol, urea)	Increase renal lithium clearance and decrease lithium concentration
Xanthine (aminophylline, caffeine, theophylline)	Increase renal lithium clearance and decrease lithium concentration
Carbonic anhydrase inhibitors (acetazolamide)	Increase renal lithium clearance
Angiotensin-converting enzyme (ACE) inhibitors	Reports of reduced lithium clearance, increased concentrations, and toxicity
Calcium channel inhibitors	Case reports of neurotoxicity; no consistent pharmacokinetic interactions
Miscellaneous	
Succinylcholine, pancuronium	Reports of prolonged neuromuscular blockade
Metronidazole	Increased lithium concentration
Methyldopa	Few reports of neurotoxicity
Sodium bicarbonate	Increased renal lithium clearance
Iodides	Additive antithyroid effects
Propranolol	Used for lithium tremor. Possible slight increase in lithium concentration

ketoprofen (Orudis), oxyphenbutazone (Oxalid), ibuprofen (Motrin, Advil, Nuprin), piroxicam (Feldene), and naproxen (Naprosyn). Aspirin and sulindac (Clinoril) do not affect lithium concentrations.

The coadministration of lithium and quetiapine (Seroquel) may cause somnolence but is otherwise well tolerated. The coadministration of lithium and ziprasidone (Zeldox) may modestly increase the incidence of tremor. The coadministration of lithium and calcium channel inhibitors should be avoided because of potentially fatal neurotoxicity.

A person taking lithium who is about to undergo ECT should discontinue taking lithium 2 days before beginning ECT, to reduce the risk of delirium resulting from the coadministration of these two treatments.

LABORATORY INTERFERENCES

Lithium is not known to interfere with any laboratory tests. However, lithium treatment does affect a number of commonly obtained laboratory values (Table 19–5).

TABLE 19–5
POSSIBLE EFFECTS OF LITHIUM ON LABORATORY VALUES

Laboratory Value	Possible Effect of Lithium
White blood cells (WBCs)	Increased count
Serum glucose	Increased level
Serum magnesium	Increased level
Serum potassium	Decreased level
Serum uric acid	Decreased level
Serum thyroxine	Decreased level
Serum cortisol	Decreased AM levels
Serum parathyroid hormone	Increased level due to adenoma
Serum calcium	Increased level due to parathyroid hormone level
Serum phosphorus	Decreased level due to increased parathyroid hormone level

From Doupe A, Szuba M: Lithium and other antimanic agents. In: *The Handbook of Psychiatry*. Residents of the UCLA Department of Psychiatry. Year Book Medical Publishers, Chicago, 1990, with permission.

DOSAGE AND CLINICAL GUIDELINES

Initial Medical Workup

Before a clinician administers lithium, the patient should have a routine laboratory workup and physical examination. The laboratory tests should include serum creatinine concentration (or a 24-hour urine creatinine if the clinician has any reason to be concerned about renal function), electrolytes, thyroid function (TSH, T_3, and T_4), a complete blood count (CBC), ECG, and a pregnancy test in women of childbearing age.

Dosage Recommendations

Lithium formulations include 150-, 300-, and 600-mg lithium carbonate capsules (Eskalith, Lithonate, and generic), 300-mg lithium carbonate tablets (Lithotabs), 450-mg controlled-release lithium carbonate capsules (Eskalith CR), and 8-mEq/mL lithium citrate syrup.

If a person has previously been treated with lithium and the previous dosage is known, then the same dosage should be used for the current episode unless changes in the person's pharmacokinetic parameters have affected lithium clearance. The starting dosage for most adults is 300 mg of the regular-release formulation three times daily. The starting dosage for elderly persons or persons with renal impairment should be 300 mg once or twice daily. An eventual dosage between 900 and 1200 mg a day usually produces a therapeutic plasma concentration of 0.6 to 1 mEq/L, and a daily dose of 1200 to 1800 mg usually produces a therapeutic concentration of 0.8 to 1.2 mEq/L. Maintenance dosing can be given either in two or three divided doses of the regular-release formulation or in a single dosage of the sustained-release formulation equivalent to the combined daily dosage of the regular-release formulation. The use of divided doses reduces gastric upset and avoids single high-peak lithium concentrations. There are no data to show a difference in clinical efficacy between the regular- and sustained-release formulations.

Serum and Plasma Concentrations

Serum and plasma concentrations of lithium are the standard methods of assessing lithium concentrations, and they serve as the basis for titrating the dosages. Lithium concentrations should be determined routinely every 2 to 6 months and promptly in persons suspected to be noncompliant with the prescribed dosages, in persons who exhibit signs of toxicity, and during dosage adjustments. Although reports have noted the measurement of lithium concentrations in saliva, tears, and red blood cells, these methods have no clinical superiority to analysis of serum or plasma.

A consensus method for sample collection specifies that the person must be at steady-state lithium dosing (usually after 5 days of constant dosing), preferably using a twice- or-thrice-daily dosing regimen, and that the blood sample must be drawn 12 hours (plus or minus 30 minutes) after a given dose. Lithium concentrations 12 hours postdose in persons treated with sustained-release preparations are generally about 30 percent higher than the corresponding concentrations obtained from those taking the regular-release preparations. Because available data are based on a sample population following a multiple-dosage regimen, regular-release formulations given at least twice daily should be used for initial determination of the appropriate dosages.

Two technical considerations should be considered if laboratory values do not seem to correspond to clinical status. First, collection of blood in a tube with a lithium-heparin anticoagulant can give results falsely elevated by as much as 1 mEq/L. Second, aging of the lithium ion–selective electrode can cause inaccuracies of up to 0.5 mEq/L. Once the daily dose has been set, it is reasonable to change to the sustained-release formulation given once daily.

The most common guidelines are 1.0 to 1.5 mEq/L for the treatment of acute mania and 0.4 to 0.8 mEq/L for maintenance treatment. Biological variations in regulation of mood and in lithium metabolism bolster the universal maxim "treat the patient, not the laboratory results." A small number of persons will not achieve therapeutic benefit with a lithium concentration of 1.5 mEq/L yet will have no signs of toxicity. For such persons, titration of the lithium dosage to achieve a concentration above 1.5 mEq/L may be warranted. If there is no response after 2 weeks at a concentration that is beginning to cause adverse effects, then the person should taper off lithium use over 1 to 2 weeks and should try other mood-stabilizing drugs. Other therapeutic options include carbamazepine, valproate, other anticonvulsants, thyroid hormones, ECT, calcium channel inhibitors, monoamine oxidase inhibitors, dopamine receptor antagonists, and SDAs.

Patient Education

Persons taking lithium should be advised that changes in the body's water and salt content can affect the amount of lithium excreted, resulting in either increases or decreases in lithium concentrations. Excessive sodium intake (e.g., a dramatic dietary change) lowers lithium concentrations. Conversely, too little sodium (e.g., fad diets) can lead to potentially toxic concentrations of lithium. Decreases in body fluid (e.g., excessive perspiration) can lead to dehydration and lithium intoxication.

For a more detailed discussion of this topic, see Jefferson JW, Griest JH: Lithium, Sec 31.18, p 2377, in CTP/VII.

20

Mirtazapine

Mirtazapine (Remeron) is as effective as amitriptyline (Elavil, Endep) in lifting mood, yet it lacks the anticholinergic effects of the tricyclic antidepressants and the gastrointestinal (GI) and anxiogenic effects of the selective serotonin reuptake inhibitors (SSRIs).

CHEMISTRY

The molecular structure of mirtazapine is shown in Figure 20–1.

PHARMACOLOGICAL ACTIONS

Mirtazapine is rapidly and completely absorbed from the GI tract. Peak concentration is achieved within 2 hours of ingestion. Plasma clearance may be slowed up to 30 percent in persons with impaired hepatic function and up to 50 percent in those with impaired renal function. Clearance may be up to 40 percent slower in elderly males and up to 10 percent slower in elderly females. The mean elimination half-life is 20 to 40 hours, and steady-state levels are achieved within about 5 days. A clinical response may require 2 to 4 weeks.

Mirtazapine acts as an antagonist of central presynaptic α_2-adrenergic receptors within the central nervous system, where it has a net effect of increasing synaptic levels of noradrenaline and serotonin. It is a potent antagonist of serotonin 5-HT$_2$ and 5-HT$_3$ receptors but has little effect on 5-HT$_1$ receptors. This appears to bias the activation of serotonin receptors in favor of the 5-HT$_1$ family, whose activation is thought to reduce anxiety and depression. Mirtazapine is a potent antagonist of histamine H$_1$ receptors and is a moderately potent antagonist at α_1-adrenergic and muscarinic-cholinergic receptors.

THERAPEUTIC INDICATIONS

Mirtazapine is effective for the treatment of depression. It is highly sedating, in the same range as amitriptyline, clomipramine (Anafranil), and trazodone (Desyrel), and is thus useful for treatment of sleep disturbances. However, some of the sedating effects generally lessen within the first week of treatment. In direct comparison, it causes somewhat less somnolence, weight gain, and constipation than does amitriptyline and less headache and nausea than does fluoxetine (Prozac). It also appears to reduce somatic and psychological symptoms of anxiety and agitation.

PRECAUTIONS AND ADVERSE REACTIONS

The most common adverse effect of mirtazapine is somnolence, which may occur in over 50 percent of persons (Table 20–1). Therefore, when persons start to take

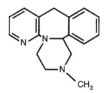

Figure. 20-1. The molecular structure of mirtazapine.

mirtazapine, they should exercise caution when driving or operating dangerous machinery. This adverse effect may be minimized by giving the dose before sleep. Mirtazapine also causes dizziness in 7 percent of persons. It does not appear to increase the risk for seizures. Mania or hypomania occurred in 0.2 percent of persons in clinical trials, a rate similar to that of other antidepressant drugs. Mirtazapine potentiates the sedative effects of alcohol.

Mirtazapine increases appetite in about 15 percent of patients. Mirtazapine may also increase serum cholesterol concentration to 20 percent or more above the upper limit of normal in 15 percent of persons and increase triglycerides to 500 mg/dL or more in 6 percent of persons. Elevations of alanine transaminase (ALT) levels to more than three times the upper limit of normal were seen in 2 percent of mirtazapine-treated persons, as opposed to 0.3 percent of placebo controls.

In limited premarketing experience, the absolute neutrophil count dropped to $500/mm^3$ or less within two months of onset of use in 0.3 percent of persons, some of whom developed symptomatic infections. This hematological condition was reversible in all cases and was more likely to occur when other risk factors for neutropenia were present. In postmarketing experience, increases in the frequency of neutropenia have not been reported. The manufacturer recommends instructing all persons to seek medical attention if they develop fever, chills, sore throat, mucous membrane ulceration, or other signs of infection. If a low white blood cell count is found, mirtazapine should be immediately discontinued, and the infectious disease status should be followed closely.

A small number of persons experience orthostatic hypotension while taking mirtazapine. Although no human data exist regarding effects on fetal development, mirtazapine should be used with caution during pregnancy.

Mirtazapine use by pregnant women has not been studied; because the drug may be excreted in breast milk, it should not be taken by nursing mothers. Because of the

TABLE 20-1
ADVERSE REACTIONS REPORTED WITH MIRTAZAPINE

Event	Percentage (%)
Somnolence	54
Dry mouth	25
Increased appetite	17
Constipation	13
Weight gain	12
Dizziness	7
Myalgias	5
Disturbing dreams	4

risk of agranulocytosis associated with mirtazapine use, persons should be attuned to signs of infection (see above). Because of the sedating effects of mirtazapine, persons should determine the degree to which they are affected prior to engaging in driving or other potentially dangerous activities. Other potentially sedating prescription or over-the-counter drugs and alcohol should be avoided during use of mirtazapine.

DRUG INTERACTIONS

Mirtazapine can potentiate the sedation of alcohol and benzodiazepines. Mirtazapine should not be used within 14 days of a monoamine oxidase inhibitor.

LABORATORY INTERFERENCES

No laboratory interferences have yet been described for mirtazapine.

DOSAGE AND ADMINISTRATION

Mirtazapine is available in 15- and 30-mg scored tablets. If persons fail to respond to the initial dose of mirtazapine of 15-mg before sleep, the dose may be increased in 15-mg increments every 5 days to a maximum of 45 mg before sleep. Lower dosages may be necessary in elderly persons or persons with renal or hepatic insufficiency.

For a more detailed discussion of this topic, see Claghorn JL: Mirtazapine, Sec 31.19, p 2390, in CTP/VII.

21

Monoamine Oxidase Inhibitors

The monoamine oxidase (MAO) inhibitors (MAOIs) are highly effective antidepressants and anxiolytics, but they are used less frequently than are other antidepressants because of the dietary precautions that must be followed to avoid tyramine-induced hypertensive crises. The currently available MAOIs include phenelzine (Nardil), isocarboxazid (Marplan), tranylcypromine (Parnate), and selegiline (Eldepryl). Selegiline is a selective inhibitor of MAO_B used for the treatment of parkinsonism. A newer class of reversible inhibitors of MAO_A (RIMAs) not available in the United States (e.g., moclobemide [Manerix] and befloxatone) require few dietary restrictions. Some clinicians believe that MAOIs are underused as effective antidepressant treatment.

CHEMISTRY

Isocarboxazid and phenelzine are derivatives of hydrazine, and tranylcypromine is a derivative of amphetamine. The molecular structures of phenelzine, isocarboxazid, tranylcypromine, and moclobemide are shown in Figure 21–1.

PHARMACOLOGICAL ACTIONS

Phenelzine, tranylcypromine, and isocarboxazid are readily absorbed through the gastrointestinal (GI) tract and reach peak plasma concentrations within 2 hours. Their plasma half-lives are in the range of 2 to 3 hours, whereas their tissue half-lives are considerably longer. Because they irreversibly inactivate MAOs, the therapeutic effect of a single dose of irreversible MAOIs may persist for as long as 2 weeks. The RIMA moclobemide is rapidly absorbed and has a half-life of 0.5 to 3.5 hours. Because it is a reversible inhibitor, moclobemide has a much briefer clinical effect following a single dose than do irreversible MAOIs.

MAO is an enzyme found intracellularly on the outer mitochondrial membrane, which degrades cytoplasmic monoamines, including norepinephrine, serotonin, dopamine, epinephrine, and tyramine. There are two types of MAO: MAO_A and MAO_B. MAO_A primarily metabolizes norepinephrine, serotonin, and epinephrine; dopamine and tyramine are metabolized by both MAO_A and MAO_B. MAOIs act in the central nervous system, the sympathetic nervous system, the liver, and the GI tract (Table 21–1). At dosages over 60 mg per day, tranylcypromine may inhibit the reuptake or increase the release of dopamine and norepinephrine and, to a lesser extent, serotonin.

When GI metabolism of dietary tyramine by MAOs is inactivated by an irreversible MAOI, intact tyramine can enter the circulation and exert a potent pressor effect, resulting in a hypertensive crisis. Tyramine-containing foods must therefore

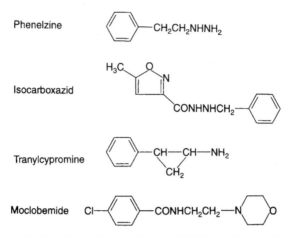

Figure. 21-1. Molecular structures of MAOIs used in psychiatry.

be avoided for 2 weeks after the last dose of an irreversible MAOI, to permit resynthesis of adequate concentrations of MAOs. In contrast, RIMAs have relatively little inhibitory activity for MAO_B, and because they are reversible, normal activity of existing MAO_A returns within 16 to 48 hours of the last dose of a RIMA. Therefore, the dietary restrictions are less stringent for RIMAs, applying only to foods containing high concentrations of tyramine, which need be avoided for only 3 days after the last dose of a RIMA.

THERAPEUTIC INDICATIONS

MAOIs are used for treatment of persons with depression, especially that associated with mood reactivity, extreme sensitivity to interpersonal loss or rejection, prominent anergia, hyperphagia, and hypersomnia—classified as atypical features in the fourth edition of *Diagnostic and Statistical Manual of Mental Disorders* (DSM-IV). MAOIs are also effective therapy for persons with features of panic disorder, posttraumatic stress disorder, anorexia nervosa, bulimia nervosa, social phobia, and pain syndromes. High dosages of tranylcypromine may be an effective treatment for

TABLE 21-1
COMPARISON OF MONOAMINE OXIDASE A AND B

Type	Location	Preferred Substrates	Selective Inhibitors
A	Central nervous system, sympathetic terminals, liver, gut, skin	Norepinephrine, serotonin, dopamine, tyramine, octopamine, tryptamine	Clorgyline
B	Central nervous system, liver, platelets	Dopamine, tyramine, tryptamine, phenylethylamine, benzylamine, N-methylhistamine	Selegiline[a] (Eldepryl)

[a] Selectivity lost at higher doses (≥10 mg/day).
From Arano GW, Hymar SE. *Handbook of Psychiatric Drug Therapy*, ed 3. Little. Brown, Boston, 1995, with permission.

persons who are refractory to the effects of other antidepressant drugs. The introduction of the selective serotonin reuptake inhibitors (SSRIs) and other antidepressants, such as bupropion (Wellbutrin), mirtazapine (Remeron), nefazodone (Serzone), and venlafaxine (Effexor), has decreased use of MAOIs for all of these psychiatric indications. The second-line status of MAOIs has less to do with considerations of efficacy than with concerns for safety.

PRECAUTIONS AND ADVERSE REACTIONS

The most frequent adverse effects of MAOIs are orthostatic hypotension, insomnia, weight gain, edema, and sexual dysfunction. The initial appearance of signs of orthostatic hypotension in the course of a cautious upward tapering of the dosage determines the maximum tolerable dosage. Treatment for orthostatic hypotension includes avoidance of caffeine, intake of 2 L of fluid per day, addition of dietary salt or adjustment of antihypertensive drugs (if applicable), support stockings, and in severe cases, treatment with fludrocortisone (Florinef), a mineralocorticoid, 0.1 to 0.2 mg a day. Orthostatic hypotension associated with tranylcypromine use can usually be relieved by dividing the daily dosage.

A rare adverse effect of MAOIs, most commonly of tranylcypromine, is a spontaneous, non-tyramine-induced hypertensive crisis occurring shortly after the first exposure to the drug. Persons experiencing such a crisis should avoid MAOIs altogether. Insomnia and behavioral activation can be treated by dividing the dose, not giving the medication after dinner, and using trazodone (Desyrel) or a benzodiazepine hypnotic if necessary. Weight gain, edema, and sexual dysfunction often do not respond to any treatment and may warrant switching to another agent. When switching from one MAOI to another, the clinician should taper and stop use of the first drug for 10 to 14 days before beginning use of the second drug.

Paresthesias, myoclonus, and muscle pains are occasionally seen in persons treated with MAOIs. Paresthesias may be secondary to MAOI-induced pyridoxine deficiency, which may respond to supplementation with pyridoxine, 50 to 150 mg orally each day. Occasionally, persons complain of feeling drunk or confused, perhaps indicating that the dosage should be reduced and then increased gradually. Reports that the hydrazine MAOIs are associated with hepatotoxic effects are relatively uncommon. MAOIs are less cardiotoxic and less epileptogenic than are the tricyclic and tetracyclic drugs.

The most common adverse effects of the RIMA moclobemide are dizziness, nausea, and insomnia or sleep disturbance. RIMAs cause fewer GI adverse effects than do SSRIs. Moclobemide does not have adverse anticholinergic or cardiovascular effects, and it has not been reported to interfere with sexual function.

MAOIs should be used with caution by persons with renal disease, cardiovascular disease, or hyperthyroidism. MAOIs may alter the dosage of a hypoglycemic agent required by diabetic persons. MAOIs have been particularly associated with induction of mania in persons in the depressed phase of bipolar I disorder and triggering of a psychotic decompensation in persons with schizophrenia. MAOIs are contraindicated during pregnancy, although data on their teratogenic risk are minimal. MAOIs should not be taken by nursing women because the drugs can pass into the breast milk.

TABLE 21–2
TYRAMINE-RICH FOODS TO BE AVOIDED IN PLANNING MAOI DIETS

High tyramine content[a] (≥2 mg of tyramine a serving)
    Cheese: English Stilton; blue cheese; white (3 years old); extra old; old cheddar; Danish blue; mozzarella; cheese snack spreads
    Fish, cured meats, sausage; pates and organs: Salami; mortadella; air-dried sausage
    Alcoholic beverages[b]: Liqueurs and concentrated after-dinner drinks
    Marmite (concentrated yeast extract)
    Sauerkraut (Krakus)
Moderate tyramine content[a] (0.5–1.99 mg of tyramine a serving)
    Cheese: Swiss Gruyere; muenster; feta; parmesan; gorgonzola; blue cheese dressing; Black Diamond
    Fish, cured meats, sausage, pâtés, and organs: Chicken liver (5 days old); bologna; aged sausage; smoked meat; salmon mousse
    Alcoholic beverages: Beer and ale (12 oz per bottle)—Amstel, Export Draft, Blue Light, Guiness Extra Stout, Old Vienna, Canadian, Miller Light, Export, Heineken, Blue Wines (per 4 oz glass)—Rioja (red wine)
Low tyramine content[a] (0.01 to >0.49 mg of tyramine a serving)
    Cheese: Brie, Camembert, Cambozola with or without rind
    Fish, cured meat, sausage, organs, and pâtés: Pickled herring; smoked fish; kielbasa sausage; chicken livers, liverwurst (<2 days old)
    Alcoholic beverages: red wines; sherry; scotch[c]
    Others: Banana or avocado (ripe or not); banana peel

[a] Any food left out to age or spoil can spontaneously develop tyramine through fermentation.
[b] Alcohol can produce profound orthostasis interacting with MAOIs, but cannot produce direct hypertensive reactions.
[c] White wines, gin, and vodka have no tyramine content.
Table by Jonathan M. Himmelhoch, M.D.

Tyramine-Induced Hypertensive Crisis

Foods rich in tyramine (Table 21–2) or other sympathomimetic amines should be avoided by persons who are taking irreversible MAOIs, to avoid significant risk of potentially life-threatening hypertension. Persons should be warned about the dangers of ingesting tyramine-rich foods while taking MAOIs, and they should be advised to continue the dietary restrictions for 2 weeks after they stop MAOI treatment, to allow the body to resynthesize the enzyme. Patients should also be warned that bee stings may cause a hypertensive crisis. The prodromal signs and symptoms of a hypertensive crisis may include headache, stiff neck, sweating, nausea, and vomiting. If these signs and symptoms occur, a person should seek immediate medical treatment. An MAOI-induced hypertensive crisis should be treated with α-adrenergic antagonists—for example, phentolamine (Regitine) or chlorpromazine (Thorazine)—which lower blood pressure within 5 minutes. A diuretic to reduce fluid load and a β-adrenergic receptor antagonist to control tachycardia may also be necessary. Acute lowering of blood pressure with use of nifedipine (Procardia) is not recommended, because a person who mistakes a headache resulting from the rebound of MAOI-induced orthostatic hypotension for a hypertensive crisis–related headache and therefore takes nifedipine runs a high risk of causing signs and symptoms of hypotensive shock. MAOIs should not be used by persons with thyrotoxicosis or pheochromocytoma. The risk of tyramine-induced hypertensive crises is relatively low for persons who are taking RIMAs, such as moclobemide and befloxatone. A reasonable dietary recommendation for persons taking RIMAs is not to eat tyramine-containing foods for a period from 1 hour before to 2 hours after taking a RIMA.

Withdrawal

Persons taking regular doses of MAOIs who cease administration abruptly may experience a self-limited discontinuation syndrome consisting of arousal, mood disturbances, and somatic symptoms. To avoid these symptoms when discontinuing use of an MAOI, dosages should be gradually tapered over several weeks.

Overdose

In general, intoxication caused by MAOIs is characterized by agitation that progresses to coma with hyperthermia, hypertension, tachypnea, tachycardia, dilated pupils, and hyperactive deep tendon reflexes. Involuntary movements may be present, particularly in the face and the jaw. There is often an asymptomatic period of 1 to 6 hours after the ingestion of the drugs before the occurrence of the symptoms of toxicity. Acidification of the urine markedly hastens the excretion of MAOIs, and dialysis can be of some use. Phentolamine or chlorpromazine may be useful if hypertension is a problem. Moclobemide alone in overdosage causes relatively mild and reversible symptoms.

The toxicity of all MAOIs is potentially increased in multidrug overdosages, especially if the overdosage includes serotonergic agents.

DRUG INTERACTIONS

The inhibition of MAO can cause severe and even fatal interactions with various other drugs (Table 21–3). In particular, because MAOIs serve to increase intrasynaptic concentrations of biogenic amine neurotransmitters, they should never be administered simultaneously with drugs with a similar effect on these neurotransmit-

TABLE 21–3
DRUGS TO BE AVOIDED DURING MAOI TREATMENT (Partial Listing)

Never use
  Antiasthmatics
  Antihypertensives (methyldopa, guanethidine, reserpine)
  Buspirone
  Levodopa
  Opioids (especially meperidine, dextromethorphan, propoxyphene, tramadol; morphine or codeine
    may be less dangerous)
  Cold, allergy, or sinus medications containing dextromethorphan or sympathomimetics
  SSRIs, clomipramine, venlafaxine, sibutramine
  Sympathomimetics (amphetamines, cocaine, methylphenidate, dopamine, metaraminol,
    epinephrine, norepinephrine, isoproterenol, ephedrine, pseudoephedrine, phenylpropanolamine)
  L-Tryptophan
Use carefully
  Anticholinergics (propanolol)
  Antihistamines
  Disulfiram
  Bromocriptine
  Hydralazine
  Sedative-hypnotics
  Terpin hydrate with codeine
  Tricyclics and tetracyclics (avoid clomipramine)

ters. This includes most antidepressants as well as precursor agents. Persons should be instructed to tell any other physicians or dentists who are treating them that they are taking an MAOI. MAOIs may potentiate the action of central nervous system depressants, including alcohol and barbiturates. MAOIs should not be coadministered with serotonergic drugs, such as SSRIs and clomipramine (Anafranil), because this combination can trigger a serotonin syndrome. The initial symptoms of a serotonin syndrome can include tremor, hypertonicity, myoclonus, and autonomic signs, which can then progress to hallucinosis, hyperthermia, and even death. Fatal reactions have occurred when MAOIs were combined with meperidine (Demerol) or fentanyl (Sublimaze).

When switching from an irreversible MAOI to any other type of antidepressant drug, persons should wait at least 14 days after the last dose of the MAOI before beginning use of the next drug, to allow replenishment of the body's MAOs. When switching from an antidepressant to an irreversible MAOI, persons should wait 10 to 14 days (or 5 weeks for fluoxetine [Prozac]) before starting use of the MAOI, to avoid drug-drug interactions. In contrast, MAO activity recovers completely 24 to 48 hours after the last dose of a RIMA.

Cimetidine (Tagamet) and fluoxetine significantly reduce the elimination of moclobemide. Modest doses of fluoxetine and moclobemide administered concurrently may be well tolerated, with no significant pharmacodynamic or pharmacokinetic interactions.

LABORATORY INTERFERENCES

The MAOIs are associated with lowering of blood glucose concentrations, which are accurately reflected by laboratory analysis. MAOIs artificially raise urinary metanephrine concentrations and may cause a false-positive test result for pheochromocytoma or neuroblastoma. MAOIs have been reported to be associated with a minimal false elevation in thyroid function test results.

DOSAGE AND CLINICAL GUIDELINES

Table 21–4 lists MAOI preparations and typical dosages. There is no definitive rationale for choosing one of the currently available irreversible MAOIs over another, although some clinicians recommend tranylcypromine because of its activating qualities, possibly associated with a fast onset of action, and its low hepatotoxic

TABLE 21–4
AVAILABLE PREPARATIONS AND TYPICAL DOSAGES OF MAOIs

Generic Name	Trade Name	Preparations	Usual Daily Dose (mg)	Usual Maximum Daily Dose (mg)
Isocarboxazid[a]	Marplan	10-mg tablets	20–40	60
Moclobemide[b]	Manerix	100, 150-mg tablets	300–600	600
Phenelzine	Nardil	15-mg tablets	30–60	90
Selegiline	Eldepryl, Atapryl	5-mg capsules, 5-mg tablets	10	30
Tranylcypromine	Parnate	10-mg tablets	20–60	60

[a] Available directly from the manufacturer.
[b] Not available in the United States.

potential. Phenelzine use should begin with a test dose of 15 mg on the first day. The dosage can be increased to 15 mg three times daily during the first week and increased by 15 mg a day each week thereafter until the dosage of 90 mg a day, in divided doses, is reached by the end of the fourth week. Tranylcypromine and isocarboxazid use should begin with a test dosage of 10 mg and may be increased to 10 mg three times daily by the end of the first week. Many clinicians and researchers have recommended upper limits of 50 mg a day for isocarboxazid and 40 mg a day for tranylcypromine. Administration of tranylcypromine in multiple small daily doses may reduce its hypotensive effects. If an MAOI trial is not successful after 6 weeks, lithium (Eskalith) or liothyronine (Cytomel) augmentation is warranted.

Hepatic transaminase serum concentrations should be monitored periodically because of the potential of hepatotoxicity, especially with phenelzine and isocarboxazid. Elderly persons may be more sensitive to MAOI adverse effects than are younger adults. MAO activity increases with age, so that MAOI dosages for elderly persons are the same as those required for younger adults. The use of MAOIs for children has had minimal study.

Moclobemide use is initiated at 300 to 450 mg a day, divided three times per day, and it may be increased to a maximum of 600 mg a day after several weeks. Dietary restrictions consist of avoidance of only large quantities of tyramine-containing foods, and the administration of moclobemide after, rather than before, tyramine-containing meals. RIMAs may be used in combination with other antidepressants with somewhat less concern for hypertensive crises, but still with caution.

For a more detailed discussion of this topic, see Kennedy SH, McKenna KF, Baker GB: Monoamine Oxidase Inhibitors, Sec 31.20, p 2397, in CTP/VII.

22

Naltrexone

The oral opioid receptor antagonists naltrexone (ReVia) and nalmefene (Revex) are effective treatments for opioid and alcohol dependence when used in combination with structured cognitive-behavioral therapy. Opioid receptor antagonists appear to reduce or eliminate the subjective "high" associated with consumption of opioids or alcohol, thus interrupting their reinforcing effects. Opioid receptor antagonists also reduce or eliminate the craving associated with withdrawal from chronic opioid or alcohol abuse.

Of these two opioid receptor antagonists, at present only oral naltrexone is Food and Drug Administration (FDA)-approved for treatment of alcohol dependence and for blockade of the effects of exogenously administered opioids. Currently, the only commercially available formulation of nalmefene is for intravenous administration, but at least one manufacturer has an oral formulation of nalmefene in clinical trials. Oral nalmefene was effective for treatment of alcohol dependence in small clinical pilot trials, and larger trials are in progress. Naloxone (Narcan), another opioid receptor antagonist, is not discussed in detail because it is available only for intravenous use.

CHEMISTRY

The molecular structure of naltrexone is shown in Figure 22–1.

PHARMACOLOGICAL ACTIONS

Oral opioid receptor antagonists are rapidly absorbed from the gastrointestinal (GI) tract, but because of first-pass hepatic metabolism, only 60 percent of a dose of naltrexone and 40 to 50 percent of a dose of nalmefene reach the systemic circulation unchanged. Peak concentrations of naltrexone and its active metabolite, 6-β-naltrexol, are achieved within 1 hour of ingestion. The half-life of naltrexone is 1 to 3 hours, and the half-life of 6-β-naltrexol is 13 hours. Peak concentrations of nalmefene are achieved in about 1 to 2 hours, and the half-life is 8 to 10 hours. Clinically, a single dose of naltrexone effectively blocks the rewarding effects of opioids for 72 hours. Traces of 6-β-naltrexol may linger for up to 125 hours after a single dose.

Naltrexone and nalmefene are competitive antagonists of opioid receptors. Understanding the pharmacology of opioid receptors can explain the difference in adverse effects caused by naltrexone and nalmefene. Opioid receptors in the body are typed pharmacologically as either μ, κ, or δ. Activation of the κ- and δ-receptors is thought to reinforce opioid and alcohol consumption centrally, whereas activation of μ-receptors is more closely associated with central and peripheral antiemetic effects. Because naltrexone is a relatively weak antagonist of κ- and δ-receptors and a po-

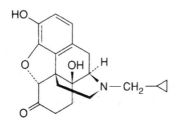

Figure. 22–1. Molecular structure of naltrexone.

tent μ-receptor antagonist, dosages of naltrexone that effectively reduce opioid and alcohol consumption also strongly block μ-receptors and therefore may cause nausea. Nalmefene, in contrast, is an equally potent antagonist of all three opioid receptor types, and dosages of nalmefene that effectively reduce opioid and alcohol consumption have no particularly increased effect on μ-receptors. Thus, nalmefene is associated clinically with few GI adverse effects.

Whereas the effects of opioid receptor antagonists on opioid use are easily understood in terms of competitive inhibition of opioid receptors, the effects of opioid receptor antagonists on alcohol dependence are less straightforward and probably relate to the fact that the desire for and effects of alcohol consumption appear to be regulated by several neurotransmitter systems, both opioid and nonopioid.

THERAPEUTIC INDICATIONS

Opioid receptor antagonists can increase the efficacy of cognitive-behavioral therapy–based opioid and alcohol abstinence programs. The combination of a cognitive-behavioral program plus use of opioid receptor antagonists is more successful than either the cognitive-behavioral program or use of opioid receptor antagonists alone.

Opioid Dependence

Patients in detoxification programs are usually weaned from potent opioid agonists such as heroin over a period of days to weeks, during which emergent adrenergic withdrawal effects are treated as needed with clonidine (Catapres). A serial protocol is sometimes used in which potent agonists are gradually replaced by weaker agonists, followed by mixed agonist-antagonists, then finally by pure antagonists. For example, an abuser of the potent agonist heroin would switch first to the weaker agonist methadone (Dolophine), then to the partial agonist buprenorphine (Buprenex) or levomethadyl acetate (ORLAAM)—commonly called LAAM—and finally, following a 7- to 10-day washout period, to a pure antagonist, such as naltrexone or nalmefene. However, even with gradual detoxification, some persons continue to experience mild adverse effects or opioid withdrawal symptoms for the first several weeks of treatment with naltrexone.

As the opioid receptor agonist potency diminishes, so do the adverse consequences of discontinuing the drug. Thus, because there are no pharmacological barriers to discontinuation of pure opioid receptor antagonists, the social environment and frequent cognitive-behavioral intervention become extremely important factors supporting continued opioid abstinence. Because of poorly tolerated adverse symptoms, most persons not simultaneously enrolled in a cognitive-behavioral program stop taking opioid receptor antagonists within 3 months. Compliance with administration of an opioid receptor antagonist regimen can also be increased with participation in a well-conceived voucher program.

Issues of medication compliance should be a central focus of treatment. If a person with a history of opioid addiction stops taking a pure opioid receptor antagonist, the person's risk of relapse into opioid abuse is exceedingly high, because reintroduction of a potent opioid agonist would yield a very rewarding subjective "high." In contrast, compliant persons do not develop tolerance to the therapeutic benefits of naltrexone, even if it is administered continuously for 1 year or longer. Individuals may undergo several relapses and remissions before achieving long-term abstinence.

Persons taking opioid receptor antagonists should also be warned that sufficiently high dosages of opioid agonists can overcome the receptor antagonism of naltrexone or nalmefene, which may lead to hazardous and unpredictable levels of receptor activation (see PRECAUTIONS AND ADVERSE REACTIONS).

Rapid Detoxification.   To avoid the 7- to 10-day period of opioid abstinence generally recommended prior to use of opioid receptor antagonists, rapid detoxification protocols have been developed. Continuous administration of adjunct clonidine—to reduce the adrenergic withdrawal symptoms—and adjunct benzodiazepines, such as oxazepam (Serax)—to reduce muscle spasms and insomnia—can permit use of oral opioid receptor antagonists on the first day of opioid cessation. Detoxification can thus be completed within 48 to 72 hours, at which point opioid receptor antagonist maintenance is initiated. Moderately severe withdrawal symptoms may be experienced on the first day, but they tail off rapidly thereafter.

Because of the potential hypotensive effects of clonidine, the blood pressure of persons undergoing rapid detoxification must be closely monitored for the first 8 hours. Outpatient rapid detoxification settings must therefore be adequately prepared to administer emergency care.

The main advantage of rapid detoxification is that the transition from opioid abuse to maintenance treatment occurs over just 2 or 3 days. The completion of detoxification in as little time as possible minimizes the risk that the person will relapse into opioid abuse during the detoxification protocol.

Ultrarapid Detoxification.   In a variant technique called "ultrarapid" opioid detoxification, the body is cleared of opioid agonist activity over a period of only a few hours by infusion of naloxone. In this controversial approach, the severe withdrawal symptoms that are triggered by the sudden naloxone-mediated reversal of opioid agonist activity are mitigated with clonidine and benzodiazepines, while the person is partially or fully anesthetized. Naltrexone or nalmefene maintenance is then initiated before the anesthesia is reversed.

Aside from the potential for morbidity and mortality associated with administration of general anesthesia, the main pitfall of ultrarapid detoxification is its high rate of relapse, most likely because naloxone-mediated opioid withdrawal does nothing to eliminate the disabling psychological need for opioids, and psychosocial support is not necessarily an integral part of the technique. Extreme caution is further warranted because the dosages of the required combination of drugs frequently affect the cardiovascular and respiratory systems adversely.

An estimated 10,000 persons worldwide have undergone anesthetized ultrarapid opioid detoxification since its introduction in the 1980s. Practitioners have been disappointed by the very high rate of relapse into opioid abuse soon after the technique is completed. Moreover, at least 10 deaths have been associated with administration of this technique. Because the known risks of the technique appear to outweigh the potential benefits, ultrarapid detoxification cannot be recommended at present.

Alcohol Dependence

Opioid receptor antagonists are also used as adjuncts to cognitive-behavioral programs for treatment of alcohol dependence. Opioid receptor antagonists reduce alcohol craving and alcohol consumption, and they ameliorate the severity of relapses. The risk of relapse into heavy consumption of alcohol attributable to an effective cognitive-behavioral program alone may be halved with concomitant use of opioid receptor antagonists.

The newer agent nalmefene has a number of potential pharmacological and clinical advantages over its predecessor naltrexone for treatment of alcohol dependence. Whereas naltrexone may cause reversible transaminase elevations in persons who take dosages of 300 mg a day (which is 6 times the recommended dosage for treatment of alcohol and opioid dependence [50 mg a day]), nalmefene has not been associated with any hepatotoxicity. Clinically effective dosages of naltrexone are discontinued by 10 to 15 percent of persons due to adverse effects, most commonly nausea. In contrast, discontinuation of nalmefene because of an adverse event is rare at the clinically effective dosage of 20 mg a day and in the range of 10 percent at excessive dosages, that is, 80 mg a day. Because of its pharmacokinetic profile, a given dosage of nalmefene may also produce a more sustained opioid antagonist effect than does naltrexone.

The efficacy of opioid receptor antagonists in reducing alcohol craving may be augmented with a selective serotonin reuptake inhibitor, although data from large trials will be needed to assess this potential synergistic effect more fully.

PRECAUTIONS AND ADVERSE REACTIONS

Because opioid receptor antagonists are used to maintain a drug-free state after opioid detoxification, great care must be taken to ensure that an adequate washout period elapses after the last dose of opioids before the first dose of an opioid receptor antagonist is taken: at least 5 days for a short-acting opioid such as heroin, and at least 10 days for longer-acting opioids such as methadone. The opioid-free state should be determined by self-report and urine toxicology screens. If any question persists of whether opioids are in the body despite a negative urine screen result, then a naloxone challenge test should be performed. Naloxone challenge is used because its opioid antagonism lasts less than 1 hour, whereas those of naltrexone and nalmefene may persist for more than 24 hours. Thus any withdrawal effects elicited by naloxone will be relatively short-lived (see DOSAGE AND CLINICAL GUIDELINES, below). Symptoms of acute opioid withdrawal include drug craving, feeling of temperature change, musculoskeletal pain, and GI distress. Signs of opioid withdrawal include confusion, drowsiness, vomiting, and diarrhea. Naltrexone and nalmefene should not taken be if naloxone infusion causes any signs of opioid withdrawal, except as part of a supervised rapid detoxification protocol.

A set of adverse effects, resembling a vestigial withdrawal syndrome, tends to affect up to 10 percent of persons who take opioid receptor antagonists. Up to 15 percent of persons taking naltrexone may experience abdominal pain, cramps, nausea, and vomiting, which may be limited by transiently halving the dosage or altering the time of administration. Adverse central nervous system effects of naltrexone, experienced by up to 10 percent of persons, include headache, low energy, insomnia, anxiety, and nervousness. Joint and muscle pains may occur in up to 10 percent of persons taking naltrexone, as may rash.

Naltrexone may cause dosage-related hepatic toxicity at dosages well in excess of 50 mg a day: 20 percent of persons taking 300 mg a day of naltrexone may experience serum aminotransferase concentrations 3 to 19 times the upper limit of normal. The hepatocellular injury of naltrexone appears to be a dose-related toxic effect rather than an idiosyncratic reaction. At the lowest dosages of naltrexone required for effective opioid antagonism, hepatocellular injury is not typically observed. However, naltrexone dosages as low as 50 mg a day may be hepatotoxic in persons with underlying liver disease, such as persons with cirrhosis of the liver due to chronic alcohol abuse. Serum aminotransferase concentrations should be monitored monthly for the first 6 months of naltrexone therapy and thereafter on the basis of clinical suspicion. Hepatic enzyme concentrations usually return to normal after discontinuation of naltrexone therapy.

If analgesia is required while a dose of an opioid receptor antagonist is pharmacologically active, opioid agonists should be avoided in favor of benzodiazepines or other nonopioid analgesics. Persons taking opioid receptor antagonists should be instructed that low dosages of opioids will have no effects, but larger dosages could overcome the receptor blockade and suddenly produce symptoms of profound opioid overdosage, with sedation possibly progressing to coma or death. Use of opioid receptor antagonists is contraindicated in persons who are taking opioid agonists, small amounts of which may be present in over-the-counter antiemetic and antitussive preparations; in persons with acute hepatitis or hepatic failure; and also in persons who are hypersensitive to the drugs.

Because naltrexone is transported across the placenta, opioid receptor antagonists should only be taken by pregnant women if a compelling need outweighs the potential risks to the fetus. It is not known whether opioid receptor antagonists are distributed into maternal milk.

Opioid receptor antagonists are relatively safe drugs, and ingestion of high doses of opioid receptor antagonists should be treated with supportive measures combined with efforts to decrease GI absorption.

DRUG INTERACTIONS

Many drug interactions involving opioid receptor antagonists have been discussed above, including those with opioid agonists associated with drug abuse, as well as those involving antiemetics and antitussives. Because of its extensive hepatic metabolism, naltrexone may affect or be affected by other drugs that influence hepatic enzyme levels. However, the clinical importance of these potential interactions is not known.

One potentially hepatotoxic drug that has been used in some cases with opioid receptor antagonists is disulfiram (Antabuse). Although no adverse effects were observed, frequent laboratory monitoring is indicated when such combination therapy is contemplated. Opioid receptor antagonists have been reported to potentiate the sedation associated with use of thioridazine (Mellaril), an interaction that probably applies equally to all low-potency dopamine receptor antagonists.

LABORATORY INTERFERENCES

No laboratory interferences have been described for opioid receptor antagonists, although relatively nonspecific immune-based toxicology screens for opioids could potentially yield positive results in persons taking only opioid receptor antagonists, because of their structural similarities to other opioids.

DOSAGE AND CLINICAL GUIDELINES

To avoid the possibility of precipitating an acute opioid withdrawal syndrome, several steps should be taken to ensure that the person is opioid free. Within a supervised detoxification setting, at least 5 days should elapse following the last dose of short-acting opioids, such as heroin, hydromorphone (Dilaudid), meperidine (Demerol), or morphine, and at least 10 days should elapse after the last dose of longer-acting opioids, such as methadone, before opioid antagonists are initiated. Briefer periods off opioids have been used in rapid detoxification protocols. To confirm that opioid detoxification is complete, urine toxicological screens should demonstrate no opioid metabolites. However, an individual may have a negative urine opioid screen result yet still be physically dependent on opioids and thus susceptible to antagonist-induced withdrawal effects. Therefore, once the urine screen result is negative, a naloxone challenge test is recommended, unless an adequate period of opioid abstinence can be reliably confirmed by observers (Table 22-1).

The initial dosage of naltrexone for treatment of opioid or alcohol dependence is 50 mg a day, which should be achieved through gradual introduction, even when the naloxone challenge test result is negative. Various authorities begin with 5, 10, 12.5, or 25 mg and titrate up to the 50-mg dosage over a period ranging from 1 hour to 2 weeks, while constantly monitoring for evidence of opioid withdrawal. Once a daily dose of 50 mg is well tolerated, it may be averaged over a week by giving 100 mg on alternate days or 150 mg every third day. Such schedules may increase compliance. The corresponding therapeutic dosage of nalmefene is 20 mg a day, divided into two equal doses. Gradual titration of nalmefene to this daily dose is probably a wise strategy, although clinical data on dosage strategies for nalmefene are not yet available.

To maximize compliance, it is recommended that ingestion of each dose be directly observed either in a facility or by family members and that random urine tests for opioid receptor antagonists and their metabolites as well as for ethanol or opioid metabolites be taken. Opioid receptor antagonists should be continued until the person is no longer considered psychologically at risk for relapse into opioid or alcohol

TABLE 22–1
NALOXONE (NARCAN) CHALLENGE TEST

The naloxone challenge test should not be performed in a patient showing clinical signs or symptoms of opioid withdrawal or in a patient whose urine contains opioids. The naloxone challenge test may be administered by either the intravenous or subcutaneous route.

Intravenous challenge: Following appropriate screening of the patient, 0.8 mg of naloxone should be drawn into a sterile syringe. If the intravenous route of administration is selected, 0.2 mg of naloxone should be injected, and while the needle is still in the patient's vein, the patient should be observed for 30 seconds for evidence of withdrawal signs or symptoms. If there is no evidence of withdrawal, the remaining 0.6 mg of naloxone should be injected, and the patient observed for an additional 20 minutes for signs and symptoms of withdrawal.

Subcutaneous challenge: If the subcutaneous route is selected, 0.8 mg should be administered subcutaneously, and the patient observed for signs and symptoms of withdrawal for 20 minutes.

Conditions and technique for observation of patient: During the appropriate period of observation, the patient's vital signs should be monitored, and the patient should be monitored for signs of withdrawal. It is also important to question the patient carefully. The signs and symptoms of opioid withdrawal include, but are not limited to the following:
  Withdrawal signs: stuffiness or running nose, tearing, yawning, sweating, tremor, vomiting, or piloerection
  Withdrawal symptoms: feeling of temperature change, joint or bone and muscle pain, abdominal cramps, and formication (feeling of bugs crawling under skin)

Interpretation of the challenge: Warning—the elicitation of the enumerated signs or symptoms indicates a potential risk for the subject, and naltrexone should not be administered. If no signs or symptoms of withdrawal are observed, elicited, or reported, naltrexone may be administered. If there is any doubt in the observer's mind that the patient is not in an opioid-free state or is in continuing withdrawal, naltrexone should be withheld for 24 hours and the challenge repeated.

abuse. This generally requires at least 6 months but may take longer, particularly if there are external stresses.

Rapid Detoxification

Rapid detoxification has been standardized using naltrexone, although nalmefene would be expected to be equally effective with fewer adverse effects. In rapid detoxification protocols, the addicted person stops opioid use abruptly and begins the first opioid-free day by taking clonidine 0.2 mg orally every 2 hours for nine doses, to a maximum dose of 1.8 mg, during which time blood pressure is monitored every 30 to 60 minutes for the first 8 hours. Naltrexone 12.5 mg is administered 1 to 3 hours after the first dose of clonidine. To reduce muscle cramps and later insomnia, a short-acting benzodiazepine, such as oxazepam 30 to 60 mg, is administered simultaneously with the first dose of clonidine, and half of the initial dose is readministered every 4 to 6 hours as needed. The maximum daily dosage of oxazepam should not exceed 180 mg. The person undergoing rapid detoxification should be accompanied home by a reliable escort. On the second day, similar doses of clonidine and the benzodiazepine are administered, but with a single dose of naltrexone 25 mg taken in the morning. Relatively asymptomatic persons may return home after 3 to 4 hours. Administration of the daily maintenance dose of naltrexone 50 mg is begun on the third day, and the dosages of clonidine and the benzodiazepine are gradually tapered off over 5 to 10 days.

For a more detailed discussion of this topic, see O'Malley SS, Krishnan-Sarin S, Rounsaville BJ: Naltrexone, Sec 31.21, p 2407, in CTP/VII.

23

Nefazodone

Nefazodone (Serzone) has antidepressant and antianxiety effects comparable to those of selective serotonin reuptake inhibitors (SSRIs), yet unlike SSRIs, nefazodone improves sleep continuity and has little effect on sexual functioning. Nefazodone is generally well tolerated. It is chemically related to trazodone (Desyrel) but causes much less sedation.

CHEMISTRY

Nefazodone is structurally related to trazodone and unrelated to the classical tricyclic and tetracyclic drugs, the monoamine oxidase inhibitors (MAOIs), SSRIs, and other currently available antidepressant drugs. Its molecular structure is shown in Figure 23–1.

PHARMACOLOGICAL ACTIONS

Nefazodone is rapidly and completely absorbed but is then extensively metabolized, so that the bioavailability of active compounds is about 20 percent of the oral dose. Its half-life is 2 to 4 hours. Steady-state concentrations of nefazodone and its principal active metabolite, hydroxynefazodone, are achieved within 4 to 5 days. Metabolism of nefazodone in the elderly, especially women, is about half that seen in younger persons, so that lowered doses are recommended for elderly persons. An important metabolite of nefazodone is methchlorophenylpiperazine (mCPP), which has some serotonergic effects and may cause migraine, anxiety, and weight loss.

Nefazodone is an inhibitor of serotonin uptake and, more weakly, of norepinephrine reuptake. Its antagonism of serotonin 5-HT_{2A} receptors is thought to lessen anxiety and depression. By both inhibiting serotonin reuptake, which raises synaptic serotonin concentrations, and blocking 5-HT_{2A} receptors, nefazodone may selectively activate 5-HT_{1A} receptors, which gives additional antidepressant and anxiolytic effects. Nefazodone is a mild antagonist of the α_1-adrenergic receptors, which predisposes some persons to orthostatic hypotension but is not sufficiently potent to produce priapism. There is no significant direct activity at α_2- and β-adrenergic, 5-HT_{1A}, cholinergic, opioid, dopaminergic, or benzodiazepine receptors.

THERAPEUTIC INDICATIONS

Nefazodone is effective for the treatment of major depression. The usual effective dose is 300 to 600 mg a day. In direct comparison with SSRIs, nefazodone is less likely to cause inhibition of orgasm or decreased sexual desire. Nefazodone is

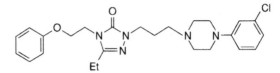

Figure. 23–1. Molecular structure of nefazodone.

also effective for treatment of panic disorder and panic with comorbid depression or depressive symptoms, of generalized anxiety disorder, and of premenstrual dysphoric disorder and for management of chronic pain. It is not effective for the treatment of obsessive-compulsive disorder. Nefazodone increases rapid eye movement (REM) sleep and increases sleep continuity. Nefazodone is also of use in patients with posttraumatic stress disorder and chronic fatigue syndrome. It may also be effective in patients who have been treatment-resistant to other antidepressant drugs.

PRECAUTIONS AND ADVERSE REACTIONS

The most common reasons for discontinuing nefazodone use are nausea, dizziness, insomnia, weakness, and agitation. Other adverse reactions reported with nefazodone are listed in Table 23–1.

Cardiovascular Effects

Some patients taking nefazodone may experience a drop in blood pressure that can cause episodes of postural hypotension. Nefazodone should therefore be used with caution by persons with underlying cardiac conditions, history of stroke or heart attack, dehydration, or hypovolemia or by persons being treated with antihypertensive medications.

TABLE 23–1
**ADVERSE REACTIONS REPORTED
WITH NEFAZODONE
(300–600 mg a day)**

Reaction	%
Headache	36
Dry mouth	25
Somnolence	25
Nausea	22
Dizziness	17
Constipation	14
Insomnia	11
Weakness	11
Lightheadedness	10
Blurred vision	9
Dyspepsia	9
Infection	8
Confusion	7
Scotomata	7

Activation of Mania

Of persons with known bipolar disorder, 1.6 percent of those treated with nefazodone experienced mania, compared with 5.1 percent of tricyclic-treated persons. The activation of mania in persons with unipolar depression was no higher with nefazodone than with placebo. Nonetheless, nefazodone, like other antidepressant medications, should be used with caution in persons with a history of manic episodes.

Other Precautions

The effects of nefazodone in human mothers are not yet as well understood as those of the SSRIs. Nefazodone should therefore be used during pregnancy only if the potential benefit to the mother outweighs the potential risks to the fetus. It is not known whether nefazodone is excreted in human breast milk. Therefore, it should be used with caution by lactating mothers. The nefazodone dosage should be lowered in persons with severe hepatic disease, but no adjustment is necessary for persons with renal disease.

DRUG INTERACTIONS AND LABORATORY INTERFERENCES

Nefazodone should not be given concomitantly with MAOIs. In addition, nefazodone has particular drug-drug interactions with the triazolobenzodiazepines triazolam (Halcion) and alprazolam (Xanax) due to the inhibition of cytochrome P450 3A4 by nefazodone. Potentially elevated levels of each of these drugs can develop after administration of nefazodone, whereas the levels of nefazodone are generally not affected. The manufacturer recommends lowering the dose of triazolam by 75 percent and the dose of alprazolam by 50 percent when given concomitantly with nefazodone.

Nefazodone may slow the metabolism of digoxin; therefore, digoxin levels should be monitored carefully in persons taking both medications. Nefazodone also slows the metabolism of haloperidol (Haldol), so that the dosage of haloperidol should be reduced in persons taking both medications. Addition of nefazodone may also exacerbate the adverse effects of lithium (Eskalith).

There are no known laboratory interferences associated with nefazodone.

DOSAGE AND CLINICAL GUIDELINES

Nefazodone is available in 50-, 200-, and 250-mg unscored tablets and 100- and 150-mg scored tablets. The recommended starting dosage of nefazodone is 100 mg twice a day, but 50 mg twice a day may be better tolerated, especially by elderly persons. To limit the development of adverse effects, the dosage should be slowly tapered up in increments of 100 to 200 mg a day at intervals of no less than 1 week per increase. The optimal dosage is 300 to 600 mg daily in two divided doses. However, some studies report that nefazodone is effective when taken once a day, especially at bedtime. Geriatric persons should receive dosages about two-thirds of the usual nongeriatric dosages, with a maximum of 400 mg a day. In common with other antidepressants, clinical benefit of nefazodone usually appears after 2 to 4 weeks of treatment. Patients with premenstrual syndrome are treated with a flexible dosage that averages about 250 mg a day.

For a more detailed discussion of this topic, see Garlow SJ, Owens MJ, Nemeroff CB: Nefazodone, Sec 31.22, p 2412, in CTP/VII.

24

Opioid Receptor Agonists: Methadone, Levomethadyl, and Buprenorphine

Opioid receptor agonists are used in psychiatry for detoxification from heroin and other opioids and in maintenance opioid detoxification programs. Maintenance therapy is used in addicted patients who are unable to remain abstinent from opioids. Persons who switch from use of heroin to one of these drugs continue to satisfy their acute physical craving for opioids but are gradually weaned from their crippling psychological dependence on heroin. The drugs in this class include methadone (Dolophine), buprenorphine (Buprenex), and levomethadyl acetate (ORLAAM), also called L-α-acetylmethadol or LAAM. The most clinical experience is available for methadone; levomethadyl and buprenorphine are relatively new and are still being evaluated in various clinical and research settings.

CHEMISTRY

The structural formulas of the synthetic opioid receptor agonists methadone, levomethadyl, and buprenorphine are shown in Figure 24–1.

PHARMACOLOGICAL ACTIONS

Methadone, levomethadyl, and buprenorphine are absorbed rapidly from the gastrointestinal (GI) tract. Hepatic first-pass metabolism significantly affects the bioavailability of each of the drugs but in markedly different ways. For methadone, hepatic enzymes reduce the bioavailability of an oral dosage by about half, an effect that is easily managed with dosage adjustments.

For levomethadyl, hepatic enzymes metabolize an oral dosage into normethyl-LAAM and dinormethyl-LAAM, which are actually several times more potent as μ-opioid receptor agonists than is levomethadyl itself.

For buprenorphine, in contrast, first-pass intestinal and hepatic metabolism eliminates oral bioavailability almost completely. For use in opioid detoxification, therefore, buprenorphine is given sublingually, in either a liquid or a tablet formulation.

The peak plasma concentrations of oral methadone are reached within 2 to 6 hours, and the plasma half-life initially is 4 to 6 hours in opioid-naive persons and 24 to 36 hours after steady dosing of any type of opioid. Methadone is highly protein bound and equilibrates widely throughout the body, which ensures little post-dosage variation in steady-state plasma concentrations.

The peak plasma concentrations of oral levomethadyl are reached within 1.5 to 2 hours, and the plasma half-lives of levomethadyl and its active metabolites range from 2 to 4 days.

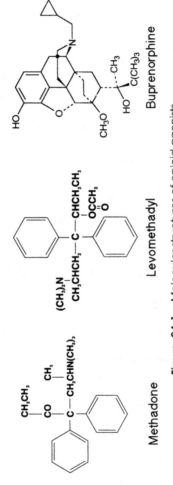

Figure. 24-1. Molecular structures of opioid agonists.

Elimination of a sublingual dosage of buprenorphine occurs in two phases, an initial phase with a half-life of 3 to 5 hours and a terminal phase with a half-life of more than 24 hours. Buprenorphine dissociates from its receptor binding site slowly, which permits an every-other-day dosing schedule.

Methadone, levomethadyl, and the active metabolites of levomethadyl act as pure agonists at μ-opioid receptors and have negligible agonist or antagonist activity at κ- or δ-opioid receptors. Buprenorphine is a partial agonist at μ-receptors, a potent antagonist at κ- receptors, and neither an agonist nor an antagonist at δ-receptors.

THERAPEUTIC INDICATIONS

Methadone

Methadone is used for short-term detoxification (7 to 30 days), long-term detoxification (up to 180 days) and maintenance (treatment beyond 180 days) of opioid-dependent individuals. For these purposes, it is only available through designated clinics called methadone maintenance treatment programs (MMTPs) and in hospitals and prisons. Methadone is a schedule II drug, which means that its administration is tightly governed by specific federal laws and regulations.

Enrollment in a methadone program reduces the risk of death by 70 percent; reduces illicit use of opioids and other substances of abuse; reduces criminal activity; reduces the risk of infectious diseases of all types, most importantly human immunodeficiency virus (HIV) and hepatitis B and C infection; and, in pregnant women, reduces the risk of fetal and neonatal morbidity and mortality. The use of methadone maintenance frequently requires lifelong treatment.

Some opioid-dependence treatment programs use a stepwise detoxification protocol in which a person addicted to heroin switches first to the strong agonist methadone, then to the weaker agonist buprenorphine, and finally to maintenance on an opioid receptor antagonist, such as naltrexone (ReVia). This approach minimizes the appearance of opioid withdrawal effects, which, if they occur, are mitigated with clonidine (Catapres). However, compliance with opioid receptor antagonist treatment is poor outside of settings using intensive cognitive-behavioral techniques. In contrast, noncompliance with methadone maintenance precipitates opioid withdrawal symptoms, which serve to reinforce use of methadone and make cognitive-behavioral therapy less than essential. Thus, some well-motivated, socially integrated former heroin addicts are able to use methadone for years without participation in a psychosocial support program.

Data pooled from many reports indicate that methadone is more effective when taken at dosages in excess of 60 mg a day. The analgesic effects of methadone are sometimes used in the management of chronic pain when less addictive agents are ineffective.

Pregnancy.   Methadone maintenance, combined with effective psychosocial services and regular obstetrical monitoring, significantly improves obstetrical and neonatal outcomes for women addicted to heroin. Enrollment of a heroin-addicted pregnant woman in such a maintenance program reduces the risk of malnutrition, infection, preterm labor, spontaneous abortion, preeclampsia, eclampsia, abruptio placenta, and septic thrombophlebitis.

The dosage of methadone during pregnancy should be the lowest effective dosage, and no withdrawal to abstinence should be attempted during pregnancy. Methadone is metabolized more rapidly in the third trimester, which may necessitate higher dosages. To avoid potentially sedating postdose peak plasma concentrations, the daily dose can be administered in two divided doses during the third trimester. Methadone treatment has no known teratogenic effects.

Neonatal Methadone Withdrawal Symptoms.   Withdrawal symptoms in newborns frequently include tremor, high-pitched cry, increased muscle tone and activity, poor sleep and eating, mottling, yawning, perspiration, and skin excoriation. Convulsions that require aggressive anticonvulsant therapy may also occur. Withdrawal symptoms may be delayed in onset and prolonged in neonates because of their immature hepatic metabolism. Women taking methadone are sometimes counseled to initiate breast-feeding as a means of gently weaning their infants from methadone dependence, but they should not breast-feed their babies while still taking methadone.

Levomethadyl

Levomethadyl is used only for maintenance treatment of opioid-dependent patients. It is not used for detoxification treatment or for analgesia. Thrice-weekly levomethadyl dosing, consisting of 100 mg on Monday, 100 mg on Wednesday, and 140 mg on Friday, is more effective for opioid maintenance than are smaller doses. Daily dosing of levomethadyl may cause overdosage.

Buprenorphine

Buprenorphine is an analgesic approved only for treatment of moderate-to-severe pain. Buprenorphine at a dosage of 8 to 16 mg a day appears to reduce heroin use. Buprenorphine also is effective in thrice-weekly dosing because of its slow dissociation from opioid receptors. The analgesic effects of buprenorphine are sometimes used in the management of chronic pain when less addictive agents are ineffective. There are some reports of depressed patients responding to buprenorphine when other agents have failed.

PRECAUTIONS AND ADVERSE REACTIONS

The most common adverse effects of opioid receptor agonists are lightheadedness, dizziness, sedation, nausea, constipation, vomiting, perspiration, weight gain, decreased libido, inhibition of orgasm, and insomnia or sleep irregularities. Opioid receptor agonists are capable of inducing tolerance as well as producing physiological and psychological dependence. Other central nervous systems (CNS) adverse effects include dizziness, depression, sedation, euphoria, dysphoria, agitation, and seizures. Delirium and insomnia have also been reported in rare cases. Occasional non-CNS adverse effects include peripheral edema, urinary retention, rash, arthralgia, dry mouth, anorexia, biliary tract spasm, bradycardia, hypotension, hypoventilation, syncope, antidiuretic hormone–like activity, pruritus, urticaria, and visual disturbances. Menstrual irregularities are common in women, especially in the first 6 months of use. Various abnormal endocrine laboratory indexes of little clinical significance may also be seen.

Most persons develop tolerance to the pharmacological adverse effects of opioid agonists during long-term maintenance, and relatively few adverse effects are experienced after the induction period.

Overdosage

The acute effects of opioid receptor agonist overdosage include sedation, hypotension, bradycardia, hypothermia, respiratory suppression, miosis, and decreased GI motility. Severe effects include coma, cardiac arrest, shock, and death. The risk of overdosage is greatest in the induction stage of treatment and in persons with slow drug metabolism due to preexisting hepatic insufficiency. Deaths have been caused during the first week of induction by methadone dosages of only 50 to 60 mg a day.

Because the therapeutic effects of levomethadyl may not appear in the first few days of treatment, addicted persons sometimes continue to administer doses of illicit opioids during this time and may experience symptoms of overdosage. Also, because of the long half-lives of levomethadyl and its active metabolites, daily dosing of levomethadyl causes excessive drug accumulation and is to be avoided in favor of thrice-weekly dosing.

The risk of overdosage with buprenorphine appears to be lower than that with methadone or levomethadyl. However, deaths have been caused by use of buprenorphine in combination with benzodiazepines.

Withdrawal Symptoms

Abrupt cessation of methadone use triggers withdrawal symptoms within 3 to 4 days, which usually reach peak intensity on the sixth day. Withdrawal symptoms include weakness, anxiety, anorexia, insomnia, gastric distress, headache, sweating, and hot and cold flashes. The withdrawal symptoms usually resolve after 2 weeks. However, a protracted methadone abstinence syndrome is possible that may include restlessness and insomnia.

The withdrawal symptoms associated with levomethadyl and buprenorphine are similar to, but less marked than, those due to methadone. In particular, buprenorphine is sometimes used to ease the transition from methadone to opioid receptor antagonists or abstinence, because of the relatively mild withdrawal reaction associated with discontinuation of buprenorphine.

DRUG-DRUG INTERACTIONS

Opioid receptor agonists can potentiate the CNS-depressant effects of alcohol, barbiturates, benzodiazepines, other opioids, low-potency dopamine receptor antagonists, tricyclic and tetracyclic drugs, and monoamine oxidase inhibitors (MAOIs). Carbamazepine (Tegretol), phenytoin (Dilantin), barbiturates, rifampin (Rimactane, Rifadin), and heavy long-term consumption of alcohol may induce hepatic enzymes, which may lower the plasma concentration of methadone or buprenorphine and thereby precipitate withdrawal symptoms. In contrast, however, hepatic enzyme induction may raise the plasma concentration of active levomethadyl metabolites and cause toxicity.

Acute opioid withdrawal symptoms may be precipitated in persons on methadone maintenance therapy who take pure opioid receptor antagonists such as naltrexone, nalmefene (Revex), and naloxone (Narcan); partial agonists such as buprenorphine; or mixed agonist-antagonists such as pentazocine (Talwin). These symptoms may be mitigated by use of clonidine, a benzodiazepine, or both.

Competitive inhibition of methadone or buprenorphine metabolism following short-term use of alcohol or administration of cimetidine (Tagamet), erythromycin, ketoconazole (Nizoral), fluoxetine (Prozac), fluvoxamine (Luvox) loratadine (Claritin), quinidine (Quinidex), and alprazolam (Xanax) may lead to higher plasma concentrations or prolonged duration of action of methadone or buprenorphine. Inhibition of levomethadyl metabolism by the same agents, however, may lead to lower plasma concentrations, delayed onset of action, or prolonged duration of action. Medications that alkalinize the urine may reduce methadone excretion.

Methadone maintenance may also increase plasma concentrations of desipramine (Norpramin, Pertofrane) and fluvoxamine. Use of methadone may increase zidovudine (Retrovir) concentrations, which increases the possibility of zidovudine toxicity at otherwise standard dosages. In vitro human liver microsome studies moreover demonstrate competitive inhibition of methadone demethylation by several protease inhibitors including ritonavir (Norvir), indinavir (Crixivan), and saquinavir (Invirase). The clinical relevance of this finding is unknown.

Fatal drug-drug interactions with the MAOIs are associated with use of the opioids fentanyl (Sublimaze) and meperidine (Demerol) but not with use of methadone, levomethadyl, or buprenorphine.

LABORATORY INTERFERENCES

Methadone, levomethadyl, and buprenorphine can be tested for separately in urine toxicology to distinguish them from other opioids. No known laboratory interferences are associated with use of methadone, levomethadyl, or buprenorphine.

DOSAGE AND CLINICAL GUIDELINES

Methadone

Methadone is supplied in 5-, 10-, and 40-mg dispersible scored tablets; 40-mg scored wafers; 5 mg/5 mL, 10 mg/5 mL, and 10 mg/mL solutions; and a 10-mg/mL parenteral form. In maintenance programs, methadone is usually dissolved in water or juice, and dose administration is directly observed to ensure compliance. For induction of opioid detoxification, an initial methadone dose of 15 to 20 mg will usually suppress craving and withdrawal symptoms. However, some individuals may require up to 40 mg a day in single or divided doses. Higher dosages should be avoided during induction of treatment to reduce the risk of acute overdosage.

Over several weeks, the dosage should be raised to at least 70 mg a day. The maximum dosage is usually 120 mg a day, and higher dosages require prior approval from regulatory agencies. Dosages above 60 mg a day are associated with much more complete abstinence from use of illicit opioids than are dosages below 60 mg a day.

The duration of treatment should not be predetermined but should be based on response to treatment and assessment of psychosocial factors. All studies of methadone maintenance programs endorse long-term treatment (i.e., several years) as more effective than short-term programs (i.e., less than 1 year) for prevention of relapse into opioid abuse. In actual practice, however, a minority of programs are permitted by policy or approved by insurers to provide even 6 months of continuous maintenance treatment. Moreover, some programs actually encourage withdrawal from methadone in less than 6 months after induction. This is quite ill conceived, because over 80 percent of persons who terminate methadone maintenance treatment eventually return to illicit drug use within 2 years. In those programs that offer both maintenance and withdrawal treatments, the overwhelming majority of participants enroll in the maintenance treatment.

Levomethadyl

Levomethadyl is supplied as a 10-mg/mL oral solution and is usually administered thrice weekly. Because of the tendency of levomethadyl to accumulate to toxic concentrations if taken daily, it should not be taken more frequently than every other day. The initial dose in persons not known to have tolerance to opioids is 20 or 40 mg. Each subsequent dose may be increased by 5 or 10 mg, and steady state for a given dosage is achieved in no less than 2 weeks. For persons already dependent on methadone, the starting dosage of levomethadyl acetate should be 1.2 to 1.3 times the dosage of methadone being replaced but not more than 120 mg. It is unnecessary to taper or overlap dosages during the crossover from methadone to levomethadyl, which can be accomplished over 2 consecutive days. Subsequent dosages of levomethadyl should be adjusted according to clinical response.

Most persons require levomethadyl doses of 60 to 90 mg, thrice weekly. The clinical dose range is 10 to 140 mg thrice weekly. The maximum recommended weekly dose is 440 mg.

Buprenorphine

Buprenorphine is supplied as a 0.3-mg/mL solution in 1-mL ampules, for use as an analgesic. Sublingual preparations of buprenorphine appropriate for use in opioid maintenance programs are not currently available in the United States. Sublingual tablet formulations of buprenorphine containing buprenorphine only or buprenorphine combined with naloxone in a 4:1 ratio are used outside of the United States for opioid maintenance treatment. Buprenorphine is not used for short-term opioid detoxification. Maintenance dosages of 8 to 16 mg thrice weekly have effectively reduced heroin use in clinical trials.

For a more detailed discussion of this topic, see Schottenfeld RS, Kleber HD: Dopamine Opioid Agonists, Sec 31.23, p 2419, in CTP/VII.

25

Orlistat

Orlistat (Xenical) is used to promote weight loss in combination with a supervised program of dietary restrictions and exercise.

CHEMISTRY

The molecular structure of orlistat is shown in Figure 25–1.

PHARMACOLOGICAL ACTIONS

Orlistat acts as a highly selective reversible inhibitor of intestinal lipase, thus preventing the breakdown of lipids and so reducing fat absorption and caloric intake. When used as recommended, orlistat inhibits dietary fat absorption by about 30 percent.

Orlistat remains in the gastrointestinal (GI) tract and is not absorbed. A single dose remains active for about 2 hours. The recommended thrice-daily dosing should be scheduled to coincide with meals.

THERAPEUTIC INDICATIONS

Orlistat is indicated for use as part of a supervised weight loss and maintenance program that includes dietary restrictions. Obesity is defined in terms of body-mass index (BMI), which is calculated by dividing weight (in kilograms) by height (in meters) squared. Orlistat is indicated for use by persons with a BMI ≥ 30 or a BMI ≥ 27 in the presence of the atherosclerosis risk factors hypertension, diabetes mellitus, or hypercholesterolemia. Orlistat is effective only while it is being taken, provided that dietary guidelines are strictly followed. When used correctly, persons lose 5 to 10 percent of their initial body weight.

PRECAUTIONS AND ADVERSE EFFECTS

GI adverse effects occur in persons taking orlistat at rates as much as 12 times those in persons taking placebo. The most common GI effects observed are oily spotting, flatus with discharge, fecal urgency, increased defecation, and fecal incontinence. Between 10 and 25 percent of persons using orlistat have one or more of these side effects; however, the incidence of these effects is reduced by 80 percent by the end of the second year of continuous use. A diet, or even one meal, high in fats increases the incidence of GI adverse effects.

Orlistat reduces the systemic absorption of the fat-soluble vitamins A, D, E, and K and of beta carotene by as much as 60 percent. The manufacturer recommends

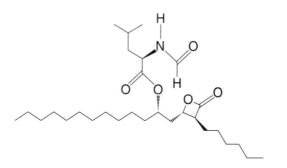

Figure. 25-1.   Molecular structure of orlistat.

supplementation with a multivitamin that contains fat-soluble vitamins at least 2 hours before or after the dosage of orlistat. Orlistat is contraindicated for use by persons with chronic malabsorption or cholestasis.

Systemic absorption of orlistat is minimal. It is not known whether orlistat is secreted into breast milk. Nevertheless, orlistat should not be taken by pregnant or nursing women.

DRUG INTERACTIONS

Theoretically, orlistat may affect the systemic absorption and therapeutic efficacy of certain lipophilic drugs such as cyclosporine (Sandimmune) or drugs such as warfarin (Coumadin) that antagonize the actions of fat-soluble vitamins.

LABORATORY INTERFERENCES

Orlistat has not been reported to interfere with any laboratory tests.

DOSAGE AND CLINICAL GUIDELINES

Pretreatment evaluation for use of orlistat should include a review of the cardiovascular system and risk factors for atherosclerosis and a complete drug history. Physical examination should include a series of at least three separate determinations of blood pressure and pulse and should focus on signs of atherosclerosis. Documentation should include evidence that the patient is obese.

Orlistat is available as a 120-mg capsule. The recommended dosage is one capsule with each of the three daily meals. The drug can be taken during or up to 1 hour after meals. Higher dosages are not associated with additional weight loss but may increase the incidence of adverse effects.

For a more detailed discussion of this topic, see Brownell KD, Wadden TA: Obesity, Sec 25.3, p 1787, in CTP/VII.

26

Other Anticonvulsants: Gabapentin, Lamotrigine, and Topiramate

Initially developed as anticonvulsant drugs, gabapentin (Neurontin), lamotrigine (Lamictal), and topiramate (Topamax) are used in psychiatry to treat bipolar disorder, anxiety disorders, agitation, pain disorders, and substance abuse. These drugs have been especially useful in the treatment of persons with bipolar disorders, since up to 50 percent of patients do not respond satisfactorily to or do not tolerate lithium (Eskalith, Lithobid), valproic acid (Depakene), or carbamazepine (Tegretol). Features that predict poor response to lithium include rapid cycling, mixed dysphoric state, and comorbid substance abuse.

CHEMISTRY

Gabapentin is chemically related to γ-aminobutyric acid (GABA) and is structurally similar to L-leucine. Lamotrigine and topiramate are each novel three-ringed compounds. Their structural formulas are shown in Figure 26–1.

PHARMACOLOGICAL ACTIONS

Gabapentin

Gabapentin is absorbed by the neutral amino acid membrane transporter system in the gut, and it crosses the blood–brain barrier. Bioavailability of 300- or 600-mg doses is 60 percent, whereas bioavailability of a 1600-mg dose is 35 percent. Because higher amounts are not absorbed, doses should not exceed 1800 mg per single dose or 5400 mg a day. Food has no effect on gabapentin absorption, and it does not bind to plasma proteins. The steady-state half-life of 5 to 9 hours is reached in 2 days if thrice-daily dosing is used. Gabapentin is not metabolized and is excreted unchanged in the urine.

Lamotrigine

Lamotrigine is completely absorbed, and its steady-state plasma half-life is 25 hours. However, the rate of lamotrigine's metabolism varies over a sixfold range, depending on which other drugs are administered concomitantly (see *Drug Interactions* below). Dosing is escalated slowly to twice-a-day maintenance dosing. Food does not affect its absorption, and it is 55 percent protein bound in the plasma; 94 percent of lamotrigine and its inactive metabolites is excreted in the urine. Lamotrigine has an anticonvulsant profile similar to that of carbamazepine and phenytoin (Dilantin).

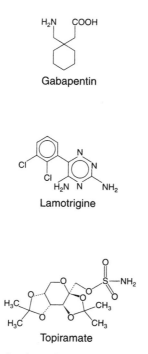

Gabapentin

Lamotrigine

Topiramate

Figure. 26-1. Molecular structure of other anticonvulsants used in psychiatry.

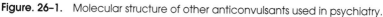

Lamotrigine inhibits dihydrofolate reductase, the enzyme responsible for generation of folic acid, which is necessary for proper fetal development. Lamotrigine modestly increases plasma serotonin concentrations and is a weak inhibitor of serotonin 5-HT$_3$ receptors.

Topiramate

Topiramate is rapidly and completely absorbed, and its steady-state half-life is 21 hours. Food does not affect its absorption. It is 15 percent protein bound in the plasma, and 70 percent of an oral dose of topiramate is excreted unchanged in the urine, together with small amounts of several inactive metabolites. Topiramate is an inhibitor of state-dependent sodium channels. It potentiates the action of GABA at a non-benzodiazepine-, non-barbiturate-sensitive GABA$_A$ receptor.

THERAPEUTIC INDICATIONS

Gabapentin, lamotrigine, and topiramate are indicated by the Food and Drug Administration (FDA) as adjuncts in the treatment of partial seizures. Gabapentin is also widely used to treat chronic pain, particularly that of polyneuropathy. In 1999, over two thirds of prescriptions for these drugs were for the nonepileptic indications listed below.

Bipolar Disorder

Each of these drugs has been used as adjunctive medication for treatment-refractory persons with bipolar disorders, including bipolar I, bipolar II, cyclothymic disorder, and bipolar disorder not otherwise specified. They appear to have both mood-stabilizing and antidepressant effects. Generally, these drugs have been added when persons have not responded satisfactorily to first-line agents, such as lithium, valproic acid, or carbamazepine. Some clinicians have used these drugs successfully as monotherapy. There are many positive case reports of lamotrigine use for patients with depressive episodes of bipolar I disorder.

Chronic Pain

Gabapentin is effective for treatment of postherpetic neuralgia and painful diabetic neuropathy, and lamotrigine has been shown to be effective for treatment of human immunodeficiency virus (HIV)-associated peripheral neuropathy and reduction of postoperative analgesic use. Other conditions responsive to gabapentin and lamotrigine include trigeminal neuralgia; central pain syndromes; compression neuropathies, such as carpal tunnel syndrome, radiculopathies, and meralgia paresthetica; and painful neuropathies due to other causes. The pain-reduction response is similar to that with selective serotonin reuptake inhibitors and tricyclic antidepressants and superior to that with intravenous and topical lidocaine (Xylocaine), carbamazepine, topical aspirin, mexiletine (Mexitil), phenytoin, topical capsaicin (Double Cap Cream), oral nonsteroidal anti-inflammatory drugs (NSAIDs), opioids, propranolol (Inderal), lorazepam (Ativan), and phentolamine (Regitine). Because of their distinct mechanisms of action and absence of interactions, gabapentin and antidepressants are often used in combination for treatment of neuropathic pain.

Other Indications

Gabapentin appears to reduce the frequency and intensity of explosive outbursts in persons with dyscontrol disorders, including children, persons with dementia, and persons with traumatic brain injury. It is also an effective treatment for social phobia and panic disorder in some persons. Because of its mildly sedating properties, gabapentin can treat insomnia and agitation due to withdrawal from benzodiazepines, alcohol, and cocaine. Gabapentin is also an effective treatment for tremor and parkinsonism.

Lamotrigine has antipsychotic effects in persons with epilepsy. This is important for persons comorbid for epilepsy and psychosis, because many antipsychotic medications lower the seizure threshold. Lamotrigine may reduce intrusive and avoidance or numbing symptoms of posttraumatic stress disorder.

Topiramate can markedly reduce appetite and is being used as a treatment for obesity and binge eating.

PRECAUTIONS AND ADVERSE REACTIONS

Gabapentin

Gabapentin is well tolerated, and the dosage can be escalated to the maintenance range within 2 to 3 days. There are almost no dose-related adverse effects, even at doses of 5 grams per day, which far exceeds the absorptive capacity of the intestines. The most frequent adverse effects of gabapentin used with other antiepileptic drugs are somnolence, dizziness, ataxia, fatigue, and nystagmus, which are usually transient.

Lamotrigine

The most common adverse effects associated with use of lamotrigine in combination with other antiepileptic drugs for treatment of epilepsy are dizziness, ataxia, somnolence, headache, diplopia, blurred vision, nausea, vomiting, and rash. Lamotrigine accumulates in melanin-rich tissues including the pigmented retina. The long-term effect on vision is unknown.

Skin Conditions. Lamotrigine is significantly associated with development of potentially life-threatening skin conditions, such as toxic epidermal necrolysis and Stevens-Johnson syndrome, in 0.1 percent of adults and 1 to 2 percent of children. These are more likely to appear if the starting dosage is too high, if the dosage is escalated too rapidly, or during concomitant administration of valproic acid. Most cases appear after 2 to 8 weeks of therapy, but cases have been reported in the absence of any of the above risk factors. The character of the rash is not a clue to the severity of the condition. Thus, lamotrigine use should be discontinued immediately upon development of any rash or other sign of hypersensitivity reaction. This may not prevent subsequent development of life-threatening rash or permanent disfiguration.

Topiramate

The most common non-dose-related adverse effects of topiramate used in combination with other antiepileptic drugs include psychomotor slowing; speech and language problems, especially word-finding difficulties; somnolence; dizziness; ataxia; nystagmus; and paresthesias. The most common dose-related adverse effects are fatigue, nervousness, poor concentration, confusion, depression, anorexia, anxiety, mood problems, weight loss, and tremor. Some 1.5 percent of persons taking topiramate develop renal calculi, a rate ten times that associated with placebo. Patients at risk for calculi should be encouraged to drink plenty of fluids.

DRUG INTERACTIONS

Gabapentin

Gabapentin has no significant hepatic cytochrome P450 or pharmacodynamic interactions. Antacids containing aluminum hydroxide and magnesium hydroxide

(Maalox) decrease gabapentin absorption by 20 percent if administered concurrently but negligibly if administered 2 hours prior to the dose of gabapentin.

Lamotrigine

Lamotrigine has significant, well-characterized drug interactions involving other anticonvulsants. Lamotrigine decreases the plasma concentration of valproic acid by 25 percent; may increase the concentration of the epoxide metabolite of carbamazepine; and may increase the incidence of carbamazepine-induced dizziness, diplopia, ataxia, and blurred vision. It has no effect on phenytoin concentrations. Lamotrigine concentrations are decreased 40 to 50 percent with concomitant administration of carbamazepine, phenytoin, or phenobarbital, whereas lamotrigine concentration is at least doubled with concurrent administration of valproic acid. Sertraline (Zoloft) also increases plasma lamotrigine concentrations, but to a lesser extent than does valproic acid. Combinations of lamotrigine and other anticonvulsants have complex effects on the time of peak plasma concentration and the plasma half-life of lamotrigine.

Topiramate

Topiramate has a few well-characterized drug interactions with other anticonvulsant drugs. Topiramate may increase phenytoin concentrations up to 25 percent and valproic acid concentrations 11 percent; it does not affect the concentrations of carbamazepine or its epoxide, phenobarbital (Luminal), or primidone. Topiramate concentrations are decreased by 40 to 48 percent with concomitant administration of carbamazepine or phenytoin and by 14 percent with concurrent administration of valproic acid. Topiramate also slightly decreases digoxin (Lanoxin) bioavailability and the efficacy of estrogenic oral contraceptives. Addition of topiramate, a weak inhibitor of carbonic anhydrase, to other inhibitors of carbonic anhydrase, such as acetazolamide (Diamox) or dichlorphenamide (Daranide), may promote development of renal calculi and is to be avoided.

LABORATORY INTERFERENCES

Gabapentin can cause false-positive readings with the Ames N-Multistix SG dipstick test for urinary protein. Lamotrigine and topiramate do not interfere with any laboratory tests.

DOSAGE AND CLINICAL GUIDELINES

Gabapentin

Gabapentin is available as 100-, 300-, and 400-mg capsules and as 600- and 800-mg tablets. The starting dose of gabapentin is 300 mg three times a day, and the dose can be rapidly titrated up to a maximum of 1800 mg three times a day over a period of a few days. Efficacy is broadly dose dependent, and most people achieve satis-

TABLE 26–1
LAMOTRIGINE DOSING (mg/day)

Treatment	Weeks 1–2	Weeks 3–4	Weeks 4–5
Lamotrigine monotherapy	25	50	100–200 (500 maximum)
Lamotrigine plus carbamazepine	50	100	200–500 (700 maximum)
Lamotrigine plus valproate	25 every other day	25	50–200 (200 maximum)

factory benefit within the range of 600 to 900 mg three times a day. Rapid advancement of the dosage and high doses are limited by sedation, which is usually mild. Although abrupt discontinuation of gabapentin does not cause withdrawal effects, use of all anticonvulsant drugs should be gradually tapered.

Lamotrigine

Lamotrigine is available as unscored 25-, 100-, 150-, and 200-mg tablets. The major determinant of lamotrigine dosing is minimization of the risk of rash. Lamotrigine should not be taken by anyone under the age of 16 years. Because valproic acid markedly slows the elimination of lamotrigine, concomitant administration of these two drugs necessitates a much slower titration (Table 26–1). People with renal insufficiency should aim for a lower maintenance dosage. Appearance of any type of rash necessitates immediate discontinuation of lamotrigine administration. Lamotrigine should usually be discontinued gradually, over 2 weeks, unless a rash emerges, in which case it should be discontinued over 1 to 2 days.

Topiramate

Topiramate is available as unscored 25-, 100-, and 200-mg tablets. To reduce the risk of adverse cognitive and sedating effects, topiramate dosage is titrated gradually over 8 weeks to a maximum of 200 mg twice a day. Higher doses are not associated with increased efficacy. Persons with renal insufficiency should reduce doses by half.

For a more detailed discussion of this topic, see Sussman N: Other Anticonvulsants, Sec 31.7c, p 2299, in CTP/VII.

27

Reboxetine

Reboxetine (Vestra) is an effective antidepressant of a novel pharmacological class that selectively inhibits norepinephrine reuptake but has little effect on serotonin reuptake. It is thus the pharmacodynamic mirror image of the selective serotonin reuptake inhibitors (SSRIs), which inhibit the reuptake of serotonin but not of norepinephrine.

CHEMISTRY

Reboxetine is structurally related to fluoxetine (Prozac). The structural formula of reboxetine is shown in Figure 27–1.

Pharmacological Actions

Reboxetine is rapidly absorbed and reaches peak plasma concentrations in 2 hours. Food does not affect the rate of absorption. The half-life is 13 hours, which permits twice-daily dosing. Steady-state concentrations are achieved in 5 days. Reboxetine is extensively metabolized in the liver (primarily via the cytochrome P450 3A4 isoenzyme) and mostly excreted in the urine.

Reboxetine selectively inhibits norepinephrine reuptake, with little inhibition of serotonin or dopamine reuptake. It is highly selective for norepinephrine and lacks direct effects on serotonin metabolism. Reboxetine has a low affinity for muscarinic or cholinergic receptors and does not interact with α_1-, α_2-, or β-adrenergic; serotonergic; dopaminergic; or histaminic receptors.

THERAPEUTIC INDICATIONS

Reboxetine is effective for treatment of acute and chronic depressive disorders, such as major depression and dysthymia. Reboxetine is as effective as imipramine (Tofranil) and may be more effective than fluoxetine for treatment of persons with severe depression. Reboxetine promotes sleep but is not associated with daytime somnolence. Patients show improvement in energy, interest, and concentration and a decrease in anxiety.

Reboxetine can also produce relatively rapid improvement in symptoms of social phobia. Social impairments, particularly those revolving around negative self-perception and low level of social activity, appear to respond positively to reboxetine.

PRECAUTIONS AND ADVERSE REACTIONS

Reboxetine is overall as well tolerated as SSRIs. The most common adverse effects are urinary hesitancy, headache, constipation, nasal congestion, perspiration,

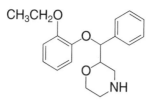

Figure. 27–1. Molecular structure of reboxetine.

dizziness, dry mouth, decreased libido, and insomnia. Urinary hesitancy may respond to augmentation with doxazosin (Cardura). Tremor and cardiovascular adverse effects, which might be anticipated with a drug that influences the adrenergic system, are unusual. Reboxetine is less likely to cause anxiety or nausea or to inhibit sexual functioning than are SSRIs. Limited data suggest that reboxitine, like fluoxetine, may rarely cause the syndrome of inappropriate secretion of antidiuretic hormone (SIADH). In long-term use, persons taking reboxetine experience no more adverse effects than those taking a placebo. Reboxetine at 4 mg twice a day does not produce psychomotor slowing and does not act synergistically with alcohol. Reboxetine is not cardiotoxic and does not increase the risk of seizures.

No data exist on the effects of reboxetine on embryonic and fetal development, and it is not known whether reboxetine is secreted into breast milk. Currently, it should not be taken by women who are pregnant or breast-feeding.

DRUG INTERACTIONS

Reboxetine has few significant drug interactions and does not inhibit hepatic metabolic enzymes. Until further data are available, reboxetine should not be taken concurrently with monoamine oxidase inhibitors (MAOIs).

LABORATORY INTERFERENCE

Reboxetine is not known to interfere with any clinical laboratory tests.

DOSAGE AND CLINICAL GUIDELINES

Reboxetine is available in 4-mg scored tablets. The usual starting dosage is 4 mg twice a day. For most patients an increase in dosage is not necessary. However, if needed, the dosage may be increased to a total of 10 mg a day in two divided doses after 3 weeks. In elderly persons and persons with severe renal impairment therapy may be initiated at 2 mg twice a day and increased to a maximum of 6 mg a day in two divided doses after 3 weeks.

Because reboxetine and SSRIs act on nonoverlapping neurotransmitter systems, some clinicians combine them for treatment of persons whose depression does not respond to either agent alone.

For a more detailed discussion of this topic, see DeBattista C, Schatzberg AF: Other Pharmacological and Biological Therapies, Sec 31.33, p 2521, in CTP/VII.

28

Selective Serotonin Reuptake Inhibitors

Selective serotonin reuptake inhibitors (SSRIs) are first-line agents for treatment of depression, obsessive-compulsive disorder (OCD), and panic disorder, as well as many other disorders. Currently, five SSRIs are available. Fluoxetine (Prozac) was introduced in 1988, and it has since become the single most widely prescribed antidepressant in the world. In the subsequent years, sertraline (Zoloft) and paroxetine (Paxil) have become nearly as widely prescribed as fluoxetine. Fluvoxamine (Luvox) has gained its own smaller niche, particularly for treating OCD. Citalopram (Celexa) has been used in Europe since 1989 and was introduced into the United States in 1998, where it has already gained acceptance.

Clomipramine (Anafranil) is another serotonin-specific drug sometimes considered in the same category as SSRIs. However, because its structure and adverse effect profile are more similar to those of the tricyclic antidepressant drugs, it is discussed with the tricyclic and tetracyclic drugs (see Chapter 35).

CHEMISTRY

The SSRIs share almost no molecular features, which explains why certain individuals may respond to one SSRI but not to another. The structural formulas of citalopram, fluoxetine, fluvoxamine, paroxetine, and sertraline are shown in Figure 28–1.

PHARMACOLOGICAL ACTIONS

Pharmacokinetics

As suggested by their diverse chemical structures, the SSRIs possess significantly different pharmacokinetic profiles (Table 28–1). The major difference is their wide range in steady-state half-lives. Fluoxetine has the longest half-life, 2 to 3 days; its active metabolite has a half-life of 7 to 9 days. The half-life of sertraline is 26 hours, and its less active metabolite has a half-life of 3 to 5 days. The half-lives of the other three, which do not have metabolites with significant pharmacological activity, are 35 hours for citalopram, 21 hours for paroxetine, and 15 hours for fluvoxamine. All SSRIs are well absorbed after oral administration and have their peak effects in the range of 4 to 8 hours.

All SSRIs are metabolized in the liver by the cytochrome P450 (CYP) enzymes. CYP 3A4 N-demethylates sertraline, citalopram, and fluvoxamine. The most clinically significant drug-drug interactions result from inhibition of CYP enzymes, and these drugs may raise serum concentrations of a number of other drugs that are also metabolized by CYP 2D6, such as tricyclic antidepressants and ven-

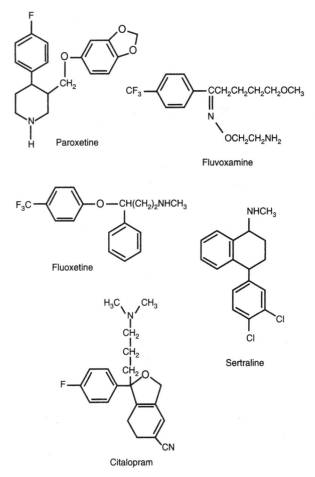

Figure 28-1. Molecular structures of SSRIs.

lafaxine (Effexor). When coadministering drugs that are principally metabolized by the same CYP enzyme, it is clinically prudent to begin with small doses and increase doses slowly and cautiously.

TABLE 28-1
PHARMACOKINETIC PROFILES OF THE SSRIs

Drug	Time to Peak Plasma Concentration	Half-Life	Half-Life Metabolite	Time to Steady State (days)	Plasma-Protein Binding (%)
Fluoxetine	6–8 h	4–6 days	4–16 days	28–35	95
Fluvoxamine	3–8 h	15 h	—	5–7	80
Paroxetine	5–6 h	21 h	—	5–10	95
Sertraline	4.5–8.5 h	26 h	62–104 h	5–7	95
Citalopram	4 h	35 h	3 h	7	80

The administration of the SSRIs with food has little effect on absorption and often reduces the incidence of SSRI-associated nausea and diarrhea.

Pharmacodynamics

The clinical benefits of SSRIs are attributed to the selective inhibition of serotonin reuptake, with little effect on reuptake of norepinephrine or dopamine. Often, adequate clinical activity is achieved at starting dosages, whereas higher dosages increase the risk of adverse effects. The same degree of clinical benefits often can be achieved either through steady use of a low dose or through more rapid dose escalation. However, the clinical response varies considerably from person to person.

Citalopram is the most selective inhibitor of serotonin reuptake, with very little inhibition of norepinephrine or dopamine reuptake and very low affinities for serotonin 5-HT$_{1A}$ or 5-HT$_{2A}$; dopamine D$_1$ or D$_2$; α_1-,α_2-, or β-adrenergic; histamine H$_1$; γ-aminobutyric acid (GABA); muscarinic or nicotinic cholinergic; or benzodiazepine receptors. The other SSRIs have a similar profile, except that fluoxetine weakly inhibits norepinephrine reuptake and binds to 5-HT$_{2C}$ receptors, sertraline weakly inhibits norepinephrine and dopamine reuptake, and paroxetine has significant anticholinergic activity at higher dosages and binds to nitric oxide synthase.

THERAPEUTIC INDICATIONS

Depression

Fluoxetine, sertraline, paroxetine, and citalopram are indicated for treatment of depression. SSRIs are first-line agents for depression in the general population, the elderly, and the medically ill as well as during pregnancy. SSRIs are as effective as any other class of antidepressants for mild and moderate depression. For severe depression and melancholia, several studies have found that the efficacy of serotonin-norepinephrine reuptake inhibitors, such as venlafaxine, mirtazapine, or tricyclic drugs, often exceeds that of SSRIs. However, recent evidence suggests that sertraline is more effective than the other SSRIs for treatment of severe depression with melancholia. It is appropriate to initiate antidepressant therapy with SSRIs for all degrees of depression.

Direct comparison of the benefits of specific SSRIs has not shown any one to be generally superior to the others. However, there can be considerable diversity in response to the various SSRIs within a given individual. Over 50 percent of people who respond poorly to one SSRI will respond favorably to another. Thus before shifting to non-SSRI antidepressants, it is most reasonable to try other agents in the SSRI class for persons who did not respond to the first SSRI.

Studies have shown SSRIs to have a similar efficacy but markedly more favorable adverse effect profile than the tricyclic antidepressants. These studies have also shown that some nervousness or agitation, sleep disturbances, gastrointestinal (GI) symptoms, and sexual side effects are more common in SSRI-treated patients than in tricyclic-treated patients.

Some clinicians have attempted to select a particular SSRI for a specific person on the basis of the drug's unique adverse effect profile. For example, thinking that fluoxetine is a most activating and stimulating SSRI, they may think it a better choice for an abulic person than paroxetine which is presumed to be a sedating SSRI. These differences, however, usually vary from person to person, even if present after the first few weeks of therapy.

Augmentation Strategies. In depressed persons with a partial response to an SSRI, augmentation strategies have generally not proven superior to simply increasing the SSRI dosage. However, one such drug combination, an SSRI plus bupropion (Wellbutrin), has marked added benefits. The noradrenergic and dopaminergic actions of bupropion dovetail nicely with the serotonergic actions of the SSRIs and pose a low risk of pharmacodynamic interactions. The addition of bupropion can elicit an antidepressant response in up to 70 percent of SSRI nonresponders. Bupropion has the additional advantage of tending to counteract the antiorgasmic adverse effects of SSRIs. Similarly, augmentation of SSRI therapy with the selective norepinephrine reuptake inhibitor reboxetine (Vestra) may be more effective than use of either drug alone.

Some evidence indicates that with lithium (Eskalith), levothyroxine (Synthroid), sympathomimetics, pindolol (Visken), or clonazepam (Klonopin) can also augment the antidepressant effects of SSRIs.

Suicide. SSRIs markedly reduce the risk of suicide. In the late 1980s, a widely publicized report suggested an association between fluoxetine use and violent acts, including suicide, but many subsequent reviews have clearly refuted this association. A few patients, however, become especially anxious and agitated when given fluoxetine. The appearance of these symptoms in a suicidal persons could conceivably aggravate the seriousness of the suicidal ideation. In addition, suicidal persons may attempt to act out their suicidal thoughts more effectively as they rise out of their depression. Thus, potentially suicidal persons should be closely monitored during the first few weeks they are taking SSRIs.

Antidepressant drugs are an essential component of the current treatment of suicidally depressed persons. A recent assessment of the use of drugs for treatment of persons with a history of prior suicide attempts concluded that a large majority received inadequate dosages of antidepressants.

Depression during Pregnancy and Postpartum. Many studies, including one that followed children into their early school years, have failed to find any perinatal complications, congenital fetal anomalies, decreases in global intelligence quotient (IQ), language delays, or specific behavioral problems attributable to the use of fluoxetine during pregnancy. Emerging data for sertraline, paroxetine, and fluvoxamine suggest that taking these agents during pregnancy also does not increase the risk of major congenital malformations.

Prospective studies have found that the risk of relapse into depression when a newly pregnant mother is taken off SSRI use is severalfold higher than the risk to the fetus of exposure to SSRIs. Since maternal depression is an independent risk factor for fetal morbidity, the balance of the data clearly indicates that SSRI use should be continued without interruption during pregnancy. SSRIs may produce a self-limited neonatal withdrawal syndrome that begins several hours after birth, may persist for days to a few weeks, and consists of jitteriness and mild tachypnea. The syndrome is rare and does not interfere with feeding.

Postpartum depression (with or without psychotic features) affects a small percentage of mothers. Some clinicians start administering SSRIs if the postpartum blues extend beyond a few weeks or if a woman becomes depressed during pregnancy. The head start afforded by starting SSRI administration during pregnancy if a woman is at risk for postpartum depression also protects the newborn, toward whom the woman may have harmful thoughts after parturition.

Studies using sensitive radioimmune and chromatographic techniques have not detected SSRIs in the plasma of babies breast-feeding from mothers who are taking SSRIs. In one study, however, a breast-fed infant was reported to have a plasma concentration of sertraline equal to one-half of the maternal concentration; however, this infant showed no abnormal behaviors. Further studies are needed.

Depression in the Elderly and Medically Ill.   Behavioral disturbances in the elderly, particularly those with medical illnesses, require a thorough diagnostic evaluation to rule out delirium or dementia. Diagnosis and treatment of depression significantly reduces the risk of excessive physical morbidity, myocardial infarction, prolonged hospitalization, and death.

The ideal antidepressant in this population would have no cognitive, cardiotoxic, anticholinergic, antihistaminergic, or α-adrenergic adverse effects. Of the SSRIs, only paroxetine has some anticholinergic activity, though this is clinically relevant only at higher doses. All SSRIs are useful for elderly, medically frail persons. They are less well tolerated by people with preexisting GI symptoms.

Chronic Depression.   Several studies have shown that nortriptyline (Aventyl, Pamelor) and monthly interpersonal psychotherapy markedly reduced the rate of relapse of depression over a 3-year period. Similar results have been reported with sertraline and would be expected with other SSRIs.

The natural history of major depression consists of waxing and waning of symptoms over periods lasting several months. Many studies indicate that discontinuation of SSRIs only 6 months after a depressive episode is associated with a high rate of relapse. It is therefore prudent for a person with chronic depression to continue taking SSRIs for at least 1 year and preferably longer. SSRIs are well tolerated in long-term use.

Depression in Children.   Children of depressed adults are at increased risk of depression. Case reports and small series have reported that SSRIs reduce childhood depressive symptoms and may prevent efforts by children and adolescents to self-medicate their sadness with alcohol or illicit drugs.

The adverse effect profile of SSRIs in children includes GI symptoms, insomnia, motor restlessness, social disinhibition, and hypomania or mania. It is therefore critical to determine that the child is truly depressed and to begin with small doses of SSRIs. There are anecdotal reports of successful treatment of children with depression together with another disorder (e.g., attention-deficit/hyperactivity disorder [ADHD]) when SSRIs are combined with other psychotropic drugs.

Anxiety Disorders

Obsessive-Compulsive Disorder.   Fluvoxamine, paroxetine, sertraline, and fluoxetine are indicated for treatment of OCD in persons over the age of 18. Fluvoxamine and sertraline have also been approved for treatment of pediatric OCD (ages 6 to 17). About 50 percent of persons with OCD begin to show symptoms in childhood or adolescence, and over half of these respond favorably to medication. Beneficial responses can be dramatic. Long-term data support the model of OCD as a genetically determined, lifelong condition that is best treated continuously with drugs and cognitive-behavioral therapy from the onset of symptoms in childhood throughout the lifespan.

In general, effective SSRI dosages for OCD are higher than those required to treat depression. Fluoxetine is effective for OCD at 20, 40, and 60 mg a day, with a dose-dependent gradation of response. The 60-mg dose is significantly more effective than the 20-mg dose. Response of OCD to sertraline is less clearly dose dependent, with efficacy demonstrated at dosages from 50 to 200 mg a day. Paroxetine is effective at 40 and 60 mg; 20 mg is not better than placebo. Response can be seen in the first few weeks of treatment, but 15 to 20 percent of persons respond only after prolonged treatment.

Comorbid depressive symptoms respond significantly better to SSRIs than to clomipramine, nortriptyline, or amitriptyline (Elavil, Endep). Comorbid tics, as in tic disorders and Tourette's syndrome, respond to the addition of dopamine receptor antagonists or serotonin-dopamine receptor antagonists such as risperidone (Risperdal). In contrast, clozapine (Clozaril) and buspirone (BuSpar) can worsen tics. There appears to be no role for lithium augmentation for OCD treatment. The combination of SSRIs and clomipramine is potentially hazardous because of the potential for cardiotoxicity.

Panic Disorder.   Paroxetine and sertraline are indicated for treatment of panic disorder, with or without agoraphobia. These agents work less rapidly than do the benzodiazepines alprazolam (Xanax) or clonazepam, but they are better tolerated in long-term use and do not cause dependence. Citalopram, fluvoxamine, and fluoxetine also may reduce spontaneous or induced panic attacks. Because fluoxetine can initially heighten anxiety symptoms, persons with panic disorder must begin taking small dosages (5 mg a day) and raise the dosage slowly. SSRIs are far superior to benzodiazepines for treatment of panic disorder with comorbid depression.

SSRIs are effective for childhood panic symptoms. If it is well tolerated, SSRI treatment of childhood panic disorder should be continued at least for 1 year. Additional benefit and maintenance of remission would be expected from continuation well into adulthood.

Social Phobia.   Paroxetine is an effective agent in the treatment of social phobia. Paroxetine reduces both symptoms and disability. This response rate was comparable to that seen with the monoamine oxidase inhibitor (MAOI) phenelzine (Nardil), the previous standard treatment. SSRIs are safer to use than MAOIs or benzodiazepines. All SSRIs are probably effective for social phobia.

Posttraumatic Stress Disorder.   Pharmacotherapy for posttraumatic stress disorder (PTSD) must target specific symptoms in three clusters: reexperiencing, avoidance, and hyperarousal. For long-term treatment, SSRIs appear to have a broader spectrum of therapeutic effects on specific PTSD symptom clusters than do tricyclic antidepressants and MAOIs. Benzodiazepine augmentation is useful in the acute symptomatic state. SSRIs are associated with marked improvement of both intrusive and avoidant symptoms.

Other Anxiety Disorders.   SSRIs may be useful for the treatment of specific phobias, generalized anxiety disorder, and separation anxiety disorder. A thorough, individualized evaluation is the first approach, with particular attention to identifying conditions amenable to drug therapy. In addition cognitive-behavioral or other psychotherapies can be added for greater efficacy.

Bulimia Nervosa and Other Eating Disorders

Fluoxetine is indicated for treatment of bulimia, which is best done in the context of psychotherapy. Doses of 60 mg a day are significantly more effective than 20 mg a day. In several well-controlled studies, fluoxetine 60 mg a day was superior to placebo in reducing binge eating and induced vomiting. Some experts recommend an initial course of cognitive-behavioral therapy alone. If there is no response in 3 to 6 weeks, then fluoxetine administration is added. The appropriate duration of treatment with fluoxetine and psychotherapy has not been determined.

Fluvoxamine was not effective at a statistically significant level in one double-blind, placebo-controlled trial for inpatients with bulimia.

Anorexia Nervosa. Fluoxetine has been used in inpatient treatment of anorexia nervosa to attempt to control comorbid mood disturbances and obsessive-compulsive symptoms. However, at least two careful studies, one of 7 months and one of 24 months, failed to find that fluoxetine affected the overall outcome and the maintenance of weight. Effective treatments for anorexia include cognitive-behavioral, interpersonal, psychodynamic, and family therapies in addition to a trial with SSRIs.

Obesity. Fluoxetine, in combination with a behavioral program, has been shown to be only modestly beneficial for weight loss. A significant percentage of all persons who take SSRIs, including fluoxetine, lose weight initially but later may gain weight. However, all SSRIs may cause initial weight gain.

DEXFENFLURAMINE. The market recall of the serotonin-releasing agent dexfenfluramine (Redux) in September 1997 raised concern about the long-term consequences of SSRI use. Specifically, since both dexfenfluramine and SSRIs increase serotonin activity in some way, would SSRIs cause the same heart-valve defects, primary pulmonary hypertension, and loss of serotonergic fibers caused by dexfenfluramine?

All available evidence indicates that SSRIs do not cause the same adverse consequences caused by dexfenfluramine. Dexfenfluramine causes a massive release of serotonin throughout the body, particularly from nerve terminals, far in excess of that required for neurotransmission. The resulting elevated plasma serotonin concentration is thought to contribute to the cardiac and pulmonary damage. In contrast, SSRIs prolong the activity of serotonin released into the synaptic cleft in the course of normal neurotransmission. SSRIs do not damage serotonergic fibers or raise plasma serotonin concentrations.

Clinically, SSRIs have been taken by tens of millions of people worldwide and have been subjected to intense scrutiny; they have not been associated with an increased risk of heart valve damage or pulmonary hypertension.

Premenstrual Dysphoric Disorder

Premenstrual dysphoric disorder is characterized by debilitating mood and behavioral changes in the week preceding menstruation that interfere with normal functioning. Sertraline, paroxetine, fluoxetine, and fluvoxamine have been reported to reduce the symptoms of premenstrual dysphoric disorder. Controlled trials of fluoxetine and sertraline administered either throughout the cycle or only during the luteal phase (the 2-week period between ovulation and menstruation) showed both schedules to be equally effective.

An additional observation of unclear significance was that fluoxetine was associated with changing the duration of the menstrual period by more than 4 days, either lengthening or shortening. The effects of SSRIs on menstrual cycle length are mostly unknown and may warrant careful monitoring in women of reproductive age.

Premature Ejaculation

The antiorgasmic effects of SSRIs make them useful as a treatment for men with premature ejaculation. SSRIs permit intercourse for a significantly longer period and are reported to improve sexual satisfaction in couples in which the man has premature ejaculation. Fluoxetine and sertraline have been shown to be effective for this purpose.

Paraphilias

SSRIs reduce obsessive-compulsive behavior in people with paraphilias. SSRIs diminish unconventional total sexual outlet and average time per day spent in unconventional sexual fantasies, urges, and activities. Evidence suggests a greater response for sexual obsessions than for paraphilias. The data support the hypothesis that paraphilias and related disorders are on the impulsive rather than the compulsive end of the obsessive-compulsive spectrum.

Attention-Deficit/Hyperactivity Disorder

Sympathomimetic drugs are the first-line agents for ADHD in children, followed by bupropion, then SSRIs. In adults, sympathomimetics and antidepressants are reported to be equally effective.

Autistic Disorder

Obsessive-compulsive behavior, poor social relatedness, and aggression are prominent autistic features that respond to serotonergic agents such as SSRIs and clomipramine. Sertraline and fluvoxamine have been shown in controlled and open-label trials to mitigate aggressiveness, self-injurious behavior, repetitive behaviors, some degree of language delay, and rarely lack of social relatedness in adults with autistic spectrum disorders. These agents were generally well tolerated. In contrast, a controlled trial of fluvoxamine in autistic children found it to be less well tolerated in this group. Fluoxetine has been reported to be effective for features of autism in children, adolescents, and adults.

Chronic Pain Syndromes

Neuropathic Pain. Pain due to nerve damage, typically described as tingling, numb, or burning pain, often responds quite satisfactorily to SSRIs and other antidepressants. In contrast, nonsteroidal anti-inflammatory agents and opioids have little effect on neuropathic pain. The most common causes of neuropathic pain are diabetes, trauma, herpes zoster, and chronic nerve compression.

Fibromyalgia. Pain syndromes in which the complaints of pain and distress appear excessive for the amount of demonstrable tissue injury are highly associated with comorbid affective disorders. SSRIs and older antidepressants have been reported to reduce subjective complaints of chronic pain.

Headache. Tricyclic antidepressants have long been used to reduce the frequency and intensity of both migrainous and nonmigrainous headaches. More recently, studies have shown that SSRIs are equally efficacious, with a more favorable adverse effect profile. In addition, people with chronic or recurrent headaches have a high incidence of comorbid depression and may require antidepressant drug therapy specifically to treat depression.

Concomitant use of SSRIs and drugs in the triptan class (sumatriptan [Imitrex], naratriptan [Amerge], rizatriptan [Maxalt], and zolmitriptan [Zomig]) may rarely result in development of a reversible serotonin syndrome (see Precautions and Adverse Reactions). However, many people use triptans while taking a low dose of an SSRI for headache prophylaxis without adverse reaction.

Psychosomatic Conditions

Mood and the propensity for panic regulate the autonomic nervous system and may trigger paroxysmal somatic events. SSRIs modulate the incidence of psychogenic symptoms. Some patients with chronic fatigue syndrome have benefited from long-term use of SSRIs, particularly fluoxetine.

Syncope. Excessive vagal tone may cause bradycardia, hypotension, and syncope. This sequence is called neurocardiogenic syncope. Medical causes of syncope to be ruled out include acute dehydration, excessive caffeine intake, overly aggressive treatment of hypertension, parkinsonism and related neurodegenerative disorders, and inadequate fluid and salt intake. Sertraline has been reported to reduce the risk of idiopathic and provoked neurocardiogenic syncope in some persons. Other SSRIs are also effective for neurocardiogenic symptoms such as dizziness.

Respiratory Conditions. The use of psychotropic medications for pulmonary disorders in people without psychiatric illness has received little attention. Airway reactivity is closely modulated by fear and panic in individuals with asthma or chronic obstructive airway disease (COPD). As many as one fourth of persons with COPD also meet criteria for panic disorder. Increased carbon dioxide (CO_2) sensitivity and dyspnea are cardinal features of both panic attacks and COPD. People with COPD often must use daily steroids and bronchodilators, which can have serious adverse effects.

In a small case series of persons with COPD sertraline use was reported to significantly decrease subjective breathlessness after 3 to 4 weeks of treatment, even in persons who did not meet criteria for diagnosable psychiatric illness. SSRIs are much better tolerated than steroids and bronchodilators. In contrast to the results with SSRIs, results have been mixed or contradictory with buspirone and tricyclic drugs in people with obstructive airway disease.

PRECAUTIONS AND ADVERSE REACTIONS

Three fourths of persons experience no side effects at low starting dosages of SS-RIs, and dosages may be increased relatively rapidly (i.e., on the order of an increase every 1 to 2 weeks) in this group. In the remaining one fourth of patients, most of the adverse effects of the SSRIs appear within the first 1 to 2 weeks, and they generally subside or resolve spontaneously if the drugs are continued at the same dosage. However, 10 to 15 percent of persons will not be able to tolerate even a low dosage of a particular SSRI and may discontinue taking the drug after only a few doses. One approach for such individuals is to fractionate the dosage over a week, with one dose every 2, 3, or 4 days. Some persons may tolerate a different SSRI or another class of antidepressant, such as a tricyclic drug or one of the other newer agents. However, some persons appear unable to tolerate even tiny doses of any antidepressant drug.

Because of the unfortunate possibility that adverse effects may reduce compliance, some clinicians administer a low dosage for the first 3 to 6 weeks of therapy and then increase gradually once a therapeutic benefit is seen. Because of the long half-life of the SSRIs, especially fluoxetine, and the even longer time it may take for the full benefit of a particular dose to be appreciated, steep increases in dose are to be avoided. For example, the lowest dosage may provide over 90 percent of the benefit of the highest dosage, if enough time is allowed. On the other hand, adverse effects are much more predictably dose dependent, and too-rapid an increase in dosage may provoke an aversive response in a sensitive person.

Sexual Dysfunction

Sexual inhibition is the most common adverse effect of SSRIs, with an incidence between 50 and 80 percent. All SSRIs appear to be equally likely to cause sexual dysfunction. The most common complaints are inhibited orgasm and decreased libido, which are dose dependent. Unlike most of the other adverse effects of SSRIs, sexual inhibition does not resolve in the first few weeks of use but usually continues as long as the drug is taken.

Treatment for SSRI-induced sexual dysfunction includes decreasing the dosage; switching to bupropion or nefazodone (Serzone), which cause much less sexual dysfunction; addition of bupropion; and addition of yohimbine (Yocon), cyroheptadine (Periactin), or dopamine receptor agonists. The combination of an SSRI with bupropion is particularly effective for both the antidepressant effect and the reduced sexual inhibition.

Recent reports have described successful treatment of SSRI-induced sexual dysfunction with sildenafil (Viagra). It is not immediately obvious why sildenafil, which works in the excitement phase of the sexual cycle, would counteract the orgasm-phase inhibition of SSRIs. Possibly, the positive reinforcement of robust sexual excitement due to sildenafil may permit a mental state more conducive to orgasm.

Gastrointestinal Adverse Effects

Sertraline, fluvoxamine, and citalopram have the highest rates of GI adverse effects, but they are also caused by fluoxetine and paroxetine. The most common GI complaints are nausea, diarrhea, anorexia, vomiting, and dyspepsia. Data indicate that the nausea and loose stools are dose related and transient, resolving usually within a few weeks. Anorexia is most common with fluoxetine, but some people gain weight while taking fluoxetine. Fluoxetine-induced appetite loss and weight loss begin as soon as the drug is taken and peak at 20 weeks, after which weight often returns to baseline.

Weight Gain.   Although most patients initially lose weight, up to one third of persons taking SSRIs will gain weight, sometimes more than 20 pounds. Paroxetine has anticholinergic activity and is the SSRI most often associated with weight gain. In some cases, weight gain results from the drug use itself or the increased appetite associated with better mood.

Headaches

The incidence of headache in SSRI trials was 18 to 20 percent, only 1 percentage point higher than the placebo rate. Fluoxetine is the most likely to cause headache. On the other hand, all SSRIs are effective prophylaxis against both migraine and tension-type headaches in many persons.

Central Nervous System Adverse Effects

Anxiety.   Fluoxetine is the SSRI most likely to cause anxiety, particularly in the first few weeks; however, these initial effects usually give way to an overall reduction in anxiety after a few weeks. Increased anxiety is caused considerably less frequently by the other SSRIs, which may be a better choice if sedation is desired, as in mixed anxiety and depressive disorders.

Insomnia and Sedation.   The major effect SSRIs exert in the area of insomnia and sedation is improved sleep resulting from treatment of depression and anxiety. However, as many as one fourth of persons taking SSRIs note either trouble sleeping or excessive somnolence. Fluoxetine is the most likely to cause insomnia, for which reason it is often taken in the morning. Sertraline and fluvoxamine are about equally likely to cause insomnia as somnolence, and citalopram and especially paroxetine are more likely to cause somnolence than insomnia. With the latter agents, persons usually report that taking the dose before retiring to bed helps them sleep better but does not cause residual daytime somnolence.

SSRI-induced insomnia can be treated with benzodiazepines, trazodone (Desyrel) (clinicians must explain the risk of priapism), or other sedating medicines. Significant SSRI-induced somnolence often requires switching to use of another SSRI or bupropion.

Vivid Dreams and Nightmares.   A minority of persons taking SSRIs report recalling extremely vivid dreams or nightmares. An individual experiencing such dreams with one SSRI may get the same therapeutic benefit without the disturbing dream images by switching to use of another SSRI. This adverse effect often resolves spontaneously over several weeks.

Seizures.   Seizures have been reported in 0.1 to 0.2 percent of all patients treated with SSRIs, an incidence comparable to that reported with other antidepressants and not significantly different from that with placebo. Seizures are more frequent at the highest doses of SSRIs (e.g., fluoxetine 100 mg a day or higher).

Extrapyramidal Symptoms.   Tremor is seen in 5 to 10 percent of persons taking SSRIs, a frequency 2 to 4 times that seen with placebo. SSRIs may rarely cause akathisia, dystonia, tremor, cogwheel rigidity, torticollis, opisthotonos, gait disorders, and bradykinesia. Rare cases of tardive dyskinesia have been reported. People with well-controlled Parkinson's disease may experience acute worsening of their motor symptoms when they take SSRIs. Extrapyramidal adverse effects are most closely associated with use of fluoxetine, particularly at dosages in excess of 40 mg per day, but may occur at any time during the course of therapy. Bruxism has also been reported, which responds to small doses of buspirone.

Anticholinergic Effects

Paroxetine has mild anticholinergic activity that causes dry mouth, constipation, and sedation in a dose-dependent fashion. However, the anticholinergic activity of paroxetine is perhaps only one fifth that of nortriptyline, and most persons taking paroxetine do not experience cholinergic adverse effects. Although not considered to have anticholinergic activity, the other SSRIs are associated with dry mouth in 15 to 20 percent of patients.

Hematological Adverse Effects

SSRIs affect platelet function and may cause increased bruisability. Paroxetine and fluoxetine are rarely associated with development of reversible neutropenia, particularly if administered concurrently with clozapine.

Electrolyte and Glucose Disturbances

SSRIs are rarely associated with a decrease in glucose concentrations; therefore, diabetic patients should be carefully monitored. Rare cases of SSRI-associated hyponatremia and the secretion of inappropriate antidiuretic hormone (SIADH) have been seen in patients treated with diuretics who are also water deprived.

Endocrine and Allergic Reactions

SSRIs can decrease prolactin levels and cause mammoplasia and galactorrhea in both men and women. Breast changes are reversible upon discontinuation of the drug, but this may take several months to occur.

Various types of rashes appear in about 4 percent of all patients; in a small subset of these patients, the allergic reaction may generalize and involve the pulmonary system, resulting rarely in fibrotic damage and dyspnea. SSRI treatment may have to be discontinued in patients with drug-related rashes.

Galactorrhea

SSRIs may cause reversible galactorrhea, presumably because of interference with regulation of prolactin secretion.

Serotonin Syndrome

Concurrent administration of an SSRI with an MAOI, L-tryptophan, or lithium can raise plasma serotonin concentrations to toxic levels, producing a constellation of symptoms called the serotonin syndrome. This serious and possibly fatal syndrome of serotonin overstimulation comprises, in order of appearance as the condition worsens, (1) diarrhea; (2) restlessness; (3) extreme agitation, hyperreflexia, and autonomic instability with possible rapid fluctuations in vital signs; (4) myoclonus, seizures, hyperthermia, uncontrollable shivering, and rigidity; and (5) delirium, coma, status epilepticus, cardiovascular collapse, and death.

Treatment of the serotonin syndrome consists of removing the offending agents and promptly instituting comprehensive supportive care with nitroglycerine, cyproheptadine, methysergide (Sansert), cooling blankets, chlorpromazine (Thorazine), dantrolene (Dantrium), benzodiazepines, anticonvulsants, mechanical ventilation, and paralyzing agents.

SSRI Withdrawal

The abrupt discontinuance of SSRI use, especially one with a shorter half-life, such as paroxetine or fluvoxamine, has been associated with a withdrawal syndrome that may include dizziness, weakness, nausea, headache, rebound depression, anxiety, insomnia, poor concentration, upper respiratory symptoms, paresthesias, and migraine-like symptoms. It usually does not appear until after at least 6 weeks of treatment and usually resolves spontaneously in 3 weeks. Persons who experienced transient adverse effects in the first weeks of taking an SSRI are more likely to experience discontinuation symptoms.

Fluoxetine is the SSRI least likely to be associated with this syndrome, because the half-life of its metabolite is more than 1 week and it effectively tapers itself. Fluoxetine has therefore been used in some cases to treat the discontinuation syndrome caused by termination of other SSRIs.

DRUG INTERACTIONS

SSRIs do not interfere with most other drugs. A serotonin syndrome (Table 28–2) can develop with concurrent administration of MAOIs, tryptophan, lithium (Eskalith), or other antidepressants that inhibit reuptake of serotonin. Fluoxetine, sertraline, and paroxetine can raise plasma concentrations of tricyclic antidepres-

TABLE 28–2
**SEROTONIN
SYNDROME**

Diarrhea
Diaphoresis
Tremor
Ataxia
Myoclonus
Hyperactive reflexes
Disorientation
Lability of mood

sants, which can cause clinical toxicity. A number of potential pharmacokinetic interactions have been described based on in vitro analyses of the CYP enzymes (see Table 1–2 in Chapter 1), but clinically relevant interactions are rare (Table 28–3).

The combination of lithium and any serotonergic drug should be used with caution, because of the possibility of precipitating seizures. SSRIs, particularly fluvoxamine, should not be used with clozapine because it raises clozapine concentrations and seizures may result. SSRIs may increase the duration and severity of zolpidem (Ambien)-induced hallucinations.

TABLE 28–3
INTERACTIONS OF DRUGS WITH THE SSRIs FLUOXETINE, FLUVOXAMINE, PAROXETINE, AND SERTRALINE

SSRI	Other Drugs	Effect	Clinical Importance
Fluoxetine	Desipramine	Inhibits metabolism	Possible
	Carbamazepine	Inhibits metabolism	Possible
	Diazepam	Inhibits metabolism	Not important
	Haloperidol	Inhibits metabolism	Possible
	Warfarin	No interaction	
	Tolbutamide	No interaction	
Fluvoxamine	Antipyrine	Inhibits metabolism	Not important
	Propranolol	Inhibits metabolism	Unlikely
	Tricyclics	Inhibits metabolism	Unlikely
	Warfarin	Inhibits metabolism	Possible
	Atenolol	No interaction	
	Digoxin	No interaction	
Paroxetine	Phenytoin	AUC increases by 12%	Possible
	Procyclidine	AUC increases by 39%	Possible
	Cimetidine	Paroxetine AUC increases by 50%	Possible
	Antipyrine	No interaction	
	Digoxin	No interaction	
	Propranolol	No interaction	
	Tranylcypromine	No interaction	Caution with combined treatment
	Warfarin	No interaction	
Sertraline	Antipyrine	Increased clearance	Not important
	Diazepam	13% decreased clearance	Not important
	Tolbutamide	16% decreased clearance	Not important
	Digoxin	No interaction	
	Lithium	No pharmacokinetic interaction	Caution with combined treatment
	Desipramine	No interaction	
	Atenolol	No pharmacodynamic interaction	

From Warrington SJ. Clinical implications of the pharmacology of serotonin reuptake inhibitors. *Int Clin Psychopharmacol*, 1982;7(Suppl 2):13, with permission.

Fluoxetine

Fluoxetine can be administered with tricyclic drugs, but the clinician should use low dosages of the tricyclic drug. Because it is metabolized by the hepatic CYP 2D6, fluoxetine may interfere with the metabolism of other drugs in the 7 percent of the population that has an inefficient isoform of this enzyme, the so-called poor metabolizers. Fluoxetine may slow the metabolism of carbamazepine (Tegretol), antineoplastic agents, diazepam (Valium), and phenytoin (Dilantin). Possibly significant drug interactions have been described for fluoxetine with benzodiazepines, antipsychotics, and lithium. Fluoxetine has no interactions with warfarin (Coumadin), tolbutamide (Orinase), or chlorthiazide (Diuril).

Sertraline

Sertraline may displace warfarin from plasma proteins and may increase the prothrombin time. The drug interaction data on sertraline support a generally similar profile to that of fluoxetine, although sertraline does not interact as strongly with the CYP 2D6 enzyme.

Paroxetine

Paroxetine has a higher risk for drug interactions than does either fluoxetine or sertraline because it is a more potent inhibitor of the CYP 2D6 enzyme. Cimetidine (Tagamet) can increase the concentration of sertraline and paroxetine, and phenobarbital (Luminal) and phenytoin can decrease the concentration of paroxetine. Because of the potential for interference with the CYP 2D6 enzyme, the coadministration of paroxetine with other antidepressants, phenothiazines, and antiarrhythmic drugs should be undertaken with caution. Paroxetine may increase the anticoagulant effect of warfarin. Coadministration of paroxetine and tramadol (Ultram) may precipitate a serotonin syndrome in elderly persons.

Fluvoxamine

Among the SSRIs, fluvoxamine appears to present the most risk for drug-drug interactions. Fluvoxamine is metabolized by the enzyme CYP 3A4, which may be inhibited by ketoconazole (Nizoral). Administration of terfenadine (no longer manufactured) to patients in whom the CYP 3A4 enzyme is inhibited may produce cardiotoxicity, which has been fatal in several cases. Fluvoxamine may increase the half-life of alprazolam (Xanax), triazolam (Halcion), and diazepam, and it should not be coadministered with these agents. Fluvoxamine may increase theophylline (Slo-Bid, Theo-Dur) levels threefold and warfarin levels twofold, with important clinical consequences; thus the serum levels of the latter drugs should be closely monitored, and the doses adjusted accordingly. Fluvoxamine raises concentrations and may increase the activity of clozapine, carbamazepine, methadone (Dolophine, Methadose), propranolol (Inderal), and diltiazem (Cardizem). Fluvoxamine has no significant interactions with lorazepam (Ativan) or digoxin (Lanoxin).

Citalopram

Citalopram is not a potent inhibitor of any CYP enzymes. Concurrent administration of cimetidine increases concentrations of citalopram about 40 percent. Citalopram does not significantly affect the metabolism of, nor is its metabolism significantly affected by, digoxin, lithium, warfarin, carbamazepine, or imipramine (Tofranil). Citalopram increases the plasma concentrations of metoprolol twofold, but this usually has no effect on blood pressure or heart rate. Data on coadministration of citalopram and potent inhibitors of CYP 3A4 or CYP 2D6 are not available.

LABORATORY INTERFERENCES

SSRIs do not interfere with any laboratory tests.

DOSAGE AND CLINICAL GUIDELINES

Fluoxetine

Fluoxetine is available in 10- and 20-mg capsules, in a scored 10-mg tablet, and as a liquid (20 mg/5 mL). For depression, the initial dosage is usually 10 or 20 mg orally each day, usually given in the morning, because insomnia is a potential adverse effect of the drug. Fluoxetine should be taken with food to minimize the possible nausea. The long half-lives of the drug and its metabolite contribute to a 4-week period to reach steady-state concentrations. As with all available antidepressants, the antidepressant effects of fluoxetine may be seen in the first weeks, but the clinician should wait until the patient has been taking the drug for 4 to 6 weeks before definitively evaluating its antidepressant activity. Several studies indicate that 20 mg is often as effective as higher doses for treating depression. The maximum dosage recommended by the manufacturer is 80 mg a day, and higher dosages may cause seizures. A reasonable strategy is to maintain a patient with 20 mg a day for 3 weeks. If the patient shows no signs of clinical improvement at that time, an increase to 20 mg may be warranted, although at least one study has found that continuing use of 20 mg a day is as effective as increasing the dosage.

To minimize the early side effects of anxiety and restlessness, some clinicians initiate fluoxetine use at 5 to 10 mg a day either with the scored 10-mg tablet or by using the liquid preparation. Alternatively, because of the long half-life of fluoxetine, its use can be initiated with an every-other-day administration schedule.

At least 2 weeks should elapse between the discontinuation of MAOI use and the administration of fluoxetine. Fluoxetine use must be discontinued for at least 5 weeks before the initiation of MAOI treatment.

The dosage of fluoxetine that is effective in other indications may differ from the 20 mg a day that is generally used for depression. A dosage of 60 mg a day has been reported to be the most effective for the treatment of obsessive-compulsive disorder, obesity, and bulimia nervosa. Fluoxetine is also marketed as Sarafem for premenstrual dysphoric disorder.

Sertraline

Sertraline is available in scored 25-, 50-, and 100-mg tablets. For the initial treatment of depression, sertraline use should be initiated with a dose of 50 mg once daily. To limit the GI effects, some clinicians begin at 25 mg a day, and increase to 50 mg a day after 3 weeks. Patients who do not respond after 1 to 3 weeks may benefit from dosage increases of 50 mg every week up to a maximum of 200 mg, given once daily. Sertraline generally is given in the evening, because it is slightly more likely to cause sedation than insomnia. However, it can be administered in the morning or the evening. Administration after eating may reduce the GI adverse effects. Sertraline concentrate is now available (1 ml = 20 mg).

Guidelines regarding the logic of dosage increases for sertraline are similar to those for fluoxetine. Several studies suggests that maintaining the dosage at 50 mg a day for many weeks may be as beneficial as rapidly increasing the dosage. Nevertheless, many clinicians maintain their patients on doses of 100 to 200 mg a day.

Paroxetine

Paroxetine is available in scored 20-mg tablets, in unscored 10-, 30-, and 40-mg tablets, and as an an orange-flavored 10 mg/5 mL oral suspension. Paroxetine use for the treatment of depression is usually initiated at a dosage of 10 or 20 mg a day. An increase in the dosage should be considered when an adequate response is not seen in 1 to 3 weeks. At that point, the clinician can initiate upward dose titration in 10-mg increments at weekly intervals to a maximum of 50 mg a day. Doses of 60, 70, and 80 mg a day have been tolerated by certain individuals but not studied in controlled trials. Persons who experience GI upset may benefit by taking the drug with food. Paroxetine should be taken initially as a single daily dose in the evening; higher dosages may be divided into two doses per day. Patients with melancholic features may require dosages exceeding 20 mg a day. The suggested therapeutic dosage range for elderly patients is 10 to 20 mg a day, as the elderly have been found to have higher mean plasma concentrations than do younger adults.

Paroxetine is the SSRI most likely to produce a discontinuation syndrome, because plasma concentrations drop rapidly in the absence of continuous dosing. To limit the development of symptoms of abrupt discontinuation, paroxetine use should be tapered gradually in increments of 10 mg a day each week until the daily dose is 10 mg, at which point its use may be stopped either directly or after an additional increment of 5 mg a day.

Fluvoxamine

Fluvoxamine is available in unscored 25-mg tablets and scored 50- and 100-mg tablets. The effective daily dosage range is 50 mg to 300 mg a day. A usual starting dosage is 50 mg once a day at bedtime for the first week, after which the dosage can be adjusted according to the adverse effects and clinical response. Dosages above 100 mg a day may be divided into twice-daily dosing. A temporary dosage reduction or slower upward titration may be necessary if nausea develops over the first 2 weeks of therapy. Fluvoxamine can also be administered as a single evening dose to minimize its adverse effects. Tablets should be swallowed with food, without chewing the tablet.

Fluvoxamine is relatively likely to cause a discontinuation syndrome.

Citalopram

Citalopram is available in 20- and 40-mg tablets and as a liquid (10 mg/5 mL). The usual starting dosage is 20 mg a day for the first week, after which it usually is increased to 40 mg a day. Some persons may require 60 mg a day, but there are no controlled trials supporting this dose. For elderly persons or persons with hepatic impairment, 20 mg a day is recommended, with an increase to 40 mg a day only if there is no response at 20 mg a day. Tablets should be taken once daily, in either the morning or the evening, with or without food.

Loss of Efficacy

Some patients report a lessened response to SSRIs with recurrence of depressive symptoms after a period of time (e.g., 4 to 6 months). The exact mechanism is unknown; however, data from an open-label trial suggest that persons with moderate-to-severe depression who respond rapidly to fluoxetine use are unlikely to experience recurrence of depression while taking fluoxetine, whereas one third of those with milder depression whose initial response to fluoxetine was slower and less robust experienced recurrence of depression within 3 months.

Potential responses to the attenuation of response to SSRIs include increasing or decreasing the dosage; tapering drug use, then rechallenging with the same medication; switching to another SSRI or non-SSRI antidepressant; and augmenting with bupropion, sympathomimetics, buspirone, lithium, anticonvulsants, naltrexone (Re-Via), or another non-SSRI antidepressant. A change in response to an SSRI should be explored in psychotherapy, which may reveal the underlying conflicts causing an increase in depressive symptoms.

For a more detailed discussion of this topic, see Kelsey JE, Nemeroff CB: Selective Serotonin Reuptake Inhibitors, Sec 31.25, p 2432, in CTP/VII.

29

Serotonin-Dopamine Antagonists: Atypical Antipsychotics

The serotonin-dopamine antagonists (SDAs), also referred to as novel or atypical antipsychotic drugs, include risperidone (Risperdal), olanzapine (Zyprexa), quetiapine (Seroquel), clozapine (Clozaril), and ziprasidone (Zeldox). These drugs improve two classes of disability typical of schizophrenia: (1) positive symptoms such as hallucinations, delusions, disordered thoughts, and agitation, and (2) negative symptoms such as withdrawal, flat affect, anhedonia, poverty of speech, catatonia, and cognitive impairment. SDAs are associated with a smaller risk of extrapyramidal symptoms than are the dopamine receptor antagonists, which eliminates the need for anticholinergic drugs with their annoying side effects.

SDAs are also effective for the treatment of mood disorders with psychotic or manic features and for behavioral disturbances associated with dementia. Olanzapine is indicated for short-term treatment of acute manic episodes associated with bipolar I disorders. All these agents are considered first-line drugs except clozapine, which causes adverse hematological effects that require weekly blood sampling.

CHEMISTRY

Clozapine is a dibenzodiazepine. Risperidone is a benzisoxazole. Olanzapine is a thienobenzodiazepine derivative of clozapine. Quetiapine is a dibenzothiazepine structurally related to clozapine. Ziprasidone is a benzisothiazolyl piperazine. The molecular structures of these compounds are shown in Figure 29–1.

PHARMACOLOGICAL ACTIONS

These drugs are called serotonin-dopamine antagonists, because they block not only dopamine receptors, as do the typical antipsychotic drugs (dopamine receptor antagonists), but also serotonin receptors. These drugs possess a diverse combination of receptor affinities, and the relative contribution of each receptor interaction to the clinical effects is unknown. Dosage changes for special populations are shown in Table 29–1.

Risperidone

Between 70 and 85 percent of risperidone is absorbed from the gastrointestinal (GI) tract, and it undergoes extensive first-pass hepatic metabolism to 9-hydroxyrisperidone, a metabolite with comparable biological activity. The combined half-

Dibenzodiazepine

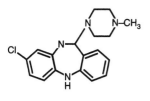

Clozapine

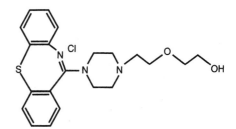

Quetiapine

Benzisoxazole

Thienobenzodiazepine

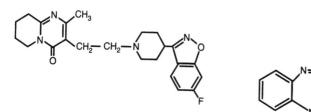

Risperidone

Olanzapine

Benzisothiazolyl piperazine

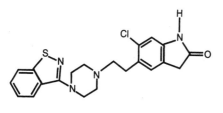

Ziprasidone

Figure 29-1. Molecular structures of serotonin-dopamine antagonists.

life of risperidone and 9-hydroxyrisperidone averages 20 hours, so that it is effective in once-daily dosing. Risperidone is an antagonist of the serotonin 5-HT$_{2A}$, dopamine D$_2$, α_1- and α_2-adrenergic, and histamine H$_1$ receptors. It has a low affinity for β-adrenergic and muscarinic cholinergic receptors. Although it is as potent an antagonist of D$_2$ receptors as is haloperidol (Haldol), risperidone

TABLE 29-1
CHANGES IN PHARMACOKINETICS: SPECIAL POPULATIONS

Drug	Elderly	Renal Impairment	Hepatic Impairment	Ethnic
Clozapine	↓↓ dosage	No Δ dosage	↓ dosage	↓ dosage women
Risperidone	↓↓ dosage	↓ dosage	↓ dosage	↓ dosage Asians?
Olanzapine	↓ dosage (35%)	No Δ dosage	No Δ dosage (preliminary)	↓ dosage women ↓ dosage Asians?
Sertindole	No Δ dosage PD concerns	No Δ dosage	↓ dosage (½)	↓ dosage women
Quetiapine	No PK Δ^a ↓ dosage 2° PD	No Δ dosage	Slight ↓ dosage	No Δ dosage
Ziprasidone	No Δ dosage	No Δ dosage	No Δ dosage	?

Abbreviations: PD, pharmacodynamic; PK, pharmacokinetic; Δ, change in.
^{a} Increased adverse reactions (α_1-blockade).
From Ereshásky L. Pharmacokinetics and drug interactions: Update for new antipsychotics. *J Clin Psychiatry*, 1996:7(Suppl):12, with permission.

is much less likely than haloperidol to cause extrapyramidal symptoms in humans.

Olanzapine

Approximately 85 percent of olanzapine is absorbed from the GI tract, and about 40 percent of the dosage is inactivated by first-pass hepatic metabolism. Peak concentrations are achieved within 6 hours, and the half-life averages 30 hours. Therefore, it is effective in once-daily dosing. Olanzapine is an effective antagonist of the 5-HT$_{2A}$; D$_1$, D$_2$, and D$_4$; α_1, muscarinic M$_1$ through M$_5$, and H$_1$ receptors.

Quetiapine

Quetiapine is rapidly absorbed from the GI tract. Peak plasma concentrations are reached in 1 to 2 hours. Steady-state half-life is about 6 hours, and optimal dosing is two or three times per day. Quetiapine is an antagonist of 5-HT$_2$ and 5-HT$_6$, D$_1$ and D$_2$, H$_1$, and α_1 and α_2 receptors. It does not block muscarinic or benzodiazepine receptors. The receptor antagonism for quetiapine is generally lower than that for other antipsychotic drugs, and it is not associated with extrapyramidal symptoms.

Clozapine

Clozapine is rapidly absorbed from the GI tract, and peak plasma levels are reached in 1 to 4 hours. The steady-state half-life of between 10 and 16 hours is usually reached in 3 to 4 days if twice-daily dosing is used. The two major metabolites have minimal pharmacological activity. Clozapine is an antagonist of 5-HT$_{2A}$; D$_1$, D$_3$, and D$_4$; and α (especially α_1) receptors. It has relatively low potency as a D$_2$-receptor antagonist. Data from positron emission tomography (PET) scanning show that 10 mg of haloperidol produces 80 percent occupancy of striatal D$_2$ receptors, whereas clinically effective dosages of clozapine occupy only 40 to 50 percent of striatal D$_2$ receptors. This difference in D$_2$ receptor occupancy is probably why clozapine does not cause extrapyramidal adverse effects.

Ziprasidone

Peak plasma concentrations of ziprasidone are reached in 2 to 6 hours. The steady-state half-life of 5 to 10 hours is reached by the third day, and twice-daily dosing is necessary. Ziprasidone is an antagonist of 5-HT_{1D}, 5-HT_{2A}, and 5-HT_{2C}; D_2, D_3, and D_4; α_1; and H_1 receptors. It has very low affinity for D_1, M_1, and α_2-receptors. Ziprasidone also has agonist activity at the serotonin 5-HT_{1A} receptors and is a serotonin reuptake inhibitor and a norepinephrine reuptake inhibitor. This suggests that it could possess antidepressant effects.

THERAPEUTIC INDICATIONS

Psychotic Disorders

SDAs are effective for treating acute and chronic psychoses such as schizophrenia and schizoaffective disorders, in both adults and adolescents. They are also effective for treating psychotic depression and for psychosis secondary to head trauma, dementia, or treatment drugs. SDAs are as good as or better than typical antipsychotics (dopamine receptor antagonists) for the treatment of positive symptoms in schizophrenia and clearly superior to dopamine receptor antagonists for the treatment of negative symptoms. Compared with persons treated with dopamine receptor antagonists, persons treated with SDAs have fewer relapses and require less-frequent hospitalization, fewer emergency room visits, less phone contact with mental health professionals, and less treatment in day programs.

Because clozapine has potentially life-threatening adverse effects, it is now appropriate only for patients with schizophrenia resistant to all other antipsychotics, and it retains a therapeutic niche for patients who are treatment resistant. Other indications for clozapine include treatment of persons with severe tardive dyskinesias and those with a low threshold for extrapyramidal symptoms. Persons who tolerate clozapine have done well on long-term therapy. The effectiveness of clozapine may be increased by augmentation with risperidone, which raises clozapine concentrations and sometimes results in dramatic clinical improvement.

Mood Disorders

SDAs are useful for the initial control of agitation during a manic episode; but they are less effective for long-term control of bipolar disorders than are lithium (Eskalith), valproate (Depakene), and carbamazepine (Tegretol). Olanzapine is FDA-approved for treatment of acute mania at dosages of 10 or 15 mg a day. In preclinical trials, olanzapine was an effective treatment for manic persons with or without psychotic features. In general, however, typical antipsychotics and benzodiazepines exert calming effects in mania more rapidly than do SDAs. Olanzapine and risperidone can be used to augment antidepressants in the acute management of major depression with psychotic features. SDAs are effective in the treatment of schizoaffective disorder, although risperidone has been reported to precipitate mania in persons with schizoaffective disorder. Olanzapine and clozapine augmentation can improve up to two thirds of persons with refractory bipolar disorder, and risperidone has been used to reduce mood swings in persons with rapid-cycling bipolar disorder. Olanzapine, but not clozapine, is effective for treatment of depressive symptoms in persons with bipolar disorders.

Other Indications

SDAs are effective for treatment of AIDS dementia, autistic spectrum disorders, dementia-related psychosis, Tourette's disorder, Huntington's disease, and Lesch-Nyhan syndrome. Risperidone and olanzapine have been used to control aggression and self-injury in children. These drugs have also been coadministered with sympathomimetics, such as methylphenidate (Ritalin) or dextroamphetamine (Dexedrine, Dextrostat), to children with attention-deficit/hyperactivity disorder who are comorbid for either opposition-defiant disorder or conduct disorder. SDAs, especially olanzapine, quetiapine, and clozapine, are useful in persons who have severe tardive dyskinesia. SDA treatment suppresses the abnormal movements of tardive dyskinesia but does not appear to worsen the movement disorder.

Treatment with olanzapine and ziprasidone decreases depressive symptoms in persons with schizophrenia to a greater extent than does haloperidol. In depressed persons without psychotic features who respond only partially to antidepressants augmentation with olanzapine can improve treatment efficacy.

Treatment with SDAs decreases the risk of suicide and water intoxication in patients with schizophrenia. Patients with treatment-resistant obsessive-compulsive disorder have responded to SDAs; however, a few persons treated with SDAs have noted treatment-emergent symptoms of obsessive-compulsive disorder. Some patients with borderline personality disorder may improve with SDAs.

ADVERSE EFFECTS

The adverse reactions reported with SDAs are listed in Table 29–2.

Risperidone

There is evidence that risperidone-induced extrapyramidal effects may be dosage dependent. Weight gain, anxiety, nausea and vomiting, rhinitis, erectile dysfunction, orgasmic dysfunction, and increased pigmentation are associated with risperidone use. The most common drug-related reasons for discontinuation of risperidone use are extrapyramidal symptoms, dizziness, hyperkinesia, somnolence, and nausea.

Olanzapine

Somnolence, dry mouth, dizziness, constipation, dyspepsia, increased appetite, and tremor are associated with olanzapine use. Olanzapine is somewhat more likely than risperidone to cause weight gain. A small number of patients (2 percent) may need to discontinue use of the drug because of transaminase elevation.

TABLE 29–2
ADVERSE EFFECTS OF ANTIPSYCHOTIC AGENTS^a

Item	Conventional Antipsychotics	Clozapine	Risperidone	Olanzapine	Quetiapine	Ziprasidone
Central nervous system						
Extrapyramidal symptoms (EPS)	0 to ++^{b,c}	0^b	0^b	0^b to +^{c}	0^b	0^b
Tardive dyskinesia	+++	0	(+)	?	?	?
Seizures	0 to +	+++	0	+	0	0
Sedation, somnolence	+ to +++	+++	+^{d}	+	+^{d}	+^{d}
Other						
Neuroleptic malignant syndrome	+	+	+	+	?	?
Orthostatic hypotension	+ to +++	0 to +++	+	+^{d}	0^d	0
QT$_c$	0 to ++	0	0 to +	0	0 to +	0
Liver transaminase increase	0 to ++	0 to +	0 to +	0 to +	0 to +	0 to +
Anticholinergic adverse effects	0 to +++	+++	0	+	0	0
Agranulocytosis	0	+++	0	0	0	0
Prolactin increase	++ to +++	0	+ to ++	0^c	0^d	0^e
Decreased ejaculatory volume	0 to +	0	0	0	0	0
Weight gain	0 to ++	+++	+	+++	+	0
Nasal congestion	0 to +	+++	0 to +	0 to +	0 to +	0

^{a} 0, None or not significantly different from placebo; +, mild; ++, moderate; +++, marked; ?, insufficient data.
^{b} Not significantly different from placebo-treated group, which may have received conventional antipsychotic before entering the study and could have EPS carried forward into the initial weeks of the investigation
^{c} Dosage-related EPS above 6 mg/day.
^{d} Transient.
^{e} Dosage-related increases within the normal range.
Modified from Casey DE. Side effect profiles of new antipsychotic agents, J Clin Psychiatry. 1996:57(Suppl):40, with permission.

Quetiapine

The most common adverse effects of quetiapine are somnolence, postural hypotension, and dizziness, which are usually transient and are best managed with initial gradual upward titration of the dosage. Quetiapine appears not to cause extrapyramidal symptoms. Quetiapine is associated with modest transient weight gain in 23 percent of persons, small increases in heart rate, constipation, and a transient rise in liver transaminases.

Clozapine

The most common drug-related adverse effects are sedation, dizziness, syncope, tachycardia, hypotension, electrocardiogram (ECG) changes, nausea, and vomiting. Leukopenia, granulocytopenia, agranulocytosis, and fever occur in about 1 percent of patients. Other common adverse effects include fatigue, sialorrhea, weight gain, various GI symptoms (most commonly constipation), anticholinergic effects, and subjective muscle weakness. The risk of seizures is about 4 percent in patients taking dosages above 600 mg a day.

Ziprasidone

In early clinical trials involving persons with schizophrenia or schizoaffective disorder, no adverse effects were reported more frequently by persons taking ziprasidone than by those taking placebo. However, the U.S. Food and Drug Administration is requiring further demonstrations of the drug's effect on QT intervals relative to other SDAs before approval can be given. The most common adverse effects in patients taking ziprasidone were somnolence, headache, dizziness, nausea, and lightheadedness. Ziprasidone has almost no significant effects outside the CNS and is associated with almost no weight gain.

Neuroleptic Malignant Syndrome

Although rare with SDAs, all antipsychotic drugs may cause neuroleptic malignant syndrome. This syndrome consists of muscular rigidity, fever, dystonia, akinesia, mutism, shifting between obtundation and agitation, diaphoresis, dysphagia, tremor, incontinence, labile blood pressure, leukocytosis, and elevated creatine phosphokinase (CPK). Neuroleptic malignant syndrome has been reported with clozapine, risperidone, and olanzapine and must be considered in the differential diagnosis of fever in a clozapine-treated person. Clozapine may be associated with reversible elevations of serum creatine phosphokinase concentrations that do not involve rhabdomyolysis and do not lead to neuroleptic malignant syndrome. Neuroleptic malignant syndrome is more likely to occur if clozapine is given together with lithium.

Tardive Dyskinesia

SDAs are much less likely than dopamine receptor antagonists to be associated with treatment-emergent tardive dyskinesias. Moreover, SDAs ameliorate the symptoms of tardive dyskinesias and are especially indicated for psychotic persons with preexisting tardive dyskinesias. Tardive dyskinesias can occur in persons treated with dopamine receptor antagonists for as little as 1 month. Therefore, long-term maintenance of psychosis with dopamine receptor antagonists has become a questionable practice. SDAs should replace dopamine receptor antagonists for chronic treatment.

Although rare, treatment-emergent cases of tardive dyskinesias have been associated with risperidone, to a lesser degree with olanzapine, and very rarely with clozapine and quetiapine. Many of these persons were previously exposed to dopamine receptor antagonists, though some only briefly. Clozapine is the drug of choice for persons with severe tardive dyskinesias. A reduction in symptoms is usually seen in 1 to 4 weeks.

Orthostatic Hypotension, Syncope, and Tachycardia

All SDAs, but most frequently quetiapine, are associated with orthostatic hypotension, particularly if the dosages are escalated rapidly. SDAs should be used with caution in persons with hypotension, diabetes mellitus, or myocardial infarction and in those who are taking antihypertensive medications. The risk of hypotension and syncope can be minimized with gradual upward titration of dosages. To determine whether the dosage can be increased, a comparison should be made between blood pressure supine and standing after 10 deep knee bends. Evidence of orthostatic hypotension includes a drop in mean arterial pressure of 20 mm Hg or more, increase in pulse rate of 20 beats per minute or more, and/or subjective dizziness. Dosage escalation should be delayed until any signs of orthostatic hypotension resolve. The tachycardia, which is due to vagal inhibition, can be treated with peripherally acting β-adrenergic antagonists, such as atenolol (Tenormin), although this treatment may aggravate the hypotensive effects of SDAs. Additional treatment measures for hypotension include avoidance of caffeine and alcohol, increased sodium intake, adequate fluid intake, support stockings, and rarely fludrocortisone (Florinef) treatment. SDAs should not be used with other drugs that may cause orthostatic hypotension, such as benzodiazepines or antihypertensives. Clozapine is associated with paradoxical hypertension in 4 percent of persons.

Cardiac Changes

Potential ECG changes include nonspecific ST-T wave changes, T wave flattening, or T wave inversions, although these changes are usually not clinically significant. Olanzapine, quetiapine, ziprasidone, and clozapine are not associated with significant changes in QT or PR intervals. Because of the variety of cardiac changes associated with SDA use, the drugs should be used with caution by persons with preexisting cardiac disease.

Agranulocytosis

Agranulocytosis is a potentially fatal condition defined as a decrease in the absolute neutrophil count (ANC), to less than $500/mm^3$ in association with infectious disease. With recommended laboratory monitoring, it occurs in 0.38 percent of all persons treated with clozapine compared with an incidence of 0.04 to 0.05 percent of persons treated with standard antipsychotics. Careful clinical monitoring of the hematological status of clozapine-treated persons can prevent fatalities by the early recognition of hematological problems and the cessation of clozapine use. Agranulocytosis can appear precipitously or gradually and most often develops in the first 6 months of treatment. Increased age and female sex are additional risk factors. Clozapine is also associated with the development of benign cases of leukocytosis (0.6 percent of persons), leukopenia (3 percent), eosinophilia (1 percent), and elevated erythrocyte sedimentation rates. Clozapine should not be used by persons with white blood cell (WBC) counts below 3500, a history of a bone marrow disorder, or a history of clozapine-induced agranulocytosis. A case report describes successful treatment of clozapine-induced neutropenia with granulocyte colony-stimulating factor (G-CSF) without discontinuation of clozapine, which was the only antipsychotic drug to which the person responded. This technique requires further study before it can be recommended.

Seizures

The risk of seizures is less than 1 percent with risperidone, olanzapine, quetiapine, and ziprasidone. About 5 percent of persons taking more than 600 mg a day of clozapine, 3 to 4 percent of persons taking 300 to 600 mg a day, and 1 to 2 percent of persons taking less than 300 mg a day, have clozapine-associated seizures. If seizures develop, clozapine use should be temporarily stopped. Anticonvulsant treatment can be initiated, and clozapine use can be resumed at about 50 percent of the previous dosage, then gradually raised again. Carbamazepine and phenytoin (Dilantin) should not be used in combination with clozapine because of their association with agranulocytosis. The plasma concentrations of other anticonvulsants must be monitored carefully because of the possibility of pharmacokinetic interactions with clozapine. Persons with preexisting seizure disorders or histories of significant head trauma are at greater risk for seizures while taking clozapine.

Hyperprolactinemia

The D_2 receptor antagonist activity of antipsychotic drugs causes a rise in prolactin levels for the duration of the therapy. Of the SDAs, risperidone is most strongly associated with hyperprolactinemia, followed by olanzapine and ziprasidone. Clozapine and quetiapine do not increase prolactin secretion.

Hyperprolactinemia can cause galactorrhea, amenorrhea, gynecomastia, and impotence.

Cognitive and Motor Impairment

All currently available SDAs cause sedation. Therefore, persons who take SDAs should exercise caution when driving or operating dangerous machinery. This adverse effect may be minimized by giving most of the dosage before sleep. Somnolence can occur in 30 percent of persons on the usual maintenance dosage of olanzapine (10 mg a day); dizziness and akathisia have also been reported in persons taking olanzapine. Somnolence due to quetiapine occurs in 18 percent of patients. Somnolence due to risperidone is dosage dependent; it is relatively infrequent at dosages below 6 mg a day, but it may occur in over 40 percent of persons taking 16 mg a day. Clozapine is associated with sedation in 40 percent of persons taking therapeutic dosages.

Body Temperature Regulation

Because SDAs alter the ability of the body to regulate temperature, persons taking them should avoid strenuous exercise, exposure to extreme heat, concomitant administration of anticholinergic drugs, and dehydration.

With clozapine, fevers 1 to 2°F above normal may develop, usually during the first month of treatment, often causing concern about the development of an infection because of agranulocytosis. Clozapine should be withheld in these cases; if the WBC count is normal, clozapine use can be reinstituted slowly at a low dosage.

Extrapyramidal Symptoms

All SDAs are much less likely than dopamine receptor antagonists to produce extrapyramidal symptoms, such as acute dystonia, parkinsonism, rabbit syndrome, and akinesia. Risperidone induces extrapyramidal symptoms in a dose-dependent manner at dosages above 6 mg a day. Olanzapine is occasionally associated with extrapyramidal symptoms at dosages above 5 mg a day. The ziprasidone-associated risk of extrapyramidal symptoms is low. Quetiapine and clozapine do not increase the risk of extrapyramidal symptoms. There are reports that risperidone, olanzapine, quetiapine, ziprasidone, and clozapine may be associated with akathisia.

Weight Gain

Risperidone, olanzapine, quetiapine, and clozapine are associated with weight gain, which can be controlled with strict adherence to a planned diet. Clozapine and olanzapine in particular may be associated with a gain of as much as 30 to 50 pounds with short-term use. Significant weight gain may induce or exacerbate diabetes mellitus, and olanzapine and clozapine should therefore be used with caution by persons who have or are at risk for diabetes. Ziprasidone appears not to cause weight gain. One approach to management of weight gain associated with use of clozapine or olanzapine is to switch over gradually to ziprasidone, quetiapine, or risperidone.

Anticholinergic Symptoms

Clozapine and, to a lesser extent, olanzapine, are associated with anticholinergic symptoms, such as dry mouth, blurred vision, constipation, and urinary retention. This may necessitate transient addition of an anticholinergic agent when switching from clozapine or olanzapine to a less anticholinergic antipsychotic drug.

Sialorrhea

Clozapine can cause sialorrhea, which may place the patient at risk for aspiration of saliva and gagging, particularly during sleep. Clozapine is thought to produce sialorrhea by inhibiting swallowing rather than by increasing salivation. Treatment options include the clonidine patch, 0.1 or 0.2 mg each week, or amitriptyline (Elavil, Endep) or clomipramine (Anafranil), 75 to 100 mg, before sleep. Anticholinergic drugs, such as atropine (Donnatal), should not be used because they can exacerbate the anticholinergic activity of clozapine. Clozapine-induced sialorrhea may resolve spontaneously in a small number of patients after several months.

Obsessive-Compulsive Symptoms

Treatment-emergent obsessive-compulsive symptoms have been reported in patients with a favorable antipsychotic response to clozapine, risperidone, and olanzapine. Controlled trials have not established a clear causal relationship. When used by persons with a prior diagnosis of obsessive-compulsive disorder, on the other hand, SDAs have been successful in augmenting the antiobsessional effects of serotonin reuptake inhibitors.

Priapism

The α-receptor antagonism of SDAs can induce priapism. There are a few isolated case reports of priapism during treatment with risperidone, olanzapine, quetiapine, and clozapine.

Genitourinary Symptoms

Enuresis, urinary frequency or urgency, and urinary hesitancy or retention have been seen with use of clozapine. These problems may respond to desmopressin (DDAVP), oxybutynin (Ditropan), or timed interruption of sleep.

Dysphagia

Antipsychotic drugs are infrequently associated with esophageal dysmotility and aspiration, which can cause aspiration pneumonia.

Transaminase Elevations and Hepatic Dysfunction

About 6 percent of persons who take quetiapine and 2 percent of those who take olanzapine have serum transaminase concentrations over three times the upper limit of normal in the first 3 weeks of treatment. This has no clinical significance and is transient; however, quetiapine and olanzapine should be used with caution by persons with underlying liver disease.

Risperidone is rarely associated with reversible hepatotoxicity in adults and children. Obesity is a risk factor for risperidone-induced hepatotoxicity. Clozapine is frequently associated with elevations of transaminase concentrations that usually resolve within 3 months and is rarely associated with serious, possibly fatal hepatotoxicity.

Cholesterol and Triglyceride Elevations

Quetiapine may cause 11 to 17 percent increases in serum cholesterol and triglyceride concentrations.

Hypothyroidism

A small number of persons taking higher dosages of quetiapine have decreased serum concentrations of total and free thyroxine. This is usually of no clinical significance.

Use in Pregnancy and Lactation

SDA use by pregnant women has not been studied, but consideration should be given to the potential of risperidone to raise prolactin concentrations, sometimes to three to four times the upper limit of the normal range. Because the drugs can be excreted in breast milk, they should not be taken by nursing mothers.

DRUG INTERACTIONS

CNS depressants, alcohol, or tricyclic drugs coadministered with SDAs may increase the risk for seizures, sedation, and cardiac effects. Antihypertensive medications may potentiate the orthostatic hypotension caused by SDAs. The coadministration of benzodiazepines and SDAs may be associated with an increased incidence of orthostasis, syncope, and respiratory depression. Risperidone, olanzapine, quetiapine, and ziprasidone can antagonize the effects of levodopa (Larodopa) and dopamine agonists. Long-term use of SDAs with drugs that induce CYP isoenzymes, such as carbamazepine, barbiturates, omeprazole (Prilosec), rifampin (Rifadin, Rifamate), or glucocorticoids, may increase the clearance of the SDAs by 50 percent or more.

Risperidone

Concurrent use of risperidone and phenytoin or serotonin reuptake inhibitors may produce extrapyramidal symptoms. Use of risperidone by persons with opioid dependence may precipitate opioid withdrawal symptoms. Addition of risperidone to the regimen of a person taking clozapine can raise clozapine plasma concentrations by 75 percent. Otherwise, risperidone has little effect on other drugs.

Olanzapine

Cimetidine (Tagamet) and warfarin (Coumadin) do not influence olanzapine metabolism. Olanzapine does not affect the metabolism of imipramine (Tofranil), desipramine (Norpramin), warfarin, diazepam (Valium), lithium, or biperiden (Akineton). Fluvoxamine (Luvox) increases serum concentrations of olanzapine.

Quetiapine

Phenytoin increases quetiapine clearance fivefold, and thioridazine (Mellaril) increases quetiapine clearance by 65 percent. Cimetidine reduces quetiapine clearance by 20 percent. Fluoxetine, imipramine, haloperidol, and risperidone do not influence quetiapine metabolism. Quetiapine reduces lorazepam (Ativan) clearance by 20 percent and does not affect lithium clearance.

Clozapine

Clozapine should not be used with any other drug that is associated with the development of agranulocytosis or bone marrow suppression. Such drugs include carbamazepine, phenytoin, propylthiouracil, sulfonamides, and captopril (Capoten). Addition of paroxetine (Paxil) may precipitate clozapine-associated neutropenia.

Lithium combined with clozapine may increase the risk of seizures, confusion, and movement disorders. Lithium should not be used in combination with clozapine by persons who have experienced an episode of neuroleptic malignant syndrome. Risperidone, fluoxetine, paroxetine, and fluvoxamine increase serum concentrations of clozapine.

Ziprasidone

Ziprasidone appears to have low potential for clinically significant drug interactions.

DOSAGE AND CLINICAL GUIDELINES

Risperidone, olanzapine, quetiapine, and ziprasidone are each appropriate for the management of an initial psychotic episode, whereas clozapine is reserved for persons refractory to all other antipsychotic drugs. If a person does not respond to the first SDA, other SDAs should be tried. Olanzapine and clozapine have some initial calming effects due to their anticholinergic activity. The SDAs are less effective sedatives for treatment of acute psychosis than are dopamine receptor antagonists or benzodiazepines. It is therefore sometimes necessary to augment an SDA with a high-potency dopamine receptor antagonist or benzodiazepine in the first few weeks of use. Lorazepam 1 to 2 mg orally (p.o.) or intramuscularly (i.m.) can be used as needed for acute agitation. SDAs usually require 4 to 6 weeks to reach full effectiveness. Once effective, dosages can be lowered as tolerated. Clinical improvement may take 6 months of treatment with SDAs in some particularly treatment-refractory persons.

Use of all SDAs must be initiated at low dosages and gradually tapered upward to therapeutic dosages. The gradual increase in dosage is necessitated by the potential development of hypotension, syncope, and sedation, which are adverse effects for which the person can usually develop tolerance if the dosage titration is gradual enough. If a person stops taking an SDA for more than 36 hours, drug use should be resumed at the initial titration schedule. After the decision to terminate olanzapine or clozapine use, dosages should be tapered whenever possible to avoid cholinergic rebound symptoms such as diaphoresis, flushing, diarrhea, and hyperactivity.

Once a clinician has determined that a trial of a SDA is warranted for a particular person, the risk and the benefits of SDA treatment must be explained to the person and the family. In the case of clozapine, an informed consent procedure should be documented in the person's chart. The patient's history should include information about blood disorders, epilepsy, cardiovascular disease, hepatic and renal diseases, and drug abuse. The presence of a hepatic or renal disease necessitates using low starting dosages of the drug. Physical examination should include supine and standing blood pressure measurements to screen for orthostatic hypotension. The laboratory examination should include an ECG; several complete blood counts (CBCs) with WBC counts, which can then be averaged; and liver and renal function tests.

Risperidone

Risperidone is available in 1-, 2-, 3-, and 4-mg tablets, and a 1-mg/mL oral solution. The initial dosage is usually 1 to 2 mg at night. The dosage can then be raised gradually (1 mg per dose every 2 or 3 days) to 4 to 6 mg at night. Risperidone was initially given twice a day, but several studies have shown equal efficacy with once-a-day dosing. Dosages above 6 mg a day are associated with a higher incidence of adverse effects. Dosages below 6 mg a day have generally not been associated with extrapyramidal symptoms, but dystonic reactions have been seen at dosages from 4 to 16 mg a day.

Olanzapine

Olanzapine is available in 2.5-, 5-, 7.5-, 10-, and 15-mg tablets. The initial dosage for treatment of psychosis is usually 5 or 10 mg and for treatment of acute mania is usually 10 or 15 mg, given once daily. A starting daily dose of 5 mg is recommended for elderly and medically ill persons and for persons with hepatic impairment or hypotension: After 1 week the dosage can be raised to 10 mg a day. Given the long half-life, 1 week must be allowed to achieve each new steady-state blood level. Dosages in clinical use range from 5 to 20 mg a day, but a beneficial response usually occurs at dosages of 10 mg a day. The higher dosages are associated with increased extrapyramidal and other adverse effects. The manufacturer recommends "periodic" assessment of transaminases during treatment with olanzapine.

Quetiapine

Quetiapine is available in 25-, 100-, and 200-mg tablets. Dosing should begin at 25 mg twice daily, and dosages can be raised by 25 to 50 mg per dose every 2 to 3 days up to a target of 300 to 400 mg a day, divided into two or three daily doses. Studies have shown efficacy in the range of 300 to 800 mg a day, with most people receiving maximum benefit at 300 to 500 mg a day.

Clozapine

Clozapine is available in 25- and 100-mg tablets. The initial dosage is usually 25 mg one or two times daily, although a conservative initial dosage is 12.5 mg twice daily. The dosage can then be raised gradually (25 mg a day every 2 or 3 days) to 300 mg a day in divided dosages, usually two or three times daily. Dosages up to 900 mg a day can be used.

Weekly WBC counts are indicated to monitor the patient for the development of agranulocytosis. Although monitoring is expensive, early indication of agranulocytosis can prevent a fatal outcome. If the WBC count is below 2000 cells per mm^3 or the granulocyte count is below 1000 per mm^3, clozapine should be discontinued, a hematological consultation should be obtained, and the obtaining of a bone marrow sample should be considered. Persons with agranulocytosis should not be reexposed to the drug. Persons can obtain the WBC count through any laboratory. Proof of monitoring must be presented to the pharmacist to obtain the medication.

Ziprasidone

Ziprasidone dosing should be initiated at 40 mg a day, divided into two daily doses. Studies have shown efficacy in the range of 80 to 160 mg a day, divided twice daily. Ziprasidone is expected to be the first SDA to be available in both oral and long-acting (depot) injectable formulations.

Switching from Typical to Atypical Antipsychotic Drugs

Although the transition from a dopamine receptor antagonist to an SDA may be made abruptly, it is probably wiser to taper off the dopamine receptor antagonist slowly while titrating up the SDA. Clozapine and olanzapine both have anticholinergic effects, and the transition from one to the other can usually be accomplished with little risk of cholinergic rebound. The transition from risperidone to olanzapine is best accomplished by tapering the risperidone off over 3 weeks while simultaneously beginning olanzapine directly at 10 mg a day. Risperidone, quetiapine, and ziprasidone lack anticholinergic effects, and the abrupt transition from a dopamine receptor antagonist, olanzapine, or clozapine to one of these agents may cause cholinergic rebound, which consists of excessive salivation, nausea, vomiting, and diarrhea. The risk of cholinergic rebound can be mitigated by initially augmenting risperidone, quetiapine, or ziprasidone with an anticholinergic drug, which is then tapered off slowly. Any initiation and termination of SDA use should be accomplished gradually.

It is wise to overlap administration of the new drug with the old drug. Of interest, some people have a more robust clinical response while taking the two agents during the transition, then regress on monotherapy with the newer drug. Little is known about the effectiveness and safety of a strategy of combining one SDA with another SDA or with a dopamine receptor antagonist.

Persons receiving regular injections of depot formulations of a dopamine receptor antagonist who are to switch to SDA use are given the first dose of the SDA on the day the next injection is due. At present, SDAs are only available in oral formulations.

Persons who developed agranulocytosis while taking clozapine can safely switch to olanzapine use, although initiation of olanzapine use in the midst of clozapine-induced agranulocytosis can prolong the time of recovery from the usual 3 to 4 days up to 11 to 12 days. It is prudent to wait for resolution of agranulocytosis before initiating olanzapine use. Emergence or recurrence of agranulocytosis has not been reported with olanzapine, even in persons who developed it while taking clozapine.

For a more detailed discussion of this topic, see van Kammen DP, Marder SR: Serotonin-Dopamine Antagonists, Sec 31.26, p 2455, in CTP/VII.

30

Sibutramine

Sibutramine (Meridia) is a novel appetite suppressant used to treat obesity and is pharmacologically similar to several antidepressant drugs, especially venlafaxine (Effexor). Sibutramine is a reuptake inhibitor of serotonin, norepinephrine, and, to a lesser extent, dopamine, but it lacks any clinical antidepressant effect.

CHEMISTRY

The structural formula of sibutramine is shown in Figure 30–1.

PHARMACOLOGICAL ACTIONS

Sibutramine is rapidly absorbed after oral administration and promptly metabolized to its active metabolites, called M_1 and M_2, which reach their peak plasma concentrations in 3 to 4 hours. The half-lives of M_1 and M_2 are 14 to 16 hours, which permits once-daily dosing.

Sibutramine's active metabolites are inhibitors of reuptake of serotonin, norepinephrine, and, to a lesser degree, dopamine. Unlike dexfenfluramine and fenfluramine (both withdrawn from the U.S. market), which promote massive systemic release of serotonin, cause cardiac and pulmonic fibrosis, and eliminate serotonergic axons in the brain, sibutramine prolongs the action of monoamines released normally into the synaptic cleft in the process of neurotransmission.

THERAPEUTIC INDICATIONS

Sibutramine is indicated for use as part of a supervised weight loss and maintenance program that includes dietary restrictions. Sibutramine is indicated for use by persons with a body-mass index (BMI) of 30 or above or a BMI of 27 or above in the presence of atherosclerosis risk factors such as hypertension, diabetes mellitus, or hypercholesterolemia. Sibutramine is effective only while it is being taken, provided that dietary guidelines are strictly followed.

Sibutramine responsiveness is defined as loss of 4 or more pounds in the first 4 weeks of use. Some 60 percent of sibutramine responders who continue to take the drug for at least 6 months will lose at least 5 percent of their initial body weight. The weight loss can be maintained for at least 12 months with continuous use of the drug. Sibutramine may also improve glucose tolerance in persons with non-insulin-dependent diabetes mellitus.

Some clinicians promote the combined use of sibutramine and phentermine (Ionamin, Adipex-P) or the use of sibutramine together with orlistat (Xenical). However, no controlled trials support these combinations.

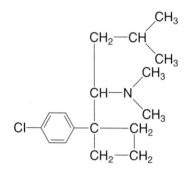

Figure 30-1. Molecular structure of sibutramine.

PRECAUTIONS AND ADVERSE EFFECTS

The most common adverse effects associated with use of sibutramine are headache, dry mouth, anorexia, insomnia, and constipation. The most serious effects associated with its use are elevations of blood pressure and pulse rate. On average, persons who take 5 to 20 mg a day of sibutramine experience a rise in mean systolic and diastolic blood pressure of 1 to 3 mm Hg and a rise in pulse rate of 4 to 5 beats per minute. The elevations in blood pressure and pulse are dose dependent and may reach clinically significant levels ($\geq$15 mm Hg systolic and $\geq$ 10 mm Hg diastolic) at dosages exceeding 10 mg a day. Because of these cardiovascular effects, sibutramine should be used cautiously by persons with a history of hypertension, atherosclerotic heart disease, myocardial infarction, congestive heart failure, arrhythmias, or stroke. It may also cause mydriasis, which could exacerbate narrow-angle glaucoma.

DRUG INTERACTIONS

Sibutramine should not be taken within 14 days of use of a monoamine oxidase inhibitor. Sibutramine could potentially precipitate a serotonin syndrome if used concurrently with serotonin specific reuptake inhibitors, tricyclic antidepressants, triptan antimigraine drugs, dihydroergotamine (D.H.T. 45), dextromethorphan (Dimetane, Sudafed), meperidine (Demerol), pentazocine (Talwin, Talacen), fentanyl (Duragesic), lithium (Eskalith), or tryptophan. However, there have been no reports of sibutramine-associated serotonin syndrome at this time. Sibutramine could raise blood pressure if used together with prescription or nonprescription preparations containing phenylpropanolamine (Triaminic, Dura-Vent, others), ephedrine (Rynatuss, others), or pseudoephedrine (numerous combination products). Ketoconazole (Nizoral), erythromycin (several), and cimetidine (Tagamet) may raise plasma concentrations of sibutramine modestly.

LABORATORY INTERFERENCES

Sibutramine has not been reported to interfere with any laboratory tests. However, a transient elevation of hepatic transaminase concentration may occur in some patients.

DOSAGE AND CLINICAL GUIDELINES

Pretreatment evaluation for use of sibutramine should include a review of the cardiovascular system and identification of risk factors for atherosclerosis as well as a complete drug history. Physical examination should include a series of at least three separate determinations of blood pressure and pulse and should focus on signs of atherosclerosis. Laboratory examination should focus on evidence for diabetes mellitus. Documentation should include evidence that the pretreatment weight falls into the category defined in the product literature as obese.

Sibutramine is available in 5-, 10-, and 15-mg capsules. The starting dosage of sibutramine is 10 mg once a day. If weight loss fails to occur after 4 weeks, then sibutramine probably will not be effective. If weight loss is less than 4 pounds in the first 4 weeks, then the dosage may be increased to 15 to 20 mg a day. If the 10-mg daily dose is not tolerated, then the dosage should be lowered to 5 mg a day.

For a more detailed discussion of this topic, see Brownell KD, Wadden TA: Obesity, Sec 25.3, p 1787, in CTP/VII.

31

Sildenafil

Sildenafil (Viagra) has revolutionized people's expectations of sexual gratification and has rapidly created its own therapeutic niche. Although indicated only for treatment of male erectile dysfunction, sildenafil has been shown to improve the sexual functioning of both men and women.

CHEMISTRY

Sildenafil is a heterocyclic piperazine derivative of zaprinast, a weak and nonselective phosphodiesterase (PDE) inhibitor. Pure sildenafil is poorly soluble in water. Its structural formula is shown in Figure 31–1.

PHARMACOLOGICAL ACTIONS

Sildenafil is fairly rapidly absorbed from the gastrointestinal (GI) tract, and its bioavailability is 40 percent. Maximum plasma concentrations of oral sildenafil are reached in 30 to 120 minutes (median, 60 minutes) in the fasting state. Because of its lipophilicity, concomitant ingestion with a high-fat meal delays the rate of absorption by up to 60 minutes and reduces the peak concentration by one quarter. Sildenafil is principally metabolized by the cytochrome P450 (CYP) 3A4 system, which may lead to clinically significant drug-drug interactions, not all of which have been documented. Excretion of 80 percent of the dose is via feces, and another 13 percent is eliminated in the urine. Elimination is reduced in persons over age 65, which results in plasma concentrations 40 percent higher than in persons aged 18 to 45. Elimination is also reduced in the presence of severe renal or hepatic insufficiency.

The principal cellular site of action of sildenafil is the enzyme PDE5, which acts on arteriolar smooth muscle cells of the corpus cavernosum of the penis. PDE5 is efficiently and selectively inhibited by sildenafil, which allows blood to fill the corpus cavernosum, causing erection to occur.

The clinician needs to be aware of the important clinical observation that sildenafil does not by itself create an erection. Rather, the mental state of sexual arousal brought on by erotic stimulation must first lead to activity in the penile nerves. Excited nerve endings then release nitric oxide into the cavernosum, triggering the erectile cascade. Sildenafil maintains the resulting erection by its enzymatic action. Thus, sildenafil permits full advantage to be taken of a sexually exciting stimulus, but it is not a substitute for foreplay and emotional arousal.

THERAPEUTIC INDICATIONS

Erectile dysfunctions have traditionally been classified as organic, psychogenic, or mixed. Over the last 20 years, the prevailing view of the cause of erectile dys-

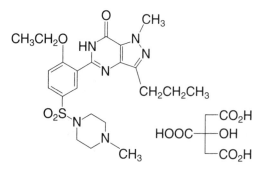

Figure 31-1. Molecular structure of sildenafil.

function has shifted away from the psychological cause toward the organic. Organic causes include diabetes mellitus, hypertension, hypercholesterolemia, cigarette smoking, peripheral vascular disease, pelvic or spinal cord injury, pelvic or abdominal surgery (especially prostate surgery), multiple sclerosis, peripheral neuropathy, and Parkinson's disease. Erectile dysfunction is often induced by alcohol and other substances of abuse and by prescription drugs.

Sildenafil is effective regardless of the baseline severity of erectile dysfunction, cause of erectile dysfunction, race, or age. Among those responding to sildenafil are men with coronary artery disease, hypertension, other cardiac disease, peripheral vascular disease, diabetes mellitus, depression, coronary artery bypass graft (CABG), radical prostatectomy, transurethral resection of the prostate, spina bifida, and spinal cord injury, as well as persons taking antidepressants, antipsychotics, antihypertensives, and diuretics.

Sildenafil has been reported to reverse selective serotonin reuptake inhibitor (SSRI)-induced anorgasmia in both men and women. There are anecdotal reports of a therapeutic effect on sexual inhibition in women as well.

PRECAUTIONS AND ADVERSE REACTIONS

The most important potential adverse effect associated with use of sildenafil is myocardial infarction (MI). The manufacturer and the U.S. Food and Drug Administration (FDA) distinguished the risk of MI due directly to sildenafil from that due to underlying conditions such as hypertension, atherosclerotic heart disease, diabetes mellitus, and other atherogenic conditions. The FDA concluded that when used according to the approved labeling, sildenafil does not by itself confer an increased risk of death. In addition to the increased oxygen demand and the stress placed on the cardiac muscle by sexual intercourse, which is facilitated by sildenafil, coronary perfusion may be severely compromised by the combined actions of sildenafil and nitrates, but not by sildenafil used alone. Any person with a history of MI, stroke, renal failure, hypertension, or diabetes mellitus and any person over the age of 70 should discuss plans to use sildenafil with an internist or a cardiologist. The cardiac evaluation should specifically address exercise tolerance and the use of nitrates.

Most deaths associated with the use of sildenafil have occurred during or after sexual intercourse and occur rarely.

Use of sildenafil is contraindicated in persons who are taking organic nitrates in any form. These medications include nitroglycerin, isosorbide mononitrate (Imdur, ISMO, Monoket), isosorbide dinitrate (Isordil, Sorbitrate), erythatyl tetranitrate, pentaerythritol tetranitrate, and sodium nitroprusside (Nipride). These agents are listed in Table 31–1. Amyl nitrate (poppers), a popular substance of abuse used by gay men to enhance the intensity of orgasm, should not be used with sildenafil. This combination has caused several deaths. Organic nitrates raise circulating nitric oxide concentrations and potentiate the nitric oxide signaling pathway that causes vasodilation. Use of 100 mg sildenafil caused an average drop in blood pressure of 10 mm Hg in normal volunteers; more-significant drops in blood pressure occur in patients concurrently taking organic nitrates. Precipitous lowering of blood pressure can reduce coronary perfusion to the point of causing MI.

Adverse effects are dose dependent, occurring at a higher rate with a dose of 100 mg than with 25 or 50 mg. The most common adverse effects are headache, flushing, and stomach pain. Other, less common adverse effects include nasal congestion, urinary tract infection, abnormal vision (colored tinge [usually blue], increased sensitivity to light, or blurred vision), diarrhea, dizziness, and rash. No cases of priapism were reported in premarketing trials. Supportive management is indicated in cases of overdosage.

No data are available on the effects of sildenafil on human fetal growth and development. However, sildenafil is never an essential treatment, and it should not be used during pregnancy.

TABLE 31–1
GENERIC AND TRADE NAMES OF SOME
COMMONLY USED ORGANIC NITRATES

Nitroglycerin
 Deponit (transdermal)
 Minitran
 Nitrek
 Nitro-Bid
 Nitrodisc
 Nitro-Dur
 Nitrogard
 Nitroglyn
 Nitrolingual Spray
 Nitrol Ointment (Appli-Kit)
 Nitrong
 Nitro-Par
 Nitrostat
 Nitro-Time
 Transderm-Nitro
Isosorbide mononitrate
 Imdur
 Ismo
 Monoket Tablets
Isosorbide dinitrate
 Dilatrate-SR
 Isordil
 Sorbitrate
Erythatyl tetranitrate
Pentaerythritol tetranitrate
Sodium nitroprusside

DRUG INTERACTIONS

The major route of sildenafil metabolism is through CYP 3A4, and the minor route is through CYP 2C9. Inducers or inhibitors of these enzymes will therefore affect the plasma concentration and half-life of sildenafil. For example, 800 mg of cimetidine (Tagamet), a nonspecific CYP inhibitor, increases plasma sildenafil concentrations by 56 percent, and erythromycin (E-mycin) increases plasma sildenafil concentrations by 182 percent. Other, stronger inhibitors of CYP 3A4 include ketoconazole (Nizoral), itraconazole (Sporanox), and mibefradil (Posicor). In contrast, rifampicin, a CYP 3A4 inducer, decreases plasma concentrations of sildenafil.

LABORATORY INTERFERENCES

No laboratory interferences have yet been described for sildenafil.

DOSAGE AND CLINICAL GUIDELINES

Sildenafil is available as 25-, 50-, and 100-mg tablets. The recommended dose of sildenafil is 50 mg taken by mouth 1 hour prior to intercourse. However, sildenafil may take effect within 30 minutes. The duration of the effect is usually 4 hours, but in healthy young men, the effect may persist for 8 to 12 hours. Based on effectiveness and adverse effects, the dose should be titrated between 25 and 100 mg. Sildenafil is recommended for use no more than once a day, although in the earliest clinical trials for treatment of angina, doses up to 50 mg every 8 hours for 10 consecutive days were generally well tolerated. The dosing guidelines for use by women, an off-label use, are the same as those for men.

Increased plasma concentrations of sildenafil may occur in persons over 65 years of age and those with cirrhosis or severe renal impairment or using CYP 3A4 inhibitors. A starting dose of 25 mg should be used in these circumstances.

An investigational nasal spray formulation of sildenafil has been developed that acts within 5 to 15 minutes of administration. This formulation is highly water soluble, and it is rapidly absorbed directly into the bloodstream. Such a formulation would permit more ease of use.

For a more detailed discussion of this topic, see Sadock VA: Normal Human Sexuality and Sexual Dysfunctions, Sec 19.1a, p 1577, in CTP/VII.

32

Sympathomimetics and Related Drugs

The sympathomimetics (also referred to as psychostimulants and analeptics) used in psychiatry include methylphenidate (Ritalin, Concerta), dextroamphetamine (Dexedrine), a combination of amphetamine and dextroamphetamine (Adderall), and pemoline (Cylert), now considered a second-line agent, because of rare but potentially fatal hepatic toxicity. The drugs are indicated for the treatment of attention-deficit/hyperactivity disorder (ADHD) and narcolepsy and are also effective in the treatment of depressive disorders in special populations (e.g., the medically ill). Both amphetamine and nonamphetamine sympathomimetics have been used as appetite suppressants. Other sympathomimetics used for appetite suppression include methamphetamine (Desoxyn), benzphetamine (Didrex), phentermine (Adipex-P, Fastin, Ionamin), diethylpropion (Tenuate), phenmetrazine (Preludin), phendimetrazine (Bontril, Adipost), and mazindol (Sanorex, Mazanor). A novel stimulant approved for treatment of narcolepsy in the United States, modafinil (Provigil), has been used as an antidepressant in France but is not used for treatment of ADHD.

CHEMISTRY

The molecular structures of dextroamphetamine, methylphenidate, pemoline, methamphetamine, phentermine, and modafinil are shown in Figure 32–1.

PHARMACOLOGICAL ACTIONS

All of these drugs are well absorbed from the gastrointestinal tract. Dextroamphetamine and Adderall reach peak plasma concentrations in 2 to 3 hours and have a half-life of about 6 hours, thereby necessitating once- or twice-daily dosing. Methylphenidate is available in immediate-release (Ritalin), sustained-release (Ritalin SR), and extended release (Concerta) formulations. Immediate-release methylphenidate reaches peak plasma concentrations in 1 to 2 hours and has a short half-life of 2 to 3 hours, thereby necessitating multiple-daily dosing. The sustained-release formulation reaches peak plasma concentrations in 4 to 5 hours and doubles the effective half-life of methylphenidate. The extended-release formulation reaches peak plasma concentrations in 6 to 8 hours and is designed to be effective for 12 hours in once-daily dosing. Pemoline reaches peak plasma concentrations in 2 to 4 hours and has a half-life of about 12 hours, and modafinil reaches peak plasma concentrations in 2 to 4 hours and has a half-life of 15 hours, thereby allowing once-daily dosing of these two agents.

Methylphenidate, dextroamphetamine, and amphetamine are indirectly acting sympathomimetics, with the primary effect of causing the release of catecholamines from presynaptic neurons. Clinical effectiveness is associated with increased release

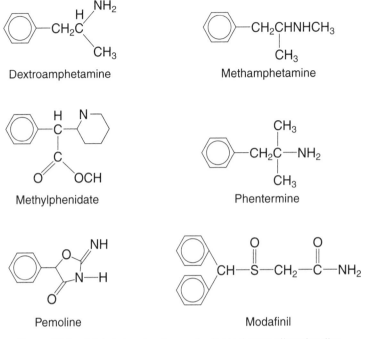

Figure 32–1. Molecular structures of selected sympathomimetics.

of both dopamine and norepinephrine. Dextroamphetamine and methylphenidate are also weak inhibitors of catecholamine reuptake and inhibitors of monoamine oxidase. Pemoline may indirectly stimulate dopaminergic activity by a poorly understood mechanism, but it has little actual sympathomimetic activity. Modafinil triggers brain activity in a pattern distinct from that of dextroamphetamine. Modafinil may inhibit the reuptake of dopamine, but its precise pharmacological site of action is unknown.

THERAPEUTIC INDICATIONS

ADHD

Sympathomimetics are the first-line drugs for treatment of ADHD in children and are effective about 75 percent of the time. Methylphenidate and dextroamphetamine are equally effective and work within 15 to 30 minutes. Pemoline requires 3 to 4 weeks to reach its full efficacy, which nevertheless may be less than that of methylphenidate and dextroamphetamine. The drugs decrease hyperactivity, increase attentiveness, and reduce impulsivity. They may also reduce comorbid oppositional behaviors associated with ADHD. Many persons take these drugs throughout their schooling and beyond. In responsive persons, use of a sympathomimetic may be a critical determinant of scholastic success.

Sympathomimetics improve the core ADHD symptoms of hyperactivity, impulsivity, and inattentiveness and permit improved social interactions with teachers, family, other adults, and peers. The success of long-term treatment of ADHD with sympathomimetics, which are efficacious for most of the various constellations of ADHD symptoms present from childhood to adulthood, supports a model in which ADHD results from a genetically determined neurochemical imbalance that requires lifelong pharmacological management.

Methylphenidate is the most commonly used initial agent, at a dosage of 5 to 10 mg every 3 to 4 hours. Dosages may be increased to a maximum of 20 mg four times daily or 1 mg/kg a day. Use of the 20-mg sustained-release formulation to achieve 6 hours of benefit and eliminate the need for dosing at school is supported by many experts, although other authorities feel it is less effective than the immediate-release formulation. Dextroamphetamine is about twice as potent as methylphenidate on a per milligram basis and provides 6 to 8 hours of benefit. Some 70 percent of nonresponders to one sympathomimetic may benefit from another. All the sympathomimetic drugs should be tried before switching to drugs of a different class. The previous dictum that sympathomimetics worsen tics and therefore should be avoided by persons with comorbid ADHD and tic disorders has been questioned more recently because of reports that small-to-moderate dosages of sympathomimetics may be well tolerated without causing an increase in the frequency and severity of the tics. Alternatives to sympathomimetics for ADHD include bupropion (Wellbutrin), venlafaxine (Effexor), guanfacine (Tenex), clonidine (Catapres), and tricyclic drugs.

Short-term use of the sympathomimetics induces a euphoric feeling; however, tolerance develops for both the euphoric feeling and the sympathomimetic activity. Importantly, tolerance does not develop for the therapeutic effects in ADHD.

Narcolepsy

Narcolepsy consists of sudden sleep attacks *(narcolepsy),* sudden loss of postural tone *(cataplexy),* loss of voluntary motor control going into (hypnagogic) or coming out of (hypnopompic) sleep *(sleep paralysis),* and hypnagogic or hypnopompic *hallucinations.* Sympathomimetics reduce narcoleptic sleep attacks and also improve wakefulness in other types of hypersomnolent states. Sympathomimetics are used to maintain wakefulness and accuracy of motor performance in persons subject to sleep deprivation, such as pilots and military personnel. Persons with narcolepsy, unlike persons with ADHD, may develop tolerance for the therapeutic effects of the sympathomimetics.

Modafinil has been studied only as an antisomnolence agent for treatment of narcolepsy and related disorders. In direct comparison with amphetamine-like drugs, modafinil is equally effective at maintaining wakefulness, with generally fewer adverse effects. Further studies are needed to determine whether modafinil improves the symptoms of ADHD.

Depressive Disorders

Sympathomimetics may be used for treatment-resistant depressive disorders, usually as augmentation of standard antidepressant drug therapy. Possible indications for use of sympathomimetics as monotherapy include depression in the elderly, who are at increased risk for adverse effects from standard antidepressant drugs; depression in medically ill persons, especially persons with acquired immune deficiency syndrome (AIDS); obtundation due to chronic use of opioids; and clinical situations in which a rapid response is important but for which electroconvulsive therapy (ECT) is contraindicated. Depressed patients with abulia and anergia may also benefit.

Dextroamphetamine may be useful in differentiating pseudodementia of depression from dementia. A depressed person generally responds to a 5-mg dose with increased alertness and improved cognition. Sympathomimetics are thought to provide only short-term benefit (2 to 4 weeks) for depression, because most persons rapidly develop tolerance for the antidepressant effects of the drugs. However, some clinicians report that long-term treatment with sympathomimetics can benefit some persons.

Encephalopathy Due to Brain Injury

Sympathomimetics increase alertness, cognition, motivation, and motor performance in persons with neurological deficits caused by strokes, trauma, tumors, or chronic infections. Treatment with sympathomimetics may permit earlier and more robust participation in rehabilitative programs. Poststroke lethargy and apathy may respond to long-term use of sympathomimetics.

Obesity

Sympathomimetics are used in the treatment of obesity because of their anorexia-inducing effects. Because tolerance develops for the anorectic effects and because of the drugs' high abuse potential, their use for this indication is limited. Of the sympathomimetic drugs, phentermine is the most widely used for appetite suppression. Phentermine was the second half of "fen-phen," an off-label combination of fenfluramine and phentermine, widely used to promote weight loss until fenfluramine and dexfenfluramine were withdrawn from commercial availability because of an association with cardiac valvular insufficiency, primary pulmonary hypertension, and irreversible loss of cerebral serotoninergic nerve fibers. The toxicity of fenfluramine is attributed to the fact that it stimulates release of massive amounts of serotonin from nerve endings, a mechanism of action not shared by phentermine. Use of phentermine alone has not been reported to cause the same adverse effects as those caused by fenfluramine or dexfenfluramine.

Careful limitation of caloric intake and judicious exercise are at the core of any successful weight loss program. Sympathomimetic drugs facilitate loss of, at most, an additional fraction of a pound per week. Sympathomimetic drugs are effective ap-

TABLE 32–1
MANAGEMENT OF COMMON STIMULANT-INDUCED ADVERSE EFFECTS IN ATTENTION-DEFICIT/HYPERACTIVITY DISORDER

Adverse Effect	Management
Anorexia, nausea, weight loss	• Administer stimulant with meals.
	• Use caloric-enhanced supplements. Discourage forcing meals.
	• If using pemoline, check liver function tests.
Insomnia, nightmares	• Administer stimulants earlier in day.
	• Change to short-acting preparations.
	• Discontinue afternoon or evening dosing.
	• Consider adjunctive treatment (e.g., antihistamines, clonidine, antidepressants).
Dizziness	• Monitor blood pressure.
	• Encourage fluid intake.
	• Change to long-acting form.
Rebound phenomena	• Overlap stimulant dosing.
	• Change to long-acting preparation or combine long- and short-acting preparations.
	• Consider adjunctive or alternative treatment (e.g., clonidine, antidepressants).
Irritability	• Assess timing of phenomena (during peak or withdrawal phase).
	• Evaluate comorbid symptoms.
	• Reduce dose.
	• Consider adjunctive or alternative treatment (e.g., lithium, antidepressants, anticonvulsants).
Dysphoria, moodiness, agitation	• Consider comorbid diagnosis (e.g., mood disorder).
	• Reduce dose or change to long-acting preparation.
	• Consider adjunctive or alternative treatment (e.g., lithium, anticonvulsants, antidepressants).

From Wilens TE, Biederman J: The stimulants. In: *The Psychiatric Clinics of North America: Pediatric Psychopharmacology,* Shaffer D, editor. Saunders, Philadelphia, 1992, with permission.

petite suppressants only for the first few weeks of use; then the anorexigenic effects tend to decrease.

PRECAUTIONS AND ADVERSE REACTIONS

The most common adverse effects associated with amphetamine-like drugs are stomach pain, anxiety, irritability, insomnia, tachycardia, cardiac arrhythmias, and dysphoria. Sympathomimetics cause a decreased appetite, although tolerance usually develops for this effect. The treatment of common adverse effects in children with ADHD is usually straightforward (Table 32–1). The drugs can also cause increases in the heart rate and the blood pressure and may cause palpitations. Less common adverse effects include the induction of movement disorders, such as tics, Tourette's disorder–like symptoms, and dyskinesias, which are often self-limited over 7 to 10 days. If a person taking a sympathomimetic develops one of these movement disorders, a correlation between the dose of the medication and the severity of the disorder must be firmly established prior to adjustments in the medication dosage. In severe cases, augmentation with risperidone (Risperdal), clonidine (Catapres), or guanfacine (Tenex) is necessary. Methylphenidate may worsen tics in one third of persons; these persons fall into two groups: those whose methylphenidate-induced tics resolve immediately upon metabolism of the dosage and a smaller group in whom methylphenidate appears to trigger tics that persist for several months but eventually resolve spontaneously.

Longitudinal studies do not indicate that sympathomimetics cause growth suppression. Sympathomimetics may exacerbate glaucoma, hypertension, cardiovascular disorders, hyperthyroidism, anxiety disorders, psychotic disorders, and seizure disorders.

High dosages of sympathomimetics can cause dry mouth, pupillary dilation, bruxism, formication, excessive ebullience, restlessness, and emotional lability. Long-term use of high dosages can cause a delusional disorder that resembles paranoid schizophrenia. Overdosages of sympathomimetics result in hypertension, tachycardia, hyperthermia, toxic psychosis, delirium, and occasionally seizures. Overdosages of sympathomimetics can also result in death, often due to cardiac arrhythmias. Seizures can be treated with benzodiazepines, cardiac effects with β-adrenergic receptor antagonists, fever with cooling blankets, and delirium with dopamine receptor antagonists.

The most limiting adverse effect of sympathomimetics is their association with psychological and physical dependence. At the doses used for treatment of ADHD, development of psychological dependence virtually never occurs. A larger concern is the presence of adolescent or adult cohabitants who might confiscate the supply of sympathomimetics for abuse or sale.

The use of sympathomimetics should be avoided during pregnancy, especially during the first trimester. Dextroamphetamine and methylphenidate pass into the breast milk, and it is not known whether pemoline or modafinil do.

A review of postmarketing experience with pemoline from 1975 to 1996 found 13 cases of acute hepatic failure, 10 of which were in children. This prompted the Food and Drug Administration (FDA) to change the package insert to recommend that pemoline no longer be considered first-line therapy for ADHD.

DRUG INTERACTIONS

The coadministration of sympathomimetics and tricyclic or tetracyclic antidepressants, warfarin (Coumadin), primidone (Mysoline), phenobarbital (Luminal), phenytoin (Dilantin), or phenylbutazone (Butazolidin) decreases the metabolism of these compounds, resulting in increased plasma levels. Sympathomimetics decrease the therapeutic efficacy of many antihypertensive drugs, especially guanethidine (Esimil, Ismelin). The sympathomimetics should be used with extreme caution with monoamine oxidase inhibitors.

LABORATORY INTERFERENCES

Dextroamphetamine may elevate plasma corticosteroid levels and interfere falsely with some assay methods for urinary corticosteroids.

DOSAGE AND ADMINISTRATION

The dosage ranges and the available preparations for sympathomimetics are presented in Table 32–2. Dextroamphetamine, methylphenidate, amphetamine, benzphetamine, and methamphetamine are schedule II drugs and in some states require

TABLE 32–2
SYMPATHOMIMETICS COMMONLY USED IN PSYCHIATRY

Generic Name	Trade Name	Preparations	Initial Daily Dose	Usual Daily Dose for ADHD[a]	Usual Daily Dose for Narcolepsy	Maximum Daily Dose
Amphetamine-dextroamphetamine	Adderall	5-, 10-, 20-, 30-mg tablets	5–10 mg	20–30 mg	5–60	Children: 40 mg Adults: 60 mg
Dextroamphetamine	Dexedrine, DextroStat	5-, 10-, 15-mg extended-release (ER) capsules; 5-, 10-mg tablets	5–10 mg	20–30 mg	5–60	Children: 40 mg Adults: 60 mg
Modafinil	Provigil	100-, 200-mg tablets	100 mg	Not used	400 mg	400 mg
Methamphetamine	Desoxyn	5-mg tablets; 5-, 10-, 15-mg ER tablets	5–10 mg	20–25 mg	Not generally used	45 mg
Methylphenidate	Ritalin, Methidate, Methylin, Attenade	5-, 10-, 20-mg tablets; 10-, 20-mg SR tablets	5–10 mg	5–60 mg	20–30 mg	Children: 80 mg Adults: 90 mg
Concerta	Concerta	18-, 36-mg ER tablets	18 mg	18–54 mg	Not yet established	54 mg
Pemoline	Cylert	18.75-, 37.5-, 75-mg tablets; 37.5 chewable tablets	37.5 mg	56.25–75 mg	Not used	112.5 mg

[a] For children 6 years of age or older.

triplicate prescriptions. Phendimetrazine and phenmetrazine are schedule III drugs, and modafinil, phentermine, diethylpropion, and mazindol are schedule IV drugs.

Pretreatment evaluation should include an evaluation of the person's cardiac function, with particular attention to the presence of hypertension or tachyarrhythmias. The clinician should also examine the person for the presence of movement disorders, such as tics and dyskinesia, because these conditions can be exacerbated by the administration of sympathomimetics. If tics are present, many experts will not use sympathomimetics, but will instead choose clonidine or antidepressants. However, recent data indicate that sympathomimetics may cause only a mild increase in motor tics and may actually suppress vocal tics. Liver function and renal function should be assessed, and dosages of sympathomimetics should be reduced for persons with impaired metabolism. In the case of pemoline, any elevation of liver enzymes is a compelling reason to discontinue the medication.

Persons with ADHD can take immediate-release methylphenidate at 8 AM, 12 noon, and 4 PM. Dextroamphetamine, Adderall, sustained-release methylphenidate, or 18 mg extended-release methylphenidate may be taken once at 8 AM. Pemoline is taken at 8 AM. The starting dose of methylphenidate ranges from 2.5 mg regular to 20 mg sustained-release in children and 90 mg daily in adults. If this is inadequate, the dosage may be increased to a maximum dosage of 80 mg. The dosage of dextroamphetamine is 2.5 to 40 mg a day up to 0.5 mg/kg a day. Pemoline is given in dosages of 18.75 to 112.5 mg a day. Liver function tests should be monitored when using pemoline. Although it is not clear that the routine liver screening can predict acute liver failure due to pemoline, it is certainly necessary to stop pemoline use if screening tests give any hint of hepatic dysfunction. Children are generally more sensitive to adverse effects than are adults. Dosing for treatment of narcolepsy and depression is comparable to that for treatment of ADHD.

The starting dosage of modafinil is 200 mg in the morning in medically healthy individuals and 100 mg in the morning in persons with hepatic impairment. Some persons take a second 100- or 200-mg dose in the afternoon. The maximum recommended daily dosage is 400 mg, although dosages of 600 to 1200 mg a day have been used safely. Adverse effects become prominent at dosages above 400 mg a day. Compared with amphetamine-like drugs, modafinil promotes wakefulness but produces both less attentiveness and less irritability. Some persons with excessive daytime sleepiness extend the activity of the morning modafinil dose with an afternoon dose of methylphenidate.

Many psychiatrists believe that amphetamine use has been overly regulated by governmental authorities. Amphetamines are listed as schedule II drugs by the U.S. Drug Enforcement Agency (DEA). In some states physicians must use triplicate prescriptions for such drugs; one copy is filed with a state government agency. Such mandates worry both patients and physicians about breaches in confidentiality, and physicians are concerned that their prescribing practices may be misinterpreted by official agencies. Consequently, some physicians may withhold prescription of sympathomimetics, even from persons who may benefit from the medications.

For a more detailed discussion of this topic, see Fawcett J: Sympathomimetics, Sec 31.27, p 2474, in CTP/VII.

33

Thyroid Hormones

Thyroid hormones—levothyroxine (Synthroid, Levothroid, Levoxine) and liothyronine (Cytomel)—are used in psychiatry either alone or as augmentation to treat persons with depression or rapid-cycling bipolar I disorder. They can convert an antidepressant-nonresponsive person into an antidepressant-responsive person. Thyroid hormones are also used as replacement therapy for persons treated with lithium (Eskalith) who have developed a hypothyroid state.

CHEMISTRY

Liothyronine and levothyroxine are the levorotatory enantiomers of the endogenous hormones triiodothyronine (T_3) and thyroxine (T_4), respectively. The molecular structures of levothyroxine and liothyronine are shown in Figure 33–1.

PHARMACOLOGICAL ACTIONS

Thyroid hormones are administered orally, and their absorption from the gastrointestinal tract is variable. Absorption is increased if the drug is administered on an empty stomach. In the brain, thyroxine crosses the blood–brain barrier and diffuses into neurons, where it is converted into triiodothyronine, which is the physiologically active form. The half-life of T_4 is 6 to 7 days, and that of T_3 is 1 to 2 days.

The mechanism of action for thyroid hormone effects on antidepressant efficacy is unknown. Thyroid hormone binds to intracellular receptors that regulate the transcription of a wide range of genes, including several receptors for neurotransmitters.

THERAPEUTIC INDICATIONS

The major indication for thyroid hormones in psychiatry is as an adjuvant to antidepressants. There is no clear correlation between the laboratory measures of thyroid function and the response to thyroid hormone supplementation of antidepressants. If a patient has not responded to a 6-week course of antidepressants at appropriate dosages, adjuvant therapy with either lithium or a thyroid hormone is an alternative. Most clinicians use adjuvant lithium before trying a thyroid hormone. Several controlled trials have indicated that liothyronine use converts about 50 percent of antidepressant nonresponders to responders.

The dosage of liothyronine is 25 or 50 μg a day added to the patient's antidepressant regimen. Liothyronine has been used primarily as an adjuvant for tricyclic drugs; however, evidence suggests that liothyronine augments the effects of all the antidepressant drugs. A trial of liothyronine supplementation should last 7 to 14

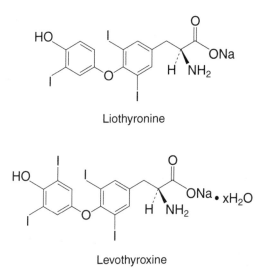

Figure 33-1. Molecular structures of liothyronine and levothyroxine.

days. If liothyronine supplementation is successful, it should be continued for 2 months, then tapered off at the rate of 12.5 mg a day every 3 to 7 days.

Thyroid hormones have not been shown to cause particular problems in pediatric or geriatric patients; however, the hormones should be used with caution in the elderly, who may have occult heart disease.

PRECAUTIONS AND ADVERSE REACTIONS

At the dosages usually used for augmentation—25 to 50 μg a day—adverse effects occur infrequently. The most common adverse effects associated with thyroid hormones are transient headache, weight loss, palpitations, nervousness, diarrhea, abdominal cramps, sweating, tachycardia, increased blood pressure, tremors, and insomnia. Osteoporosis may also occur with long-term treatment, but this has not been found in studies involving liothyronine augmentation. Overdoses of thyroid hormones can lead to cardiac failure and death.

Thyroid hormones should not be taken by persons with cardiac disease, angina, or hypertension. The hormones are contraindicated in thyrotoxicosis and uncorrected adrenal insufficiency and in persons with acute myocardial infarctions. Thyroid hormones can be administered safely to pregnant women, provided that laboratory thyroid indexes are monitored to avoid pregnancy-related hypothyroidism. Thyroid hormones are minimally excreted in the breast milk and have not been shown to cause problems in nursing babies.

DRUG INTERACTIONS

Thyroid hormones can potentiate the effects of warfarin (Coumadin) and other anticoagulants by increasing the catabolism of clotting factors. Thyroid hormones may increase the insulin requirement for diabetic persons and the digitalis requirement for persons with cardiac disease. Thyroid hormones should not be coadministered with sympathomimetics, ketamine (Ketalar), or maprotiline (Ludiomil) because of the risk of cardiac decompensation. Administration of SSRIs, tricyclic and tetracyclic drugs, lithium, or carbamazepine (Tegretol) can mildly lower serum thyroxine and raise serum thyrotropin concentrations in euthyroid persons or persons taking thyroid replacements. This interaction warrants close serum monitoring and may require an increase in the dosage or initiation of thyroid hormone supplementation.

LABORATORY INTERFERENCES

Levothyroxine has not been reported to interfere with any laboratory test other than thyroid function indexes. Liothyronine, however, suppresses the release of endogenous T_4, thereby lowering the result of any thyroid function test that depends on the measure of T_4.

DOSAGE AND CLINICAL GUIDELINES

Liothyronine is available in 5-, 25-, and 50-μg tablets. Levothyroxine is available in 12.5-, 25-, 50-, 75-, 88-, 100-, 112-, 125-, 150-, 175-, 200-, and 300-μg tablets; it is also available in a 200- and 500-μg parenteral form. The dosage of liothyronine is 25 or 50 μg a day added to the person's antidepressant regimen. Liothyronine has been used as an adjuvant for all the available antidepressant drugs. An adequate trial of liothyronine supplementation should last 2 to 3 weeks. If liothyronine supplementation is successful, it should be continued for 2 months and then tapered off at the rate of 12.5 μg a day every 3 to 7 days.

For a more detailed discussion of this topic, see Joffe RT: Thyroid Hormones, Sec 31.28, p 2478, in CTP/VII.

34

Trazodone

Trazodone (Desyrel) is effective in the treatment of depressive disorders and may be effective in the treatment of panic disorder and obsessive-compulsive disorder. Trazodone is distinctive in having more marked sedative effects than are found with other antidepressants. For this reason it is used to treat insomnia, particularly insomnia induced by selective serotonin reuptake inhibitors (SSRIs).

CHEMISTRY

Trazodone is structurally related to nefazodone (Serzone) and structurally unrelated to the SSRIs, tricyclic and tetracyclic drugs, monoamine oxidase inhibitors (MAOIs), and other currently available antidepressant drugs. The structural formula of trazodone is shown in Figure 34–1.

PHARMACOLOGICAL ACTIONS

Trazodone is readily absorbed from the gastrointestinal tract, reaches peak plasma levels in 1 to 2 hours, and has a half-life of 5 to 9 hours. Trazodone is metabolized in the liver, and 75 percent of its metabolites are excreted in the urine.

Trazodone is a weak inhibitor of serotonin reuptake and a potent antagonist of serotonin 5-HT_{2A} and 5-HT_{2C} receptors. The active metabolite of trazodone is m-chlorophenylpiperazine (mCPP), which is an agonist at 5-HT_{2C} receptors and has a half-life of 14 hours. mCPP has been associated with migraine, anxiety, and weight loss. The adverse effects of trazodone are partially mediated by α_1-adrenergic receptor antagonism.

THERAPEUTIC INDICATIONS

Depressive Disorders

The primary indication for the use of trazodone is major depressive disorder. It is as effective as the standard antidepressants in short-term and long-term treatment of major depressive disorder, although dosages of 250 to 350 mg a day may be necessary for trazodone to have therapeutic benefit comparable to that of other antidepressants. The drug is particularly effective at improving sleep quality. It increases total sleep time, decreases the number and the duration of nighttime awakenings, and decreases the amount of rapid eye movement (REM) sleep. Unlike tricyclic drugs, trazodone does not decrease stage 4 sleep. Trazodone is more useful for depressed persons with anxiety and insomnia than for those with anergia and psychomotor retardation.

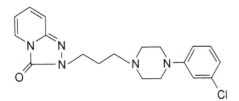

Figure 34-1. Molecular structure of trazodone.

Insomnia

Trazodone is a first-line agent for the treatment of insomnia because of its marked sedative qualities and favorable effects on sleep architecture (see above), combined with its lack of anticholinergic effects. Trazodone is effective for insomnia due to depression and that caused by use of drugs, particularly fluoxetine (Prozac), bupropion (Wellbutrin), and MAOIs. When used as a hypnotic, the usual initial dosage is 50 to 100 mg at bedtime.

Erectile Disorder

Trazodone prolongs erectile time and turgidity in some men with erectile disorder. The dosage for this indication is 150 to 200 mg a day. Trazodone usually potentiates erections resulting from sexual stimulation, but it can trigger the development of priapism in rare cases. Priapism (erection lasting over 3 hours with pain) is a medical emergency that is treated by injecting the corpora cavernosum with an α-adrenergic receptor agonist such as epinephrine (Adrenaline). The use of trazodone for treatment of male erectile dysfunction has diminished considerably since the introduction of sildenafil (Viagra) and alprostadil (Muse, Caverject).

Other Indications

Trazodone may be useful in low dosages (50 mg a day) for controlling severe agitation in children with developmental disabilities and elderly persons with dementia. At dosages above 250 mg a day, trazodone reduces the tension and apprehension associated with generalized anxiety disorder. Trazodone is not effective for treatment of psychotic symptoms, but can be used to treat depression in schizophrenia patients. Trazodone is occasionally effective for treatment of obsessive-compulsive disorder, panic disorder with or without agoraphobia, and bulimia nervosa and as prophylaxis against migraine in children.

PRECAUTIONS AND ADVERSE REACTIONS

The most common adverse effects associated with trazodone are sedation, orthostatic hypotension, dizziness, headache, and nausea. Some persons experience dry mouth or gastric irritation. The drug is not associated with anticholinergic adverse effects, such as urinary retention, weight gain, and constipation. A few case reports have noted an association between trazodone and arrhythmias in persons with pre-existing premature ventricular contractions or mitral valve prolapse. Neutropenia, usually not of clinical significance, may develop, which should be considered if persons have fever or sore throat.

Trazodone may cause significant orthostatic hypotension 4 to 6 hours after a dose is taken, especially if taken concurrently with antihypertensive agents or if a large dose is taken without food. Administration of trazodone with food slows absorption and reduces the peak plasma concentration, thus reducing the risk of orthostatic hypotension.

Trazodone causes priapism, prolonged erection in the absence of sexual stimuli, in 1 out of every 10,000 men. Trazodone-induced priapism usually appears in the first 4 weeks of treatment but may occur as late as 18 months into treatment. It can appear at dosages from 50 to 400 mg a day. In such cases, trazodone use should be discontinued and another antidepressant should be used. Painful erections or erections lasting more than 1 hour are warning signs that warrant immediate discontinuation of the drug and medical evaluation. The first step in the emergency management of priapism is intracavernosal injection of an α_1-adrenergic agonist pressor agent, such as metaraminol (Aramine) or epinephrine.

Trazodone is less likely to precipitate mania in vulnerable persons than are other antidepressant drugs.

The use of trazodone is contraindicated in pregnant and nursing women. Trazodone should be used with caution in persons with hepatic and renal diseases.

DRUG INTERACTIONS

Trazodone potentiates the central nervous system depressant effects of other centrally acting drugs and alcohol. The combination of MAOIs and trazodone should be used with caution. Concurrent use of trazodone and antihypertensives may cause hypotension. Electroconvulsive therapy (ECT) concurrent with trazodone administration should also be avoided.

LABORATORY INTERFERENCES

No known laboratory interferences are associated with the administration of trazodone.

DOSAGE AND CLINICAL GUIDELINES

Trazodone is available in 50-, 100-, 150-, and 300-mg Tablets. Once-a-day dosing is as effective as divided dosing and reduces daytime sedation. The usual starting dose is 50 mg before sleep. The dosage can be increased in increments of 50 mg every 3 days if sedation or orthostatic hypotension does not become a problem. The therapeutic range for trazodone is 200 to 600 mg a day in divided doses. Some reports indicate that dosages of 400 to 600 mg a day are required for maximal therapeutic effects; other reports indicate that 250 to 400 mg a day is sufficient. The dosage may be titrated up to 300 mg a day; then the person can be evaluated for the need for further dosage increases on the basis of the presence or the absence of signs of clinical improvement.

For a more detailed discussion of this topic, see Garlow SJ, Nemeroff CB: Trazodone, Sec 31.29, p 2482, in CTP/VII.

35

Tricyclics and Tetracyclics

The tricyclic antidepressants and the tetracyclic antidepressants (commonly abbreviated as the TCAs) are effective treatments for persons with a wide range of disorders, including depression, panic disorder, generalized anxiety disorder, posttraumatic stress disorder, obsessive-compulsive disorder, eating disorders, and pain syndromes. With the current availability of several less toxic alternatives, including the selective serotonin reuptake inhibitors (SSRIs), bupropion (Wellbutrin), nefazodone (Serzone), venlafaxine (Effexor), trazodone (Desyrel), and mirtazapine (Remeron), the TCAs are no longer widely used for these indications.

CHEMISTRY

The structural formulas of the TCAs are shown in Figure 35–1.

PHARMACOLOGICAL ACTIONS

Absorption from oral administration of most TCAs is complete, and there is significant metabolism from the first-pass effect. Peak plasma concentrations occur within 2 to 8 hours, and the half-lives of the TCAs vary from 10 to 70 hours; nortriptyline (Aventyl, Pamelor), maprotiline (Ludiomil), and particularly protriptyline (Vivactil) can have longer half-lives. The long half-lives allow all the compounds to be given once daily; 5 to 7 days are needed to reach steady-state plasma concentrations. Imipramine pamoate (Tofranil) is a depot form of the drug for intramuscular (i.m.) administration; indications for the use of this preparation are limited.

TCAs undergo hepatic metabolism by the cytochrome P450 enzyme system. Clinically relevant drug interactions may result from competition for enzyme P450 (CYP) 2D6 between TCAs and quinidine, cimetidine (Tagamet), fluoxetine (Prozac), sertraline (Zoloft), paroxetine (Paxil), phenothiazines, carbamazepine (Tegretol), and the type IC antiarrhythmics propafenone (Rythmol) and flecainide (Tambocor). Concomitant administration of TCAs and these inhibitors may slow the metabolism and raise the plasma concentrations of TCAs. Additionally, genetic variations in the activity of CYP 2D6 may account for up to a 40-fold difference in plasma TCA concentrations in different persons. The dosage of the TCA may need to be adjusted to correct changes in the rate of hepatic TCA metabolism.

TCAs block the reuptake of norepinephrine and serotonin and are competitive antagonists at the muscarinic acetylcholine, histamine H_1, and α_1- and α_2-adrenergic receptors (Table 35–1). Amoxapine (Asendin), nortriptyline, desipramine (Norpramin, Pertofrane), and maprotiline have the least anticholinergic activity; doxepin (Adapin, Sinequan) has the most antihistaminergic activity; clomipramine (Anafranil) is the most serotonin-selective of the TCAs. A metabolite of amoxapine

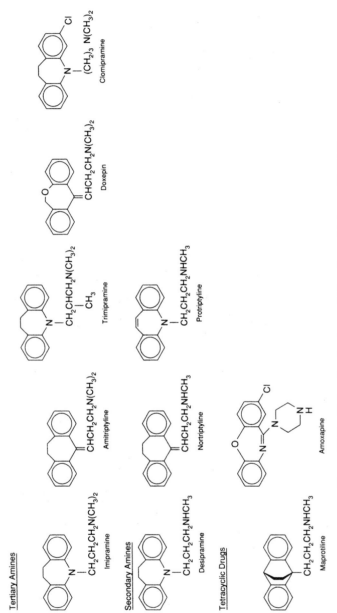

Figure 35–1. Molecular structures of tricyclic and tetracyclic drugs.

TABLE 35-1
NEUROTRANSMITTER EFFECTS OF TRICYCLIC AND TETRACYCLIC DRUGS

Drug	Reuptake Blockade		Receptor Blockade		
	NE	5-HT	Muscarinic ACh	H$_1$	H$_2$
Imipramine	+	+	++	±	±
Desipramine	+++	±	±	−	−
Trimipramine	±	±	++	++	?
Amitriptyline	±	++	+++	++	++
Nortriptyline	++	±	+	±	±
Protriptyline	+++	±	+	+++	−
Amoxapine	++	±	+	±	?
Doxepin	+	±	++	+++	+
Maprotiline	+++	−	+	±	?
Clomipramine	±	++	+	?	?

NE, norepinephrine; 5-HT, serotonin; ACh, acetylcholine; H$_1$, histamine type 1; and H$_2$, histamine type 2.

has potent dopamine-blocking activity, thus causing antipsychotic-like neurological and endocrinological adverse effects.

THERAPEUTIC INDICATIONS

Each of these indications is also an indication for SSRIs, which have widely replaced the TCAs in clinical practice. However, TCAs represent a possible alternative for persons who cannot adapt to the anxiety or gastrointestinal adverse effects of the SSRIs.

Major Depressive Disorder

The treatment of a major depressive episode and the prophylactic treatment of major depressive disorder are the principal indications for using TCAs. The drugs are also effective in the treatment of depression in persons with bipolar I disorder. Melancholic features, prior major depressive episodes, and a family history of depressive disorders increase the likelihood of a therapeutic response. All available TCAs are equally effective in the treatment of depressive disorders. In the case of an individual person, however, one tricyclic or tetracyclic may be effective, whereas another one may be ineffective. The treatment of a major depressive episode with psychotic features almost always requires the coadministration of an antipsychotic drug and an antidepressant.

TCAs appear to be more likely to induce mania in susceptible persons than are SSRIs and bupropion.

Panic Disorder with Agoraphobia

Imipramine is the TCA most studied for panic disorder with agoraphobia, but other TCAs are also effective when taken at the usual antidepressant dosages. Because of the potential initial anxiogenic effects of the TCAs, starting dosages should be small, and the dosage should be titrated upward slowly.

Generalized Anxiety Disorder

The use of doxepin for the treatment of anxiety disorders is approved by the Food and Drug Administration (FDA). Some research data show that imipramine may also be useful, and some clinicians use a chlordiazepoxide-amitriptyline combination (Limbitrol) for mixed anxiety and depressive disorders.

Obsessive-Compulsive Disorder

Obsessive-compulsive disorder appears to respond specifically to clomipramine and the SSRIs. Improvement is usually seen in 2 to 4 weeks, but a gradual improvement may continue for the first 4 to 5 months of treatment. None of the other TCAs appears to be nearly as effective as clomipramine for treatment of this disorder. Clomipramine may also be a drug of choice for depressed persons with marked obsessive features.

Eating Disorders

Both anorexia nervosa and bulimia nervosa have been successfully treated with imipramine, desipramine, and clomipramine; other TCAs may also be effective.

Pain

Chronic neuropathic pain may be directly ameliorated by TCAs. In addition, TCAs can treat the comorbid mood disorders typical of many persons with chronic pain.

Other Disorders

Childhood enuresis is often treated with imipramine. Peptic ulcer disease can be treated with doxepin, which has marked antihistaminergic effects. Other indications for TCAs are narcolepsy, nightmare disorder, and posttraumatic stress disorder. The drugs are sometimes used for treatment of children and adolescents with attention-deficit/hyperactivity disorder, sleepwalking disorder, separation anxiety disorder, and sleep terror disorder. Clomipramine has also been used to treat premature ejaculation, movement disorders, and compulsive behavior in children with autistic disorders; however, because TCAs have caused sudden death in several children and adolescents their use is best avoided in this population.

PRECAUTIONS AND ADVERSE REACTIONS

Table 35–2 lists the adverse-effect profiles of the TCAs.

TABLE 35–2
SIDE EFFECT PROFILE OF TRICYCLIC AND TETRACYCLIC ANTIDEPRESSANTS

	Anticholinergic Effects	Sedation	Orthostatic Hypotension	Seizures	Conduction Abnormalities
Tertiary amines					
Amitriptyline	+ + + +	+ + + +	+ + +	+ + +	+ + + +
Clomipramine	+ + + +	+ + + +	+ + +	+ + +	+ + + +
Doxepin	+ + +	+ + + +	+ +	+ + +	+ +
Imipramine	+ + +	+ + +	+ + + +	+ + +	+ + + +
Trimipramine	+ + + +	+ + + +	+ + +	+ + +	+ + + + +
Secondary amines					
Desipramine	+ +	+ +	+ + +	+ +	+ + +
Nortriptyline	+ + +	+ + +	+	+ +	+ + +
Protriptyline	+ + +	+	+ +	+ +	+ + + +
Tetracyclics					
Amoxapine	+ + +	+ +	+	+ + +	+ +
Maprotiline	+ +	+ + +	+ +	+ + + +	+ + +

+ + + +, high; + + +, moderate; + +, low; +, very low.

Psychiatric Effects

A major adverse effect of all TCAs and other antidepressants is the possibility of inducing a manic episode in both persons with bipolar I disorder and those without a history of bipolar I disorder. This is more likely to occur if there is a history of substance-induced mania. SSRIs and bupropion are considered less likely to precipitate a manic episode than are TCAs. TCAs may also exacerbate psychotic disorders in susceptible persons. At high plasma concentrations, TCAs can cause confusion or delirium.

Anticholinergic Effects

Anticholinergic effects are common with TCAs and often limit the tolerable dosage to relatively low ranges. Some persons may develop a tolerance for the anticholinergic effects with continued treatment. Amitriptyline (Elavil), imipramine, trimipramine (Surmontil), and doxepin are the most anticholinergic drugs; amoxapine, nortriptyline, and maprotiline are less anticholinergic; and desipramine may be the least anticholinergic. Anticholinergic effects include dry mouth, constipation, blurred vision, delirium, and urinary retention. Sugarless gum, candy, or fluoride lozenges can alleviate the dry mouth. Bethanechol (Urecholine), 25 to 50 mg three or four times a day, may reduce urinary hesitancy and may be helpful in erectile dysfunction when the drug is taken 30 minutes before sexual intercourse. Narrow-angle glaucoma can also be aggravated by anticholinergic drugs, and the precipitation of glaucoma requires emergency treatment with a miotic agent. TCAs should be avoided in persons with narrow-angle glaucoma, and an SSRI should be substituted. Severe anticholinergic effects can lead to a central nervous system (CNS) anticholinergic syndrome with confusion and delirium, especially if TCAs are administered with dopamine receptor antagonists or anticholinergic drugs. Some clinicians have used i.m. or intravenous (i.v.) physostigmine (Antilirium, Eserine) to diagnose and treat anticholinergic delirium.

Cardiac Effects

When administered in their usual therapeutic dosages, the TCAs may cause tachycardia, flattened T waves, prolonged QT intervals, and depressed ST segments in the electrocardiographic (ECG) recording. Imipramine has a quinidine-like effect at therapeutic plasma concentrations and may reduce the number of premature ventricular contractions. Because the drugs prolong conduction time, their use in persons with preexisting conduction defects is contraindicated. In persons with a history of any type of heart disease, TCAs should be used only after SSRIs or other newer antidepressants have been found ineffective, and if used, they should be introduced at low dosages, with gradual increases in dosage and monitoring of cardiac functions. All TCAs can cause tachycardia, which may persist for months and is one of the most common reasons for drug discontinuation, especially in younger persons. At high plasma concentrations, as seen in overdoses, the drugs become arrhythmogenic.

Other Autonomic Effects

Orthostatic hypotension is the most common cardiovascular autonomic adverse effect. It can result in falls and injuries in affected persons. Nortriptyline may be the drug least likely to cause this problem. Orthostatic hypotension is treated with avoidance of caffeine, intake of at least 2 L of fluid per day, and addition of salt to the diet unless the person is being treated for hypertension. In persons taking antihypertensive agents, reduction of the dosage may reduce the risk of orthostatic hypotension. Other possible autonomic effects are profuse sweating, palpitations, and increased blood pressure. Although some persons respond to fludrocortisone (Florinef), 0.02 to 0.05 mg twice a day, substitution of an SSRI is preferable to addition of a potentially toxic mineralocorticoid such as fludrocortisone. TCA use should be discontinued several days before elective surgery because of the occurrence of hypertensive episodes during surgery in persons receiving TCAs.

Sedation

Sedation is a common effect of TCAs and may be welcomed if sleeplessness has been a problem. The sedative effect of TCAs is a result of anticholinergic and antihistaminergic activities. Amitriptyline, trimipramine, and doxepin are the most sedating agents; imipramine, amoxapine, nortriptyline, and maprotiline are less sedating; and desipramine and protriptyline are the least sedating agents.

Neurological Effects

In addition to the sedation induced by TCAs and the possibility of anticholinergic-induced delirium, two TCAs—desipramine and protriptyline—are associated with psychomotor stimulation. Myoclonic twitches and tremors of the tongue and the upper extremities are common. Rare effects include speech blockage, paresthesia, peroneal palsies, and ataxia.

Amoxapine is unique in causing parkinsonian symptoms, akathisia, and even dyskinesia because of the dopaminergic blocking activity of one of its metabolites. Amoxapine may also cause neuroleptic malignant syndrome in rare cases. Maprotiline may cause seizures when the dosage is increased too quickly or is kept at high levels for too long. Clomipramine and amoxapine may lower the seizure threshold more than other drugs in the class. As a class, however, the TCAs have a relatively low risk for inducing seizures, except in persons who are at risk for seizures (e.g., persons with epilepsy and those with brain lesions). Although TCAs can still be used by such persons, the initial dosages should be lower than usual, and subsequent dosage increases should be gradual.

Allergic and Hematological Effects

Exanthematous rashes are seen in 4 to 5 percent of all persons treated with maprotiline. Jaundice is rare. Agranulocytosis, leukocytosis, leukopenia, and eosinophilia are rare complications of TCA treatment. However, a person who has a sore throat or a fever during the first few months of TCA treatment should have a complete blood count (CBC) done immediately.

Hepatic Effects

TCAs often produce a benign and self-limited rise in serum transaminase concentrations. TCAs can also produce a fulminant acute hepatitis, probably due to immune hypersensitivity, in 0.1 to 1 percent of persons.

Other Adverse Effects

Weight gain is common, which frequently cannot be managed solely with dietary restrictions. Fluoxetine, bupropion, or nefazodone are much less likely to cause weight gain than are TCAs. Amoxapine exerts a dopamine receptor antagonist effect and may cause hyperprolactinemia, impotence, galactorrhea, anorgasmia, and ejaculatory disturbances. Other TCAs have also been associated with gynecomastia and amenorrhea. Inappropriate secretion of antidiuretic hormone has also been reported with TCAs. Other effects include nausea, vomiting, and hepatitis. Bupropion, nefazodone, and mirtazapine have all been associated with significantly fewer sexual adverse effects than TCAs or SSRIs.

Precautions

The TCAs may cause a withdrawal syndrome in newborns, consisting of tachypnea, cyanosis, irritability, and poor sucking reflex. The drugs do pass into breast milk, but at concentrations that are usually undetectable in the infant's plasma. The drugs should be used with caution in persons with hepatic and renal diseases. TCAs should not be administered during a course of electroconvulsive therapy (ECT), primarily because of the risk of serious adverse cardiac effects.

DRUG INTERACTIONS

Monoamine Oxidase Inhibitors

TCAs should not be taken within 14 days of administration of a monoamine oxidase inhibitor (MAOI).

Antihypertensives

TCAs block the neuronal reuptake of guanethidine (Esimil, Ismelin), which is required for antihypertensive activity. The antihypertensive effects of β-adrenergic receptor antagonists (e.g., propranolol (Inderal) and clonidine (Catapres) may also be blocked by TCAs. The coadministration of a TCA and α-methyldopa (Aldomet) may cause behavioral agitation.

Antiarrhythmic Drugs

The antiarrhythmic properties of TCAs can be additive to those of quinidine, an effect that is further exacerbated by the inhibition of TCA metabolism by quinidine.

Dopamine Receptor Antagonists

Concurrent administration of TCAs and dopamine receptor antagonists increases the plasma concentrations of both drugs. Desipramine plasma concentrations may rise twofold during concurrent administration with perphenazine (Trilafon). Dopamine receptor antagonists also add to the anticholinergic and sedative effects of the TCAs.

CNS Depressants

Opioids, alcohol, anxiolytics, hypnotics, and over-the-counter cold medications have additive effects by causing CNS depression when coadministered with TCAs. Persons should be advised to avoid driving or using dangerous equipment if sedated by TCAs.

Sympathomimetics

Tricyclic drug use with sympathomimetic drugs may cause serious cardiovascular effects.

Oral Contraceptives

Birth control pills may decrease TCA plasma concentrations through the induction of hepatic enzymes.

Other Drug Interactions

TCA plasma concentrations may also be increased by concurrent use of acetazolamide (Diamox), acetylsalicylic acid, cimetidine, thiazide diuretics, fluoxetine, and sodium bicarbonate. Plasma concentrations may be lowered by ascorbic acid, ammonium chloride, barbiturates, cigarette smoking, carbamazepine, chloral hydrate, lithium (Eskalith), and primidone (Mysoline). Plasma concentrations of desipramine and possibly also nortriptyline may rise threefold to fourfold when administered concurrently with fluoxetine and paroxetine.

LABORATORY INTERFERENCES

Laboratory interferences with the TCAs have not been reported.

DOSAGE AND CLINICAL GUIDELINES

Persons who intend to take TCAs should undergo routine physical and laboratory examination, including a complete blood count, a white blood cell (WBC) count with differential, and serum electrolytes with liver function tests. An ECG should be obtained for all persons, especially women over 40 and men over 30. TCAs are contraindicated in persons with a QT_c greater than 450 milliseconds. The initial dose should be small and should be raised gradually. Because of the availability of highly effective alternatives to TCAs, a newer agent should be used if there is any medical condition that may interact adversely with the TCAs.

The elderly and children are more sensitive to TCA adverse effects than are young adults. In children, the ECG should be regularly monitored during use of a TCA.

The available preparations of TCAs are presented in Table 35–3. The dosages for the TCAs varies among the drugs (Table 35–4). Imipramine, amitriptyline, doxepin, desipramine, clomipramine, and trimipramine use can be started at 75 mg a day. Di-

TABLE 35–3
TRICYCLIC AND TETRACYCLIC ANTIDEPRESSANT PREPARATIONS

	Tablets	Capsules	Parenteral	Solution
Imipramine	10, 25, 50 mg	75, 100, 125, 150 mg	12.5 mg/mL	—
Desipramine	10, 25, 50, 75, 100, 150 mg	25, 50 mg	—	—
Trimipramine	—	25, 50, 100 mg	—	—
Amitriptyline	10, 25, 50, 75, 100, 150 mg	—	10 mg/mL	—
Nortriptyline	—	10, 25, 50, 75 mg	—	10 mg/5 mL
Protriptyline	5, 10 mg	—	—	—
Amoxapine	25, 50, 100, 150 mg	—	—	—
Doxepin	—	10, 25, 50, 75, 100, 150 mg	—	10 mg/mL
Maprotiline	25, 50, 75 mg	—	—	—
Clomipramine	—	25, 50, 75 mg	—	—

TABLE 35–4
GENERAL INFORMATION FOR THE TRICYCLIC AND TETRACYCLIC ANTIDEPRESSANTS

Generic Name	Trade Name	Usual Adult Dosage Range (mg a day)	Therapeutic Plasma Concentrations (μg per mL)
Imipramine	Tofranil	150–300	150–300[a]
Desipramine	Norpramin, Pertofrane	150–300	150–300[a]
Trimipramine	Surmontil	150–300	?
Amitriptyline	Elavil, Endep	150–300	100–250[b]
Nortriptyline	Pamelor, Aventyl	50–150	50–150[a] (maximum)
Protriptyline	Vivactil	15–60	75–250
Amoxapine	Asendin	150–400	?
Doxepin	Adapin, Sinequan	150–300	100–250[a]
Maprotiline	Ludiomil	150–230	150–300[a]
Clomipramine	Anafranil	130–250	?

[a] Exact range may vary among laboratories.
[b] Includes parent compound and desmethyl metabolite.

vided doses at first reduce the severity of the adverse effects, although most of the dosage should be given at night to help induce sleep if a sedating drug such as amitriptyline is used. Eventually, the entire daily dose can be given at bedtime. Protriptyline and less-sedating drugs should be given at least 2 to 3 hours before a person goes to sleep. The dosage can be raised to 150 mg a day the second week, 225 mg a day the third week, and 300 mg a day the fourth week. A common clinical mistake is to stop increasing the dosage when the person is taking less than 250 mg a day and does not show clinical improvement. Doing so can result in a further delay in obtaining a therapeutic response, disenchantment with the treatment, and premature discontinuation of drug use. The clinician should routinely assess the person's pulse and orthostatic changes in blood pressure while the dosage is being increased.

Nortriptyline use should be started at 50 mg a day and raised to 150 mg a day over 3 or 4 weeks unless a response occurs at a lower dosage, such as 100 mg a day. Amoxapine use should be started at 150 mg a day and raised to 400 mg a day. Protriptyline use should be started at 15 mg a day and raised to 60 mg a day. Maprotiline has been associated with an increased incidence of seizures if the dosage is raised too quickly or is maintained at too high a level. Maprotiline use should be started at 75 mg a day and maintained at that level for 2 weeks. The dosage can be increased over 4 weeks to 225 mg a day but should be kept at that level for only 6 weeks and then be reduced to 175 to 200 mg a day.

Persons with chronic pain may be particularly sensitive to adverse effects when TCA use is started. Therefore, treatment should begin with low dosages that are raised in small increments. However, persons with chronic pain may experience relief on long-term low-dosage therapy, such as amitriptyline or nortriptyline at 10 to 75 mg a day.

TCAs should be avoided in children, except as a last resort. Dosing guidelines in children for imipramine include initiation at 1.5 mg/kg a day. The dosage can be titrated to no more than 5 mg/kg a day. In enuresis the dosage is usually 50 to 100 mg a day taken at bedtime. Clomipramine use can be initiated at 50 mg a day and increased to no more than 3 mg/kg a day or 200 mg a day.

When TCA treatment is discontinued, the dosage should first be decreased to three-fourths the maximal dosage, for a month. At that time, if no symptoms are present, drug use can be tapered by 25 mg (5 mg for protriptyline) every 2 to 3 days.

The slow tapering process is indicated for most psychotherapeutic drugs; in the case of most TCAs, slow tapering avoids a cholinergic rebound syndrome consisting of nausea, upset stomach, sweating, headache, neck pain, and vomiting. This syndrome can be treated by reinstituting a small dosage of the drug and tapering more slowly than before. Several case reports note the appearance of rebound mania or hypomania after the abrupt discontinuation of TCA use.

Plasma Concentrations and Therapeutic Drug Monitoring

Research has defined the dose-response curves for a number of the TCAs when given to treat depressive disorders. Clinical determinations of plasma concentrations should be conducted after 5 to 7 days on the same dosage of medication and 8 to 12 hours after the last dose. Because of variations in absorption and metabolism, there may be a 30- to 50-fold difference in the plasma concentrations in persons given the same dosage of a TCA. The therapeutic ranges for plasma concentrations have been determined (Table 35–4). Nortriptyline is unique in its association with a therapeutic window; that is, plasma concentrations below 50 ng/mL or above 150 ng/mL may reduce its efficacy. Clinicians must follow the directions for collection from the testing laboratory and have confidence in the assay procedure used at a particular laboratory.

The use of plasma concentrations in clinical practice is still an evolving skill. Plasma concentrations may be useful in confirming compliance, assessing reasons for drug failures, and documenting effective plasma concentrations for future treatment. Clinicians should always treat the person and not the plasma concentration. Some persons have adequate clinical responses with seemingly subtherapeutic plasma concentrations, and other persons only respond at supratherapeutic plasma concentrations, without experiencing adverse effects. The latter situation, however, should alert the clinician to monitor the person's condition with, for example, serial ECG recordings.

Overdose Attempts

Overdose attempts with TCAs are serious and can often be fatal. Prescriptions for these drugs should be nonrefillable and for no longer than a week at a time for patients at risk for suicide. Amoxapine may be more likely than the other TCAs to result in death when taken in overdose. The newer antidepressants are safer in overdose.

Symptoms of overdose include agitation, delirium, convulsions, hyperactive deep tendon reflexes, bowel and bladder paralysis, dysregulation of blood pressure and temperature, and mydriasis. The patient then progresses to coma and perhaps respiratory depression. Cardiac arrhythmias may not respond to treatment. Because of the long half-lives of TCAs, the patients are at risk of cardiac arrhythmias for 3 to 4 days after the overdose, so they should be monitored in an intensive care medical setting.

For a more detailed discussion of this topic, see Nelson JC: Tricyclics and Tetracyclics, Sec 31.30, p 2491, in CTP/VII.

36

Valproate

Valproate (Depakene, Depakote) is used to treat bipolar I disorder and is equal in efficacy and safety to lithium (Eskalith). Valproate is also used for treatment of schizoaffective disorders, impulse-control disorders, and behavioral agitation. Valproate is an effective treatment for several types of epilepsy and an effective prophylaxis against migraine headaches.

CHEMISTRY

Available formulations include valproic acid (Depakene); divalproex sodium (Depakote), a 1:1 mixture of valproic acid and sodium valproate; and sodium valproate injection (Depacon). Each of these is therapeutically equivalent, because at physiological pH, valproic acid dissociates into valproate ion. Valproate is also called valproic acid because it is rapidly converted to the acid form in the stomach. The structural formula of valproate is shown in Figure 36–1.

PHARMACOLOGICAL ACTIONS

All valproate formulations are rapidly and completely absorbed after oral administration. The steady-state half-life of valproate is about 8 to 17 hours, and clinically effective plasma concentrations can usually be maintained with dosing one to four times a day. Protein binding becomes saturated and concentrations of therapeutically effective free valproate increase at serum concentrations above 50 to 100 μg/mL.

The therapeutic effects of valproate in bipolar I disorder may be mediated by as yet undefined effects of the drug on the γ-aminobutyric acid (GABA) neurotransmitter system.

THERAPEUTIC INDICATIONS

Bipolar I Disorder

Acute episodes. Valproate effectively controls manic symptoms in about two thirds of persons with acute mania. Valproate also reduces overall psychiatric symptoms and the need for supplemental doses of benzodiazepines or dopamine receptor antagonists. Persons with mania usually respond 1 to 4 days after valproate serum concentrations rise above 50 μg/mL. Using gradual dosing strategies, this serum concentration may be achieved within 1 week of initiation of dosing, but newer, rapid oral loading strategies achieve therapeutic serum concentrations in 1 day and can control manic symptoms within 5 days. The short-term antimanic effects of val-

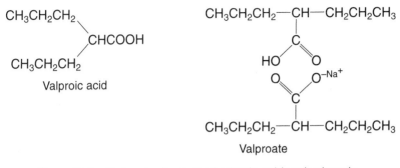

Figure 36-1. Molecular structure of valproic acid and valproate.

proate can be augmented with addition of lithium, carbamazepine (Tegretol), or dopamine receptor antagonists. Serotonin-dopamine antagonists and gabapentin (Neurontin) may also potentiate the effects of valproate, albeit less rapidly. Because of its more favorable profile of cognitive, dermatological, thyroid, and renal adverse effects, valproate is preferred to lithium for treatment of acute mania in children and elderly persons.

Valproate alone is less effective for the short-term treatment of depressive episodes in bipolar I disorder than for treatment of manic episodes. Among depressive symptoms, valproate is more effective for treatment of agitation than dysphoria.

Prophylaxis.   Valproate is effective in the prophylactic treatment of bipolar I disorder, resulting in fewer, less severe, and shorter manic episodes. In direct comparison, valproate is at least as effective as lithium and is better tolerated than lithium. Compared with lithium, valproate may be particularly effective in persons with rapid-cycling and ultrarapid-cycling bipolar disorders, dysphoric or mixed mania, and mania due to a general medical condition and in persons who have comorbid substance abuse or panic attacks or who have not had complete favorable responses to lithium treatment. Addition of valproate to lithium may be more effective than use of lithium alone.

In persons with bipolar I disorder, maintenance valproate treatment markedly reduces the frequency and severity of manic episodes but is only mildly to moderately effective in the prophylactic treatment of depressive episodes.

The prophylactic effectiveness of valproate can be augmented by addition of lithium, carbamazepine, dopamine receptor antagonists, serotonin-dopamine antagonists, antidepressant drugs, gabapentin, or lamotrigine (Lamictal).

Schizoaffective Disorder

Valproate is effective in treating the short-term phase of the bipolar type of schizoaffective disorder, but valproate alone is generally less effective in schizoaffective disorder than in bipolar I disorder. Valproate may be an effective adjunct agent for use with lithium, carbamazepine, or a serotonin-dopamine antagonist by persons with schizoaffective disorder. Valproate alone is ineffective for treatment of psychotic symptoms.

Other Mental Disorders

Valproate can be effective for treatment of intermittent explosive disorder, kleptomania, and other behavioral dyscontrol syndromes, particularly if these disorders are comorbid with bipolar symptoms. Valproate can effectively control physical aggression, restlessness, agitation, and, to a lesser degree, verbal aggression associated with dementia, organic brain diseases, or traumatic brain injury, although it should be considered for use only after therapeutic trials of benzodiazepines and serotonin-dopamine antagonists have failed. Valproate may be effective alone or in combination with other psychotropic drugs in treatment of other mental disorders, including major depressive disorder; panic disorder; posttraumatic stress disorder; obsessive-compulsive disorder; bulimia nervosa; alcohol and sedative, hypnotic, or anxiolytic (particularly benzodiazepine) withdrawal; symptoms of borderline personality disorder; and cocaine detoxification.

PRECAUTIONS AND ADVERSE REACTIONS

Valproate treatment is generally well tolerated and safe and is less likely than lithium to trigger medication discontinuation because of adverse effects. The common adverse effects associated with valproate (Table 36–1) are those affecting the gastrointestinal system, such as nausea, vomiting, dyspepsia, and diarrhea. The gastrointestinal effects are generally most common in the first month of treatment, particularly if the dosage is increased rapidly. Unbuffered valproic acid (Depakene) is more likely to cause gastrointestinal symptoms than are the enteric-coated "sprinkle" or the delayed-release divalproex sodium formulations. Gastrointestinal symp-

TABLE 36–1
ADVERSE EFFECTS OF VALPROATE

Common
  Gastrointestinal irritation
  Nausea
  Sedation
  Tremor
  Weight gain
  Hair loss
Uncommon
  Vomiting
  Diarrhea
  Ataxia
  Dysarthria
  Persistent elevation of hepatic transaminases
Rare
  Fatal hepatotoxicity (primarily in pediatric patients)
  Reversible thrombocytopenia
  Platelet dysfunction
  Coagulation disturbances
  Edema
  Hemorrhagic pancreatitis
  Agranulocytosis
  Encephalopathy and coma
  Respiratory muscle weakness and respiratory failure

toms may respond to histamine H_2 receptor antagonists. Other common adverse effects involve the nervous system, such as sedation, ataxia, dysarthria, and tremor. Valproate-induced tremor may respond well to treatment with β-adrenergic receptor antagonists or gabapentin. Treatment of the other neurological adverse effects usually requires lowering the valproate dosage.

Weight gain is a common adverse effect, especially in long-term treatment, and can best be treated by strict limitation of caloric intake. Hair loss may occur in 5 to 10 percent of all persons treated, and rare cases of complete loss of body hair have been reported. Some clinicians have recommended treatment of valproate-associated hair loss with vitamin supplements that contain zinc and selenium. Five to 40 percent of persons experience a persistent but clinically insignificant elevation in liver transaminases to three times the upper limit of normal, which is usually asymptomatic and resolves after discontinuation of the drug. Other rare adverse events include effects on the hematopoietic system, including thrombocytopenia and platelet dysfunction, occurring most commonly at high dosages and resulting in the prolongation of bleeding times. High dosages of valproate (above 1000 mg a day) may rarely produce mild-to-moderate hyponatremia, most likely because of some degree of the syndrome of secretion of inappropriate antidiuretic hormone (SIADH), which is reversible upon lowering of the dosage. Overdoses of valproate can lead to coma and death.

The two most serious adverse effects of valproate treatment affect the pancreas and the liver. Risk factors for potentially fatal hepatotoxicity include young age (less than 3 years), concurrent use of phenobarbital, and the presence of neurological disorders, especially inborn errors of metabolism. The rate of fatal hepatotoxicity in persons who have been treated with only valproate is 0.85 per 100,000 persons; no persons over the age of 10 years are reported to have died from fatal hepatotoxicity. Therefore, the risk of this adverse reaction in adult psychiatric persons seems low. Nevertheless, if symptoms of lethargy, malaise, anorexia, nausea and vomiting, edema, and abdominal pain occur in a person treated with valproate, the clinician must consider the possibility of severe hepatotoxicity. A modest increase in liver function test results does not correlate with the development of serious hepatotoxicity. Rare cases of pancreatitis have been reported; they occur most often in the first 6 months of treatment, and the condition occasionally results in death. Pancreatic function can be assessed and followed with serum amylase concentrations.

Valproate should not be used by pregnant or nursing women. The drug is associated with neural tube defects (e.g., spina bifida) in about 1 to 2 percent of all women who take valproate during the first trimester of the pregnancy. The risk of valproate-induced neural tube defects can be reduced with daily folic acid supplements (1 to 4 mg a day) taken continuously for at least 3 months prior to conception and throughout pregnancy. Women who require valproate therapy should therefore inform their physicians if they intend to become pregnant. Infants breast-fed by mothers taking valproate develop serum valproate concentrations 1 to 10 percent of maternal serum concentrations, and no data suggest that this poses a risk to the infant. Thus, valproate is relatively contraindicated in nursing mothers. Clinicians should not administer the drug to persons with hepatic diseases. Rare cases of polycystic ovary disease have been reported in woman using valproate.

TABLE 36–2
INTERACTIONS OF VALPROATE WITH OTHER DRUGS

Drug	Interactions Reported with Valproate
Lithium	Increased tremor
Antipsychotics	Increased sedation; increased extrapyramidal effects; delirium and stupor (single report)
Clozapine	Increased sedation; confusional syndrome (single report)
Carbamazepine	Acute psychosis (single report); ataxia, nausea, lethargy (single report); may decrease valproate serum concentrations
Antidepressants	Amitriptyline and fluoxetine may increase valproate serum concentrations
Diazepam	Serum concentration increased by valproate
Clonazepam	Absence status (rare; reported only in patients with preexisting epilepsy)
Phenytoin	Serum concentration decreased by valproate
Phenobarbital	Serum, concentration increased by valproate; increased sedation
Other CNS depressants	Increased sedation
Anticoagulants	Possible potentiation of effect

DRUG INTERACTIONS

Valproate is commonly coadministered with lithium, carbamazepine, and dopamine receptor antagonists. The only consistent drug interaction with lithium, if both drugs are maintained in their respective therapeutic ranges, is the exacerbation of drug-induced tremors, which can usually be treated with β-receptor antagonists. The combination of valproate and dopamine receptor antagonists may result in increased sedation, as can be seen when valproate is added to any central nervous system (CNS) depressant (e.g., alcohol), and increased severity of extrapyramidal symptoms, which usually respond to treatment with the usual antiparkinsonian drugs. Valproate can usually be safely combined with carbamazepine or serotonin-dopamine antagonists. The plasma concentrations of carbamazepine, lamotrigine, diazepam (Valium), amitriptyline (Elavil), nortriptyline (Pamelor), and phenobarbital (Luminal) may be increased when these drugs are coadministered with valproate, and the plasma concentrations of phenytoin (Dilantin) and desipramine (Norpramin) may be decreased when they are combined with valproate. The plasma concentrations of valproate may be decreased when the drug is coadministered with carbamazepine and may be increased when coadministered with guanfacine (Tenex), amitriptyline, or fluoxetine (Prozac). Valproate can be displaced from plasma proteins by carbamazepine, diazepam, and aspirin. Persons who are treated with anticoagulants (e.g., aspirin and warfarin [Coumadin]) should also be monitored when valproate use is initiated, to assess the development of any undesired augmentation of the anticoagulation effects. Interactions of valproate with other drugs are listed in Table 36–2.

LABORATORY INTERFERENCES

Valproate was reported to cause an overestimation of serum free fatty acids in almost half of the persons tested. Valproate was also reported to elevate urinary ketone estimations falsely and to result in falsely abnormal thyroid function test results.

TABLE 36–3
VALPROATE PREPARATIONS AVAILABLE IN THE UNITED STATES

Generic Name	Trade Name, Form (doses)	Time to Peak
Valproate sodium injection	Depacon Injection (100 mg valproic acid/mL)	1 h
Valproic acid	Depakene, syrup (250 mg/5 mL)	1–2 h
	Depakene, capsules (250 mg)	1–2 h
Divalproex sodium	Depakote, delayed-released tablets (125, 250, 500 mg)	3–8 h
Divalproex sodium coated particles in capsules	Depakote, sprinkle capsules (125 mg)	Compared with divalproex tablets, divalproex sprinkle has earlier onset and slower absorption, with slightly lower peak plasma concentration

DOSAGE AND CLINICAL GUIDELINES

Pretreatment evaluation should routinely include white blood cell (WBC) and platelet counts, hepatic transaminase concentrations, and pregnancy testing, if applicable. Additional testing should include amylase and coagulation studies if baseline pancreatic disease or coagulopathy is suspected.

Valproate is available in a number of formulations (Table 36–3). For treatment of acute mania, an oral loading strategy of initiation with 20 to 30 mg/kg a day can be used to accelerate control of symptoms. This is usually well tolerated but can cause excessive sedation and tremor in elderly persons. Agitated behavior can be rapidly stabilized with intravenous infusion of valproate. If acute mania is absent, it is best to initiate drug treatment gradually, to minimize the common adverse effects of nausea, vomiting, and sedation. The dose on the first day should be 250 mg administered with a meal. The dosage can be raised up to 250 mg orally three times daily over the course of 3 to 6 days. Trough plasma concentrations can be assessed in the morning before the first daily dose is administered. Therapeutic plasma concentrations for the control of seizures range between 50 and 150 μg/mL, but concentrations up to 200 μg/mL are usually well tolerated. It is reasonable to use the same range for the treatment of mental disorders; most of the controlled studies have used 50 to 100 μg/mL. Most persons attain therapeutic plasma concentrations on a

TABLE 36–4
RECOMMENDED LABORATORY TESTS DURING VALPROATE THERAPY

Prior to treatment
  Standard chemistry screen with special attention to liver function tests
  Complete blood count, including white cell and platelet count
During treatment
  Liver function tests at 1 month, then every 3 to 24 months if no abnormalities are found
  Complete blood work with platelet count at 1 month, then every 3 to 24 months if findings are normal
If liver function test results become abnormal
  Mild transaminase elevation (less than three times normal): monitoring every 1 to 2 weeks; if stable and patient is responding to valproate, results are monitored monthly to every 3 months
  Pronounced transaminase elevation (more than three times normal): dosage reduction or discontinuation of valproate; increase dose or rechallenge if transaminases normalize and if the patient is a valproate responder

dosage between 1200 and 1500 mg a day in divided doses. Once a person's symptoms are well controlled, the full daily dose can be taken all at once before sleep.

WBC and platelet counts and hepatic transaminase concentrations should be obtained 1 month after initiation of therapy and every 6 to 24 months thereafter. However, because even frequent monitoring may not predict serious organ toxicity, it is more prudent to reinforce the need for prompt evaluation of any illnesses when reviewing the instructions to patients. Asymptomatic elevation of transaminase concentrations up to three times the upper limit of normal are common and do not require any change in dosage. Table 36–4 lists the recommended laboratory tests for valproate treatment.

For a more detailed discussion of this topic, see McElroy SL, Pope HG, Keck PE: Valproate, Sec 31.7b, p 2289, in CTP/VII.

37

Venlafaxine

Venlafaxine (Effexor) is an effective antidepressant drug that may have a faster onset of action than other antidepressant drugs when the dosage is increased rapidly. Venlafaxine is among the most efficacious drugs for treatment of severe depression with melancholic features. Venlafaxine is the first nonbenzodiazepine drug, other than buspirone (Buspar), to be approved by the Food and Drug Administration (FDA) for treatment of generalized anxiety disorder.

CHEMISTRY

Venlafaxine is structurally distinct from other antidepressant drugs. The structural formula of venlafaxine is shown in Figure 37–1.

PHARMACOLOGICAL ACTIONS

Venlafaxine is well absorbed from the gastrointestinal tract. The extended-release formulations of venlafaxine (Effexor XR) and O-desmethylvenlafaxine reach peak plasma concentrations in 5.5 hours and 9 hours, respectively. Venlafaxine has a half-life of about 3.5 hours, and O-desmethylvenlafaxine has a half-life of 9 hours.

Venlafaxine is a potent inhibitor of serotonin and norepinephrine reuptake, and a weak inhibitor of dopamine reuptake. Venlafaxine does not have activity at muscarinic, nicotinic, histaminergic, opioid, or adrenergic receptors, and it is not active as a monoamine oxidase inhibitor. It is metabolized in the liver by cytochrome P450 (CYP) isoenzyme 2D6.

THERAPEUTIC INDICATIONS

Depression

Venlafaxine is used for the treatment of major depressive disorder. Severely depressed persons may respond within 2 weeks to 200 mg a day of venlafaxine, which is somewhat sooner than the 2- to 4-week period usually required for the serotonin-specific reuptake inhibitors. Therefore, high-dosage venlafaxine may become a preferred drug to use for seriously ill persons when a rapid response is desired. In studies directly comparing fluoxetine (Prozac) with venlafaxine for the treatment of seriously depressed persons with melancholic features, venlafaxine has consistently been the superior agent in terms of rate of response, percent response, and completeness of response. Direct comparisons of venlafaxine and sertraline (Zoloft), which is the most effective SSRI for treatment of seriously depressed persons with melancholic features, have not been described.

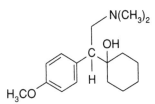

Figure 37-1. Molecular structure of venlafaxine.

Generalized Anxiety Disorder

The extended-release formulation of venlafaxine is approved for treatment of generalized anxiety disorder. In clinical trials, dosages of 75 to 225 mg a day were effective against insomnia, poor concentration, restlessness, irritability, and excessive muscle tension related to generalized anxiety disorder.

Other Indications

Case reports and uncontrolled studies have indicated that venlafaxine may be beneficial in the treatment of obsessive-compulsive disorder, panic disorder, agoraphobia, social phobia, and attention-deficit/hyperactivity disorder. It has also been used in chronic pain syndromes with good effect.

PRECAUTIONS AND ADVERSE REACTIONS

Venlafaxine has generally been reported to be well tolerated. The most common adverse reactions are nausea, somnolence, dry mouth, dizziness, nervousness, constipation, asthenia, anxiety, anorexia, blurred vision, abnormal ejaculation or orgasm, erectile disturbances, and impotence. The incidence of nausea is reduced considerably with use of the extended-release capsules.

Abrupt discontinuation of venlafaxine use may produce a discontinuation syndrome consisting of nausea, somnolence, and insomnia. Therefore, venlafaxine use should be tapered gradually over 2 to 4 weeks.

The most potentially worrisome adverse effect associated with venlafaxine is an increase in blood pressure in some persons, particularly those who are treated with more than 300 mg a day. In clinical trials a mean increase of 7.2 mm Hg in diastolic blood pressure was observed in persons who were receiving 375 mg a day of venlafaxine, in contrast to no significant change in persons receiving 75 or 225 mg a day. Thus, the drug should be used cautiously by persons with preexisting hypertension and then only at lower dosages.

Information concerning use of venlafaxine by pregnant and nursing women is not available at this time. Clinicians should avoid the use of venlafaxine by pregnant and nursing women until more clinical experience has been gained.

DRUG INTERACTIONS

Cimetidine (Tagamet) appears to inhibit the first-pass hepatic metabolism of venlafaxine and to raise the levels of the unmetabolized drug. However, since the metabolite is mainly responsible for the therapeutic effect, this interaction is of concern only in persons with preexisting hypertension or hepatic disease, in whom this combination should be avoided. Venlafaxine may raise plasma concentrations of concurrently administered haloperidol (Haldol). As is true of all antidepressant medications, venlafaxine should not be used within 14 days of the use of monoamine oxidase inhibitors, and it may potentiate the sedative effects of other drugs that act on the central nervous system.

LABORATORY INTERFERENCES

Data are not currently available on laboratory interferences with venlafaxine.

DOSAGE AND ADMINISTRATION

Venlafaxine is available in 25-, 37.5-, 50-, 75-, and 100-mg tablets and 37.5-, 75-, and 150-mg extended-release capsules. The tablets should be given in two or three daily doses, and the extended-release capsules are to be taken in a single dose before sleep up to a maximum of 225 mg a day. The tablets and the extended-release capsules are equally potent, and persons stabilized with one can switch to an equivalent dosage of the other. The usual starting dosage in depressed persons is 75 mg a day, given as tablets in two to three divided doses or as extended-release capsules in a single dose before sleep. Some persons require a starting dosage of 37.5 mg for 4 to 7 days to minimize adverse effects, particularly nausea, prior to titration up to 75 mg a day. In persons with depression, the dosage can be raised to 150 mg a day, given as tablets in two or three divided doses or as extended-release capsules once at night, after an appropriate period of clinical assessment at the lower dosage (usually 2 to 3 weeks). The dosage can be raised in increments of 75 mg a day every 4 or more days. Moderately depressed persons probably do not need dosages above 225 mg a day, whereas severely depressed persons may require 300 to 375 mg a day for a satisfactory response. Rapid antidepressant response—within 1 to 2 weeks—may result from administration of dosages of 200 mg per day from the beginning. The maximum dosage of venlafaxine is 375 mg a day. The dosage of venlafaxine should be halved in persons with significantly diminished hepatic or renal function. If discontinued, venlafaxine use should be gradually tapered over 2 to 4 weeks.

For a more detailed discussion of this topic, see Beauclair L, Radoi-Andraous D, Chounard G: Selective Serotonin-Noradrenaline Reuptake Inhibitors, Sec 31.24, p 2427, in CTP/VII.

38

Yohimbine

Yohimbine (Yocon, Aphrodyne) is an α_2-adrenergic receptor antagonist that is used as a treatment for both idiopathic and medication-induced male sexual dysfunction. Currently, sildenafil (Viagra) and alprostadil (Muse, Caverject) are universally considered more efficacious for this indication than yohimbine.

CHEMISTRY

Yohimbine hydrochloride is derived from an alkaloid found in *Rubaceae* and related trees and in the *Rauwolfia serpentina* plant. Its molecular structure is shown in Figure 38–1.

PHARMACOLOGICAL ACTIONS

Yohimbine is erratically absorbed following oral administration, with bioavailablity ranging from 7 to 87 percent. There is extensive hepatic first-pass metabolism. Yohimbine affects the sympathomimetic autonomic nervous system by increasing plasma concentrations of norepinephrine. The half-life of yohimbine is 0.5 to 2 hours.

Yohimbine is an antagonist of α_2-receptors located both presynaptically and postsynaptically on noradrenergic neurons. α_2-Receptors are also located on synaptic terminals of some serotonergic neurons. Stimulation of presynaptic α_2-receptors results in a decrease in the release of neurotransmitters from the neuron; therefore, blockade of the receptors results in an increase in the release of neurotransmitters. Both norepinephrine and serotonin are involved in the physiology of male sexual response. Clinically, yohimbine produces increased parasympathetic (cholinergic) tone.

THERAPEUTIC INDICATIONS

In psychiatry yohimbine has been used to treat medical, psychogenic, and substance-induced erectile dysfunction. Penile erection has been linked to cholinergic activity and to α_2-adrenergic blockade, which theoretically results in increased penile inflow of blood or decreased penile outflow of blood or both. Urologists have used yohimbine for the diagnostic classification of certain types of male impotence.

Yohimbine is reported to help counteract the loss of sexual desire and the orgasmic inhibition caused by some serotonergic antidepressants (e.g., selective serotonin reuptake inhibitors). It has not been found useful in women for these indications.

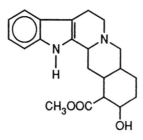

Figure 38-1.   Molecular structure of yohimbine.

PRECAUTIONS AND ADVERSE EFFECTS

The side effects of yohimbine include anxiety, elevated blood pressure and heart rate, increased psychomotor activity, irritability, tremor, headache, skin flushing, dizziness, urinary frequency, nausea, vomiting, and sweating. Patients with panic disorder show heightened sensitivity to yohimbine and experience increased anxiety, increased blood pressure, and increased plasma 3-methoxy-4-hydroxyphenyl-glycol (MHPG).

Yohimbine should be used with caution in female patients and should not be used in patients with renal disease, cardiac disease, glaucoma, or a history of gastric or duodenal ulcer.

DRUG INTERACTIONS

Yohimbine blocks the effect of clonidine (Catapres), gaunfacine (Tenex), and other α_2-receptor agonists.

LABORATORY INTERFERENCES

No known laboratory interferences are associated with yohimbine use.

DOSAGE AND CLINICAL GUIDELINES

Yohimbine is available in 5.4-mg tablets. The dosage of yohimbine in the treatment of impotence is approximately 18 mg a day given in doses that range from 2.7 to 5.4 mg three times a day. In the event of significant adverse effects, dosage should first be reduced, then gradually increased again. Yohimbine should be used judiciously in psychiatric patients because it may have an adverse effect on their mental status. Because yohimbine has no consistent effects on erectile dysfunction, its use remains controversial.

For a more detailed discussion of this topic, see DeBattista C, Shatzberg AF: Other Pharmacological and Biological Therapies, Sec 31.33, p 2521, in CTP/VII.

39

Drug Augmentation Therapy

Combination drug therapy is often used to achieve optimal response in the treatment of mental disorders. Reasons for use of combination therapy include nonresponse, partial response, delay in onset of response, intolerance of side effects, and the presence of comorbid disorders (Table 39–1).

Drug combination strategies may involve the combination of two or more agents with the same therapeutic indication. For example, there may be simultaneous use of two different classes of antidepressants (e.g., a selective serotonin reuptake inhibitor [SSRI] and bupropion (Wellbutrin). Another strategy consists of the addition of a second agent with an unrelated indication. One such combination is the addition of thyroid hormone to an antidepressant.

Some drugs are extensively and almost exclusively used in an adjunct role. Antiparkinsonian drugs, for example, are routinely prescribed in psychiatry to treat extrapyramidal side effects of dopamine receptor agonists. Benzodiazepine agonists are used in combination with other drugs more often than they are used alone. Coadministration of benzodiazepine agonists may improve treatment outcome by enhancing the effects of the primary medication or may represent efforts to manage particular symptoms, such as anxiety and insomnia, that accompany most psychiatric disorders.

While complex combination therapy is common, it has not been systematically studied. Often-used strategies are either discovered by accident or are based on the application of theoretical neurochemical synergies. Each of these interventions should be considered only when conventional treatment has failed and in the context of clinical circumstances. Each additional agent increases the possibility of an adverse interaction. It also gives a message that the person being treated may interpret—often correctly—as desperation. In terms of compliance, the more medications that are used, the more reluctant a patient may be to continue treatment.

Primary considerations when using drug augmentation include the potential for enhanced response and possible risks. It is wise to inform patients of the risks and benefits involved with drug combinations (Table 39–2) and to document clearly the rationale for using a combination strategy.

Described below are selected combination strategies that are used in the treatment of common mental disorders.

DEPRESSION

Most antidepressants have been described as being part of a successful combination strategy (Table 39–3). It should be noted that no antidepressant augmentation strategy has been proven more effective than another. In the absence of standard algorithms for choice of augmentation agent, such factors as the level of supporting

TABLE 39-1
REASONS FOR COMBINING MEDICATIONS

Nonresponse	Comorbidity
Partial response	Mitigation of side effects
Delay in onset of response	

evidence, safety, tolerability, or concerns about special cautions or clinical monitoring should be considered (Table 39–4).

Antidepressant Supplementation

It is a standard warning that other antidepressants should not be used in combination with a monoamine oxidase inhibitor (MAOI) or within 2 to 4 weeks of discontinuing MAOI use. However, it has been the practice, in extremely refractory cases of depression, to combine an MAOI with a TCA. MAOI-TCA combinations are used with greater comfort in the United Kingdom than in the United States. If this strategy is selected, use of both drugs is started concurrently or use of the TCA is started before that of the MAOI. MAOIs should not be added to ongoing therapy with another class of antidepressant. Given the risks involved, and the lack of data that show this combination to be more effective than other approaches, the reluctance of American clinicians to use MAOI-TCA combinations is understandable. MAOIs and SSRIs should not be combined because of the risks of hypertension and serotonin syndrome.

Clinical studies show that there is an enhanced response rate when noradrenergic TCAs, such as desipramine (Norpramin, Pertofrane) and nortriptyline (Aventyl, Pamelor), are used with an SSRI. The risks of this approach include potentially dangerous increases in TCA plasma concentrations, caused by inhibition of hepatic metabolism, and an overall increase in adverse effects. The section on drug interactions in Chapter 1 of this book describes the types of pharmacokinetic interactions that may underlie these effects. Among the SSRIs, sertraline (Zoloft) and citalopram (Celexa) are least likely to increase TCA plasma concentrations. It is advisable to obtain TCA plasma concentrations whenever SSRI-TCA combinations are used.

TABLE 39-2
ADVANTAGES AND DISADVANTAGES OF DRUG AUGMENTATION OR COMBINATION

Advantages
  Novel mechanisms
  Treatment of residual symptoms
  Continuity of treatment
  Reduced side effects
  Treatment of comorbid disorders
Disadvantages
  Off-label use
  Lack of extensive database
  Medicolegal concerns
  Drug interactions
  Possible increase in severity or frequency of side effects
  Reduced compliance because of complexity, apprehension
  Cost

TABLE 39–3
ANTIDEPRESSANT COMBINATIONS

MAOI + TCA
TCA + SSRI
SSRI + bupropion
SSRI + venlafaxine
Venlafaxine + bupropion
Nefazodone + bupropion
Nefazodone + SSRI
Mirtazapine + bupropion
Mirtazapine + SSRI

Venlafaxine (Effexor) may be used instead of a TCA because of its lack of TCA-like cardiovascular effects and its favorable cytochrome P450 (CYP) profile.

SSRIs may also be combined with bupropion, which has no independent effects on serotonergic neurotransmission. This combination exemplifies the broad-spectrum approach to antidepressant drug combinations, since this mixture contains agents that are selective for different neurotransmitters. There is a strong theoretical argument for this strategy, mainly that there is targeting of all the monoamine systems that have been implicated in the pathophysiology of depression. A few case series have reported improved rates of response with addition of bupropion to ongoing treatment with fluoxetine (Prozac), sertraline (Zoloft), and paroxetine (Paxil).

TABLE 39–4
CLINICAL CONSIDERATIONS FOR SELECTING ANTIDEPRESSANT AUGMENTATION STRATEGIES

Treatment	Level of Supporting Evidence	Safety	Tolerability	Cautions or Special Monitoring
Lithium	+++	++	++	Lithium levels, thyroid function, and renal function monitoring
Thyroid	+++	++	++	Thyroid function monitoring
Buspirone	++	+++	+++	No specific safety concerns or need for special laboratory monitoring
Pindolol	++	+	++	Blood pressure and heart rate monitoring; caution in patients with asthma, severe allergies, and cardiac conduction problems
Dopamine agonists and stimulants	+	+	+	Abuse, regulatory concerns; activation, nausea, blood pressure changes
Anticonvulsants	+	+	++	Pharmacokinetic interactions
Antidepressant combinations	+	+	+	Safety varies according to combination; risk of drug interactions requires plasma monitoring

+++, Very positive; ++, positive; +, problematic.

Another reason to combine antidepressant drugs is the mitigation of side effects. Mirtazapine (Remeron) is especially well suited for blocking some common SSRI side effects. Its serotonin 5-HT$_3$ antagonist properties reduce nausea and diarrhea, while its histamine H$_1$ antagonist properties help to normalize sleep. Bupropion may be useful to counteract sedation caused by other drugs.

Lithium

Controlled trials support the clinical experience that lithium (Eskalith) augmentation of a variety of antidepressants converts 30 to 65 percent of nonresponders into responders. Dosages of 600 to 1200 mg a day (or blood levels of 0.4 to 0.8 mmol) have been used to augment antidepressant response. Serum lithium levels do not appear to be tightly correlated with responsiveness of depressive symptoms to lithium augmentation.

Thyroid Hormones

The addition of small doses (25 to 50 μg) of the thyroid hormone liothyronine (Cytomel) has been used to augment response to TCAs and MAOIs. Fewer controlled studies have been conducted than with lithium. Liothyronine augmentation of TCAs was shown to be effective in approximately 50 to 60 percent of patients. The efficacy of liothyronine augmentation of MAOIs and the SSRI fluoxetine (Prozac) has been limited to evaluation of case reports, but preliminary evidence suggests that liothyronine may be effective with a wide range of antidepressants. Although levothyroxine (Levoxyl, Levothroid, Synthroid) is a precursor of liothyronine, levothyroxine appears less effective as an augmenting agent. Doses of 25 to 50 μg have been used to augment antidepressant response.

Sympathomimetics

Sympathomimetics, such as dextroamphetamine (Dexedrine) and methylphenidate (Ritalin), have long been used in patients with depression. Persons who do not respond to SSRIs, TCAs, and even MAOIs may be treated successfully with the addition of methylphenidate or dextroamphetamine. Persons who exhibit sluggishness, apathy, and fatigue despite otherwise good antidepressant response, or perhaps because of their primary antidepressant may benefit from the addition of a sympathomimetic. It should be noted that there are no controlled studies of sympathomimetic augmentation therapy. Also, abuse potential makes use of sympathomimetics a less desirable strategy than other options.

Pindolol

Pindolol (Visken) is an antagonist of β-adrenergic receptors and 5-HT$_{1A}$ serotonin receptors. Pindolol has been reported to reduce the latency period of antidepressant response in persons with depression and in persons who are resistant to treatment with SSRIs. In controlled studies, however, pindolol has been no more effective than placebo.

Benzodiazepines

Augmentation with a benzodiazepine during the first weeks of antidepressant treatment may provide a more rapid anxiolytic response. Drawbacks include sedation, psychomotor impairment, small risk of withdrawal phenomena, and long-term dependence if the benzodiazepine, especially alprazolam (Xanax), is used for more than 2 months.

Buspirone

Case reports and open-label clinical trials have noted positive responses to buspirone (BuSpar) augmentation at dosages between 20 and 50 mg a day. The addition of buspirone to nefazodone (Serzone) or fluvoxamine (Luvox) may result in higher than expected plasma levels of buspirone. It is thus best to lower the initial dosage of buspirone (e.g., to 2.5 mg twice daily) when it is used in combination with nefazodone or fluvoxamine. Buspirone has been reported to reverse SSRIs-induced bruxism and sexual dysfunction.

Dopamine Receptor Antagonists and Other Antipsychotic Agents

Persons with depression who exhibit psychotic symptoms may benefit from the addition of drugs that are used primarily to treat schizophrenia. These include dopamine receptor antagonists and the serotonin-dopamine antagonists (SDAs), such as risperidone (Risperdal), olanzapine (Zyprexa), and quetiapine (Seroquel). There have also been reports of nonpsychotic depressed patients, unresponsive to conventional treatment, deriving benefit from this strategy.

BIPOLAR DISORDER

Many patients with bipolar disorder cannot be stabilized with a single mood stabilizer. Combination therapy is thus common in the management of bipolar disorders. Typically, patients take a primary mood stabilizer, such as lithium, carbamazepine (Tegretol), divalproex (Depakote), or a combination of these drugs (Table 39–5).

In addition, a dopamine receptor agonist, a serotonin-dopamine antagonist (SDA), or clonazepam (Klonopin) may be used simultaneously, particularly during the treatment of acute mania. In addition, patients with depressed phase bipolar disorder may be treated with an antidepressant.

Lamotrigine (Lamictal) is an anticonvulsant that is increasingly being used alone and as an adjunct in the treatment of bipolar disorders. Case reports and clinical trials suggest that it has both mood-stabilizing and antidepressant activity. Potentially life-threatening rashes are associated with use of the drug. The risk of rash is concentration dependent, especially early in treatment, and occurs more often when lamotrigine is administered along with valproic acid (Depakene). The coadministration of lamotrigine and valproic acid increases lamotrigine concentrations, necessitating a reduction in lamotrigine dosage.

TABLE 39-5
**MOOD STABILIZER COMBINATIONS IN
REFRACTORY BIPOLAR DISORDER**

Lithium + divalproex
Lithium + gabapentin
Lithium + tiagabine
Divalproex + carbamazepine
Divalproex + gabapentin
Divalproex + topiramate
Carbamazepine + gabapentin

Other anticonvulsant drugs, such as gabapentin (Neurontin), topiramate (Topamax), and tiagabine (Gabitril), are also being used as adjuncts in the treatment of bipolar disorders. However, in contrast to lamotrigine, currently no significant drug interaction concerns have been noted with these drugs. Topiramate may offer a particular advantage when combined with other mood stabilizers in that it may both enhance efficacy and also counteract drug-induced weight gain, although it may also impair cognition.

OBSESSIVE-COMPULSIVE DISORDER (OCD)

SSRIs and clomipramine (Anafranil) are the only proven treatments for OCD, but only 40 percent of patients respond to these agents. Few patients demonstrate complete remission with monotherapy while using these drugs. Commonly used add-on agents include valproate, gabapentin and clonazepam. SDAs have recently been reported to be effective. Comorbid tics may require the coadministration of an SDA, pimozide (Orap) or haloperidol (Haldol). Buspirone may be useful in some patients. Patients with body dysmorphic disorder, which has been broadly conceptualized as a form of obsessive-compulsive disorder and which responds to treatment with SSRIs, may also respond to buspirone augmentation. Patients who have a partial response to the antidepressant before the augmentation show the best response following the addition of buspirone.

SCHIZOPHRENIA

Two different antipsychotic drugs may be combined for the purpose of enhancing efficacy. Usually these combinations result from attempts to make a transition from one agent to another, in which the patient shows improvement in the midst of the conversion. Some clinicians choose to leave well enough alone and maintain the patient on the combination.

The most common combination involving a dopamine receptor antagonist is the addition of an antiparkinsonian agent. The use of these drugs, which treat movement disorders caused by typical antipsychotics and by risperidone, is discussed in other sections of this book.

SSRIs are used to treat secondary depression in persons with schizophrenia already stabilized on a neuroleptic as well as for the treatment of residual negative symptoms with some patients exhibiting improvement, including reduction in positive and negative symptoms and decreased frequency of aggressive incidents. Reported adverse effects of SSRI–dopamine receptor antagonist treatment include worsening of psychosis and aggressiveness and worsening of extrapyramidal symptoms.

The effects of combining an SSRI with a dopamine receptor antagonist may result from pharmacokinetic interactions. For example, fluoxetine may produce a 65 percent elevation in fluphenazine concentrations and a 20 percent increase in haloperidol concentrations.

Patients may experience either improvement or worsening of psychosis when clozapine (Clozaril) and SSRIs are combined. Special caution is needed when combining some SSRIs with clozapine. Seizure is a serious, concentration-dependent side effect of clozapine, and SSRIs can significantly elevate concentrations of clozapine and its primary metabolite. Fluvoxamine may be more likely than other SSRIs to produce marked increases in these plasma concentrations.

ATTENTION-DEFICIT/HYPERACTIVITY DISORDER (ADHD)

The combination of clonidine (Catapres) with sympathomimetics is sometimes helpful in treating children with ADHD who are unresponsive to other interventions. A potential benefit of combining clonidine with sympathomimetics is improvement of sleep difficulties. For this purpose, daily dosages range from 0.05 to 0.8 mg of clonidine.

Sudden deaths have been reported in children taking the clonidine-methylphenidate combination. The mechanism causing these deaths has not been identified, and evidence that these deaths were related to this combination of drugs is still viewed as tenuous. Electrocardiograms (ECGs) should be obtained, whether clonidine is used alone or in combination with other drugs, if abnormalities are found during the physical examination or if there is evidence or history of preexisting heart disease. It is advisable to monitor vital signs whenever clonidine is used because of its hypotensive effects. Alternatives to the clonidine-methylphenidate combination may also be considered. Dextroamphetamine can be substituted for methylphenidate, and guanfacine (Tenex) for clonidine.

For a more detailed discussion of this topic, see Rush AJ: Mood Disorders: Treatment of Depression, Sec 14.7, p 1377; Post RM: Mood Disorders: Treatment of Bipolar Disorders, Sec 14.8, p 1385; Papp LA: Anxiety Disorders: Somatic Treatment, Sec 15.7, p 1490; Grebb JA: General Principles of Psychopharmacology, Sec 31.1, p 2235, in CTP/VII.

40

Laboratory Tests and Drug Therapy

Diagnoses in clinical psychiatry are made primarily on the basis of clinical history and mental status examination. Laboratory tests should be ordered on the basis of clinical suspicions arising from the initial evaluation. Because many systemic diseases influence mood, thought, and behavior, a complete psychiatric evaluation requires accurate diagnosis and management of all medical conditions. The laboratory tests routinely ordered at the time of hospital admission are listed in Table 40–1.

All persons with psychiatric symptoms should be carefully evaluated for abnormalities of thyroid, adrenal, renal, and hepatic function. Thyroid disease and other endocrinopathies may cause mood changes or psychosis; cancer or infectious diseases may cause depression; and infectious diseases, metabolic disorders, and structural brain insults may cause acute changes in mental status. In addition, psychiatric symptoms may be present with a wide range of chronic medical and neurological conditions, including multiple sclerosis, Parkinson's disease, Alzheimer's disease, Pick's disease, vascular dementia, human immunodeficiency virus (HIV) infection, Huntington's disease, and temporal lobe epilepsy. Any persons experiencing unexpected clinical changes suggesting drug intoxication should have appropriate urine and plasma drug screening.

Drug therapy.   Certain drug therapies require monitoring of plasma drug concentrations. Laboratory testing is essential for all persons taking lithium (Eskalith), carbamazepine (Tegretol), valproate (Depakene), or tacrine (Cognex) and may be useful for selected persons taking tricyclic and tetracyclic drugs. Clozapine (Clozaril) use requires special precautions (see below). Persons taking lithium should have thyroid function testing, persons taking valproate should have tests of hepatic and bone marrow function, and individuals taking tacrine should have hepatic function testing.

LABORATORY TESTS RELATED TO MEDICATION

Nonpsychiatric Drugs

The initial evaluation must always include a thorough assessment of prescribed and over-the-counter medications that the patient is taking. Many psychiatric syndromes can be caused by nonpsychiatric medications, for example, depression induced by a β-adrenergic receptor antagonist (or other antihypertensive agent), anticholinergic-induced delirium, and anabolic steroid-induced psychotic disorder. Often, if clinically possible, a "washout" of medications may aid diagnosis.

Psychiatric Drugs

Knowing the plasma concentrations of various drugs can help the clinician ascertain a variety of factors: (1) compliance, since low or absent plasma concentra-

TABLE 40–1
ROUTINE ADMISSION WORKUP

1. Complete blood count (CBC) with differential
2. Complete blood chemistry tests (including electrolytes, glucose, calcium, magnesium, hepatic, and renal function tests)
3. Thyroid function tests (TFTs)
4. Rapid plasma reagin (RPR) or Veneral Disease Research Laboratory (VDRL) test
5. Urinalysis
6. Urine toxicology screen
7. Electrocardiogram (ECG)
8. Chest X-ray (for patients over 35)
9. Plasma concentrations of any drugs being taken, if appropriate

tions are found in noncompliant persons; (2) pharmacodynamics, since plasma concentrations may be abnormally high or low because of metabolic inhibition (e.g., enzyme defects or liver damage), medical illness, and drug-drug interactions; (3) therapeutic drug concentrations, which can correlate with clinical improvement; and (4) toxic drug concentrations, which can account for adverse effects. Table 40–2 lists common therapeutic and toxic plasma concentrations of some drugs used in psychiatry.

Benzodiazepines.   No special tests are needed before prescribing benzodiazepines, although liver function tests are often useful. The drugs are metabolized in the liver by either oxidation or conjugation. Impaired hepatic function increases the elimination half-life of benzodiazepines that are oxidized, but it has less effect on benzodiazepines that are conjugated (oxazepam [Serax], lorazepam [Ativan], and temazepam [Restoril]). Benzodiazepines can also precipitate porphyria.

Dopamine Receptor Antagonists.   No special tests are needed, although it may be useful to have baseline liver function tests and a complete blood count (CBC). Dopamine receptor antagonists are metabolized primarily in the liver, with metabolites excreted primarily in the urine. Many metabolites are active. Peak plasma concentration is usually reached 2 to 3 hours after an oral dose is administered. Elimination half-life is 12 to 30 hours but may be much longer. Steady state requires at least a week at a constant dosage (months at a constant dosage of depot antipsychotics). Dopamine receptor antagonists cause elevation in serum prolactin levels (because of tuberoinfundibular activity). A normal prolactin level often indicates either noncompliance or nonabsorption.

Adverse effects include leukocytosis, leukopenia, impaired platelet functioning, mild anemia (both aplastic and hemolytic), and agranulocytosis. Bone marrow and

TABLE 40–2
THERAPEUTIC AND TOXIC PLASMA CONCENTRATIONS

Drug	Therapeutic Range	Toxic Levels
Amitriptyline	>120 ng/mL (but studies differ)	500 ng/mL
Bupropion	20–75 ng/mL	—
Carbamazepine	8–12 μg/mL	15 μg/mL
Clomipramine	Max 1000 ng/mL	
Desipramine	>125 ng/mL	500 ng/mL
Doxepin	150–250 ng/mL	—
Imipramine	>200–250 ng/mL	500 ng/mL
Lithium	0.6–1.2 mEq/L for maintenance	1.5–2 mEq/L
	1.0–1.5 mEq/L for acute mania	
Nortriptyline	Therapeutic window 50–150 ng/mL	500 ng/mL
Valproic acid	50–100 μg/mL	200 μg/mL

blood element adverse effects can occur abruptly, even when the dosage has remained constant. Low-potency dopamine receptor antagonists are most likely to cause agranulocytosis, which is the most common bone marrow adverse effect. They can also cause electrocardiogram (ECG) changes (not as frequently as tricyclic antidepressants) including a prolonged QT interval; flattened, inverted, or bifid T waves; and U waves. High plasma concentrations probably offer no clinical benefit and increase the risk of adverse effects.

Adverse effects may also include hypotension, sedation, lowering of the seizure threshold, anticholinergic effects, tremor, dystonia, cogwheel rigidity, rigidity without cogwheeling, akathisia, akinesia, so-called rabbit syndrome, and tardive dyskinesia.

Clozapine.   Because of the risk of agranulocytosis (1 to 2 percent), patients who are being treated with clozapine must have a baseline white blood cell (WBC) and differential count before the initiation of treatment, a WBC count every week throughout treatment, and a weekly WBC count 4 weeks after the discontinuation of clozapine (Table 40–3).

Tricyclics and Tetracyclics.   Patients should have an ECG before taking cyclic antidepressants, to assess for conduction delays, which may lead to heart block at therapeutic concentrations. Some clinicians believe that all patients receiving prolonged cyclic antidepressant therapy should have an annual ECG. At therapeutic concentrations, the drugs suppress arrhythmias through a quinidine (Duraquin)-like effect. Trazodone (Desyrel), an antidepressant unrelated to cyclic antidepressants, has been reported to cause ventricular arrhythmias and priapism, mild leukopenia, and neutropenia.

Plasma concentrations are often tested routinely when using imipramine (Tofranil), desipramine (Norpramin), or nortriptyline (Pamelor) in the treatment of depression. Knowing plasma concentrations may also be of use with patients who display a poor response at normal dosage ranges and in high-risk patients when there is an urgent need to know whether a therapeutic or toxic plasma concentration of drug has been reached. Blood concentration tests should also include measurement of active metabolites (e.g., imipramine is converted to desipramine, amitriptyline [Elavil] to nortriptyline).

Some characteristics of tricyclic drug plasma concentrations are as follows:

1. Imipramine. The percentage of favorable responses correlates with plasma concentrations in a linear manner between 200 and 250 ng/mL, but some patients may respond to a lower concentration. At concentrations above 250 ng/mL, there is no improved favorable response, and adverse effects increase.
2. Nortriptyline. The therapeutic window (the range within which a drug is most effective) is between 50 and 150 ng/mL. There is a decreased response rate at concentrations over 150 ng/mL.
3. Desipramine. Concentrations above 125 ng/mL correlate with a higher percentage of favorable responses.
4. Amitriptyline. Different studies have produced conflicting results with regard to blood concentrations.

PROCEDURE
The physician should draw the blood specimen 10 to 14 hours after the last dose, usually in the morning after a bedtime dose. Patients must be on a stable daily dosage

TABLE 40-3
CLINICAL MANAGEMENT OF REDUCED WHITE BLOOD CELL COUNT, LEUKOPENIA, AND AGRANULOCYTOSIS IN PERSONS TAKING CLOZAPINE

Problem Phase	WBC Findings	Clinical Findings	Treatment Plan
Reduced WBC	WBC count reveals a significant drop (even if WBC count is still in normal range): "significant drop" (1) drop of more than 3000 cells from prior test or (2) three or more consecutive drops in WBC counts	No symptoms of infection	1. Monitor patient closely 2. Institute twice-weekly CBC tests with differentials if deemed appropriate by attending physician 3. Clozapine therapy may continue
Mild leukopenia	WBC = 3000–3500	Patient may or may not show clinical symptoms, such as lethargy, fever, sore throat, weakness	1. Monitor patient closely 2. Institute a minimum of twice-weekly CBC tests with differentials 3. Clozapine therapy may continue
Leukopenia or granulocytopenia	WBC = 2000–3000 or granulocytes = 1000–1500	Patient may or may not show clinical symptoms, such as fever, sore throat, lethargy, weakness	1. Interrupt clozapine at once 2. Institute daily CBC tests with differentials 3. Increase surveillance, consider hospitalization 4. Clozapine therapy may be reinstituted after normalization of WBC
Agranulocytosis (uncomplicated)	WBC count <2000 or granulocytes <1000	The patient may or may not show clinical symptoms, such as fever, sore throat, lethargy, weakness	1. Discontinue clozapine at once 2. Place patient in protective isolation in a medical unit with modern facilities 3. Consider a bone marrow specimen to determine if progenitor cells are being suppressed 4. Monitor patient every 2 days until WBC and differential counts return to normal (about 2 weeks) 5. Avoid use of concomitant medications with bone marrow–suppressing potential 6. Consult with hematologist or other specialist to determine appropriate antibiotic regimen 7. Start appropriate therapy; monitor closely
Agranulocytosis (with complications)	WBC count <2000 or granulocytes <1000	Definite evidence of infection, such as fever, sore throat, lethargy, weakness, malaise, skin ulcerations, etc.	
Recovery	WBC count >4000 and granulocytes >2000	No symptoms of infection	1. Once-weekly CBC with differential counts for four consecutive normal values 2. Clozapine must not be restarted

From Sandoz Pharmaceuticals Corporation and MacKinnon RA, Yudofsky SC. *Principles of the Psychiatric Evaluation.* Lippincott, Philadelphia, 1991, with permission.

for at least 5 days for the test results to be valid. Some patients are unusually poor metabolizers of cyclic antidepressants and may have levels as high as 2000 ng/mL while taking normal doses and before showing a favorable clinical response. Such patients must be monitored very closely for cardiac side effects. Patients with levels above 500 ng/mL are generally at risk for toxic effects.

Monoamine Oxidase Inhibitors.   Patients taking monoamine oxidase inhibitors (MAOIs) are instructed to avoid foods containing tyramine (see Table 21-2 in Chapter 21) because of the danger of a potential hypertensive crisis. A baseline normal blood pressure (BP) should be recorded, and the BP should be followed during treatment. MAOIs may also cause orthostatic hypotension as a direct drug side effect unrelated to diet. Other than their potential for elevating the BP when taken with certain foods, MAOIs are relatively free of adverse effects. There are no clinical plasma concentration values available for MAOIs, although a research test involves correlating therapeutic response with the degree of platelet monoamine oxidase inhibition.

Lithium.   Patients receiving lithium should have baseline thyroid function tests, electrolyte determinations, a WBC count, renal function tests (specific gravity, blood urea nitrogen [BUN], and creatinine clearance), and a baseline ECG (Table 40–4). The rationale for these tests is that lithium can cause renal concentrating defects, hypothyroidism, and leukocytosis; sodium depletion can cause toxic lithium concentrations; and approximately 95 percent of lithium is excreted in the urine. Lithium has also been shown to cause ECG changes, including various conduction defects.

Lithium is most clearly indicated in the prophylactic treatment of mania (direct antimanic effect may take up to 2 weeks) and is commonly coupled with antipsychotics for the short-term treatment of manic episodes. Lithium itself may have antipsychotic activity as well. The maintenance concentration is 0.6 to 1.2 mEq/L, although acutely manic patients can tolerate up to 1.5 to 1.8 mEq/L. Some patients may respond at lower concentrations; others may require higher concentrations. A response below 0.4 mEq/L is probably a placebo effect. Toxic reactions may occur with concentrations above 2.0 mEq/L. Regular lithium monitoring is essential, since there is a narrow therapeutic range beyond which cardiac problems and central nervous system (CNS) effects can occur.

Blood for lithium concentration determination is drawn 8 to 12 hours after the last dose, usually in the morning after the bedtime dose. The concentration should be measured at least twice a week while stabilizing the patient and may be determined monthly thereafter.

Carbamazepine.   Prior to treatment with carbamazepine, a CBC, including platelet count, should be done. Reticulocyte count and serum iron determination are

TABLE 40–4
OTHER LABORATORY TESTING FOR PATIENTS TAKING LITHIUM

Test	Frequency
1. Complete blood count	Before treatment and yearly
2. Serum electrolytes	Before treatment and yearly
3. Fasting blood glucose	Before treatment and yearly
4. Electrocardiogram	Before treatment and yearly
5. Pregnancy testing for women of childbearing age[a]	Before treatment

[a] Take more frequently when compliance with treatment plan is uncertain.
From MacKinnon RA, Yudofsky SC. *Principles of the Psychiatric Evaluation.* Lippincott, Philadelphia, 1991, with permission.

also desirable. The tests should be repeated once during the first 3 months of treatment and every 6 months thereafter. Carbamazepine can cause aplastic anemia, agranulocytosis, thrombocytopenia, and leukopenia. Because of the minor risk of hepatotoxicity, liver function tests should be done every 6 months. The medication should be discontinued if there are any signs of bone marrow suppression as measured with periodic CBCs. The therapeutic concentration of carbamazepine is 8 to 12 μg/mL, with toxicity most often reached at 15 μg/mL.

Valproate.   Serum levels of valproic acid (Depakene) and divalproex (Depakote) are therapeutic in the range of 50 to 150 μg/mL. Above 180 μg/mL, adverse effects may occur. Serum concentrations should be determined periodically, and liver function tests should be done every 6 to 12 months.

Tacrine.   Tacrine may cause liver damage. A baseline of liver function should be established, and follow-up serum transaminase concentrations should be determined every other week for about 5 months. Patients who develop jaundice or who have bilirubin levels above 3 mg/dL must be withdrawn from use of drug.

NEUROENDOCRINE TESTS

Thyroid Function Tests

Several thyroid function tests are available, including tests for thyroxine (T_4) by competitive protein binding (T_4 [D]) and by radioimmunoassay (T_4 [RIA]) involving a specific antigen-antibody reaction. Over 90 percent of T_4 is bound to serum protein and is responsible for thyroid-stimulating hormone (TSH) secretion and cellular metabolism. Other thyroid measures include the free T_4 index (FT_4I), triiodothyronine (T_3) uptake, and total serum T_3 measured by radioimmunoassay (T_3 [RIA]). Those tests are used to rule out hypothyroidism, which can exhibit symptoms of depression. In some studies, up to 10 percent of patients complaining of depression and associated fatigue had incipient hypothyroid disease. Lithium can cause hypothyroidism and, more rarely, hyperthyroidism. Neonatal hypothyroidism results in mental retardation and is preventable if the diagnosis is made at birth.

Thyrotropin-Releasing Hormone Stimulation Test.   The thyrotropin-releasing hormone (TRH) stimulation test is indicated for patients who have marginally abnormal thyroid test results with suspected subclinical hypothyroidism, which may account for clinical depression. It is also used in patients with possible lithium-induced hypothyroidism. The procedure entails an intravenous (i.v.) injection of 500 mg of protirelin (TRH), which produces a sharp rise in serum TSH measured at 15, 30, 60, and 90 minutes. An increase in serum TSH of 5 to 25 mIU/mL above the baseline is normal. An increase of less than 7 mIU/mL is considered a blunted response, which may correlate with a diagnosis of depression. Eight percent of all patients with depression have some thyroid illness.

Dexamethasone-Suppression Test

Dexamethasone (Decadron) is a long-acting synthetic glucocorticoid with a long half-life. Approximately 1 mg of dexamethasone is equivalent to 25 mg of hydrocortisone. The dexamethasone-suppression test (DST) is used to help confirm a diagnostic impression of major depressive disorder with melancholic features (DSM-IV classification) or endogenous depression (Research Diagnostic Criteria [RDC] classification).

Procedure. The patient is given 1 mg of dexamethasone by mouth at 11 PM, and plasma cortisol is measured at 8 AM, 4 PM, and 11 PM. Plasma cortisol concentration above 5 μg/dL (known as nonsuppression) is considered abnormal (i.e., positive). Suppression of cortisol indicates that the hypothalamic-adrenal-pituitary axis is functioning properly. Since the 1930s, dysfunction of that axis has been known to be associated with stress.

The DST can be used to follow the response of a depressed person to treatment. Normalization of the DST, however, is not an indication to stop antidepressant treatment, because the DST may normalize before the depression resolves.

There is some evidence that patients with a positive DST result (especially 10 μg/dL) will have a good response to somatic treatment, such as electroconvulsive therapy (ECT) or tricyclic or tetracyclic antidepressant therapy. The problems associated with the DST include varying reports of sensitivity and specificity. False-positive and false-negative results are common and are listed in Table 40–5. The sensitivity of the DST is considered to be 45 percent in major depressive disorder and 70 percent in psychotic mood disorders. The specificity is 90 percent compared with controls and 77 percent compared with other psychiatric diagnoses.

TABLE 40–5
**CAUSES OF FALSE POSITIVE OR NEGATIVE RESULTS ON THE
DEXAMETHASONE-SUPPRESSION TEST (DST)**

False Positives	False Negatives
Cushing's syndrome	Addison's disease
Weight loss or malnutrition	Hypopituitarism
Obesity	Slow dexamethasone metabolism
Bulimia nervosa	Drugs
Pregnancy	Synthetic corticosteroids
Alcohol abuse and withdrawal	Indomethacin
Anorexia nervosa	High doses of benzodiazepines
Temporal lobe epilepsy	High doses of cyproheptadine
Dementia	
Diabetes mellitus	
Infection	
Trauma	
Recent surgery	
Advanced age	
Fever	
Carcinoma	
Renal or cardiac failure	
Renovascular hypertension	
Cerebrovascular disorder	
Antipsychotic withdrawal	
Tricyclic withdrawal	
Drugs	
High doses of estrogens	
Narcotics	
Sedative-hypnotics	
Anticonvulsants	

From Rosse RB, Rosse LH, Deutsch SI. Medical assessment and laboratory testing in psychiatry. In: *Comprehensive Textbook of Psychiatry*, ed. 6 Kaplan HI, Sadock BJ, editors. Williams & Wilkins, Baltimore, 1995.

Other Endocrine Tests

A variety of other hormones affect behavior. Exogenous hormonal administration has been shown to affect behavior, and known endocrine diseases have associated psychiatric disorders.

In addition to thyroid hormones, the hormones include the anterior pituitary hormone prolactin, growth hormone, somatostatin, gonadotropin-releasing hormone (GnRH), and the sex steroids—luteinizing hormone (LH), follicle-stimulating hormone (FSH), testosterone, and estrogen. Melatonin from the pineal gland has been implicated in mood disorder with seasonal pattern (previously called seasonal affective disorder).

Tests of Catecholamines and Neurotransmitter Metabolites

The concentration of serotonin metabolite 5-hydroxyindoleacetic acid (5-HIAA) is elevated in the urine of patients with carcinoid tumors and at times in patients who take phenothiazine medication or in persons who eat foods high in serotonin (e.g., walnuts, bananas, avocados). The amount of 5-HIAA in cerebrospinal fluid may be low in some persons who are in a suicidal depression and in those who have committed suicide in particularly violent ways. Low cerebrospinal fluid 5-HIAA concentration may be associated with violence in general. Norepinephrine and its metabolic products—metanephrine, normetanephrine, and vanillylmandelic acid (VMA)—can be measured in the urine, blood, and plasma. Plasma catecholamine concentrations are markedly elevated in pheochromocytoma, which is associated with anxiety, agitation, and hypertension. Some patients with chronic anxiety may have elevated blood norepinephrine and epinephrine concentrations. Some depressed patients have a lower urinary norepinephrine to epinephrine ratio (NE:E).

High levels of urinary norepinephrine and epinephrine have been found in some patients with posttraumatic stress disorder. The norepinephrine metabolite 3-methoxy-4-hydroxyphenylglycol (MHPG) concentration is decreased in patients with severe depressive disorders, especially in those who attempt suicide.

Renal Function Tests

Creatinine clearance detects early kidney damage and can be serially monitored to follow the course of renal disease. BUN is also elevated in renal disease. Lithium may cause renal damage, and the serum BUN and creatinine are followed in patients taking lithium. If the serum BUN or creatinine is abnormal, the patient's 2-hour creatinine clearance and ultimately the 24-hour creatinine clearance are tested.

Liver Function Tests

Total bilirubin and direct bilirubin are elevated in hepatocellular injury and intrahepatic bile stasis that can occur with phenothiazine or tricyclic medication and with alcohol and drug abuse. Certain drugs (e.g., phenobarbital [Solfoton, Luminal]) may decrease serum bilirubin concentration. Liver damage or disease, which is reflected by abnormal findings in liver function tests, may present with signs and symptoms of a cognitive disorder, including disorientation and delirium. Impaired hepatic function may increase the elimination half-lives of certain drugs, including some of the benzodiazepines, so that the drugs may stay in the system longer than they would under normal circumstances.

URINE SCREEN FOR SUBSTANCES OF ABUSE

A number of drugs may be detected in a patient's urine if the urine is tested within a specific (and variable) period of time after ingestion. Knowledge of urine drug testing is becoming crucial for practicing physicians as the controversial issue of mandatory or random drug testing becomes prevalent. Table 40-6 provides a summary of drugs of abuse that can be tested in urine.

OUTLINES OF OTHER TESTS

A. Provocation of panic attacks by sodium lactate
  1. Indications
     a. Possible diagnosis of panic disorder
     b. Lactate-provoked panic confirms presence of panic attacks
     c. Up to 72 percent of panic attacks will be lactate-provoked
     d. Has been used to induce flashbacks in patients with posttraumatic stress disorder
  2. Procedure
     a. Inject a 5 percent dextrose in water solution intravenously slowly for 28 minutes, then rapidly for 2 minutes
     b. Infuse 0.5 M racemic sodium lactate (total 10 mL/kg of body weight) over a 20-minute period or until panic occurs
  3. Physiological changes from lactate infusion include hemodilution, metabolic alkalosis (metabolized to bicarbonate), hypocalcemia (calcium bound to lactate), and hypophosphatemia (caused by increased glomerular filtration rate [GFR])

TABLE 40-6
SUBSTANCES OF ABUSE THAT CAN BE TESTED IN URINE

Substance	Length of Time Detected in Urine
Alcohol	7–12 hours
Amphetamine	48 hours
Barbiturate	24 hours (short acting)
	3 weeks (long acting)
Benzodiazepine	3 days
Cannabis	3 days to 4 weeks (depending on use)
Cocaine	6–8 hours (metabolites, 2–4 days)
Codeine	48 hours
Heroin	36–72 hours
Methadone	3 days
Methaqualone	7 days
Morphine	48–72 hours
Phencyclidine (PCP)	8 days
Propoxyphene	6–48 hours

    4. Comments
      a. Effect is a direct response to lactate or its metabolism and occurs peripherally
      b. Simple hyperventilation has not been as sensitive in inducing panic attacks
      c. Lactate-induced panic is not blocked by peripheral β-adrenergic receptor antagonists but is blocked by alprazolam (Xanax) and by tricyclic antidepressants
      d. Carbon dioxide (CO_2) inhalation precipitates panic attacks, but mechanism is thought to be central and related to CNS concentrations of CO_2, possibly as a locus ceruleus stimulant (CO_2 crosses blood–brain barrier [BBB], but bicarbonate does not)
      e. Lactate crosses the BBB through an easily saturated active transport system
      f. L-Lactate is metabolized to pyruvate

B. **Amobarbital interview.** The common use of amobarbital (Amytal), a barbiturate with a half-life of 8 to 42 hours, led to the popular name "Amytal interview" for this technique. However, other sedative drugs, particularly the benzodiazepines, are as effective as the barbiturates.
    1. Diagnostic indications—catatonia; hysterical stupor; unexplained muteness; differentiating functional and organic stupors (organic conditions should worsen, and functional conditions should improve because of decreased anxiety)
    2. Therapeutic indications (as an interview aid for disorders of repression and dissociation)
      a. Abreaction of posttraumatic stress disorder
      b. Recovery of memory in dissociative amnesia and fugue
      c. Recovery of function in conversion disorder
    3. Procedure
      a. Have patient recline in an environment in which cardiopulmonary resuscitation is readily available should hypotension or respiratory depression develop
      b. Explain to patient that medication should help him or her relax and feel like talking
      c. Insert narrow-bore needle into peripheral vein
      d. Inject a 5 percent solution of sodium amobarbital (500 mg dissolved in 10 mL of sterile water) at a rate no faster than 1 mL a minute (50 mg a minute)
      e. Conduct interview by using frequent suggestions and beginning with neutral topics; it is often helpful to prompt patient with known facts about his or her life
      f. Continue infusion until either sustained lateral nystagmus or drowsiness is noted
      g. To maintain level of narcosis, continue infusion at a rate of 0.5 to 1.0 mL per 5 minutes (25 to 50 mg/5 min)
      h. Have patient remain in reclining position for at least 15 minutes after the interview is terminated and until patient can walk without supervision
      i. Use the same method every time to avoid dosage errors

TABLE 40–7
PSYCHIATRIC INDICATIONS FOR DIAGNOSTIC TESTS

Test	Major Psychiatric Indications	Comments
Acid phosphatase	Cognitive/medical workup	Increased in prostate cancer, benign prostatic hypertrophy, excessive platelet destruction, bone disease
Adrenocorticotropic hormone (ACTH)	Cognitive/medical workup	Increased in steroid abuse; may be increased in seizures, psychoses, and Cushing's disease and in response to stress Decreased in Addison's disease
Alanine aminotransferase (ALT), (formerly called serum, glutamic-pyruvic transaminase (SGPT))	Cognitive/medical workup	Increased in hepatitis, cirrhosis, liver metastases Decreased in pyridoxine (vitamin B_6) deficiency
Albumin	Cognitive/medical workup	Increased in dehydration Decreased in malnutrition, hepatic failure, burns, multiple myeloma, carcinomas
Aldolase	Eating disorders Schizophrenia	Increased in patients who abuse ipecac (e.g., bulimia nervosa patients), some patients with schizophrenia
Alkaline phosphatase	Cognitive/medical workup Use of psychotropic medications	Increased in Paget's disease, hyperparathyroidism, hepatic disease, hepatic metastases, heart failure, phenothiazine use Decreased in pernicious anemia (vitamin B_{12} deficiency)
Ammonia, serum	Cognitive/medical workup	Increased in hepatic encephalopathy, liver failure, Reye's syndrome; also increases with GI hemorrhage and severe congestive heart failure
Amylase, serum	Eating disorders	May be increased in bulimia nervosa
Antinuclear antibodies	Cognitive/medical workup	Found in systemic lupus erythematosus (SLE) and drug-induced lupus (e.g., secondary to phenothiazines, anticonvulsants); SLE can be associated with delirium, psychosis, mood disorder
Aspartate aminotransferase (AST) (formerly SGOT)	Cognitive/medical workup	Increased in heart failure, hepatic disease, pancreatitis, eclampsia, cerebral damage, alcoholism Decreased in pyridoxine (vitamin B_6) deficiency and terminal stages of liver disease
Bicarbonate, serum	Panic disorder Eating disorders	May be elevated in patients with bulimia nervosa, in laxative abuse, in psychogenic vomiting
Bilirubin	Cognitive/medical workup	Increased in hepatic disease
Blood urea nitrogen (BUN)	Delirium Use of psychotropic medications	Elevated in renal disease, dehydration Elevations associated with lethargy, delirium If elevated, can increase toxic potential of psychiatric medications, especially lithium and amantadine (Symmetrel)
Bromide, serum	Dementia Psychosis	Bromide intoxication can cause psychosis, hallucinations, delirium Part of dementia workup, especially when serum chloride is elevated

continues

TABLE 40–7—continued

Test	Major Psychiatric Indications	Comments
Caffeine level, serum	Anxiety/panic disorder	Evaluation of patients with suspected caffeinism (caffeine intoxication)
Calcium (Ca), serum	Cognitive/medical workup	Increased in hyperparathyroidism, bone metastases
	Mood disorders	Increase associated with delirium, depression, psychosis
	Psychosis	Decrease associated with depression, irritability, delirium, chronic laxative abuse
	Eating disorders	Decrease in hypoparathyroidism, renal failure
Carotid ultrasound	Dementia	Occasionally included in dementia workup, especially to rule out vascular dementia
Catecholamines, urinary and plasma	Panic attacks	Primary value is in search for possible infarct causes
	Anxiety	Elevated in pheochromocytoma
Cerebrospinal fluid (CSF)	Cognitive/medical workup	Increased protein and cells in infection, positive VDRL in neurosyphilis, bloody CSF in hemorrhagic conditions
Ceruloplasmin, serum; copper, serum	Cognitive/medical workup	Low in Wilson's disease (hepatolenticular disease)
Chloride (Cl), serum	Eating disorders	Decreased in patients with bulimia nervosa and psychogenic vomiting
	Panic disorder	Mild elevation in hyperventilation syndrome, panic disorder
Cholecystokinin (CCK)	Eating disorders	Compared with controls, blunted in bulimia nervosa patients after eating meal (may normalize after treatment with antidepressants)
CO_2 inhalations; sodium bicarbonate infusion	Anxiety/panic attacks	Panic attacks produced in subgroup of patients
Coombs' test, direct and indirect	Hemolytic anemias secondary to psychotropic medications	Evaluation of drug-induced hemolytic anemias, such as those induced by chlorpromazine, phenytoin, levodopa, and methyldopa
Copper, urine	Cognitive/medical workup	Elevated in Wilson's disease
Cortisol (hydrocortisone)	Cognitive/medical workup	Excessive level may indicate Cushing's disease associated with anxiety, depression, and a variety of other conditions
	Mood disorders	
Creatine phosphokinase (CPK)	Use of antipsychotics	Increased in neuroleptic malignant syndrome, intramuscular injection, rhabdomyolysis (secondary to substance abuse), patients in restraints, patients experiencing dystonic reactions; asymptomatic elevations seen with use of antipsychotics
	Use of restraints	
	Substance abuse	
Creatine, serum	Cognitive/medical workup	Elevated in renal disease (see BUN)
Dopamine (DA) (levodopa stimulation of dopamine)	Depression	Inhibits prolactin
		Test used to assess functional integrity of dopaminergic system, which is impaired in Parkinson's disease, depression
Doppler ultrasound	Erectile disorder	Carotid occlusion, transient ischemic attack (TIA), reduced penile blood flow in erectile disorder
	Cognitive/medical workup	
Echocardiogram	Panic disorder	10–40% of patients with panic disorder show mitral valve prolapse

Test	Category	Notes
Electroencephalogram (EEG)	Cognitive/medical workup	Seizures, brain death, lesions; shortened REM latency in depression
		High-voltage activity in stupor; low-voltage fast activity in excitement; in functional nonorganic cases (e.g., dissociative states), alpha activity is present in the background, which responds to auditory and visual stimuli
		Biphasic or triphasic slow bursts seen in dementia due to Creutzfeldt-Jakob disease
Epstein-Barr virus (EBV); cytomegalovirus (CMV)	Cognitive/medical workup	Part of herpesvirus group
	Anxiety	EBV is causative agent for infectious mononucleosis, which can present with depression, fatigue, and personality change
	Mood disorders	CMV can produce anxiety, confusion, mood disorders
		EBV may be associated with chronic mononucleosis-like syndrome associated with chronic depression and fatigue
Erythrocyte sedimentation rate (ESR)	Cognitive/medical workup	An increase in ESR represents a nonspecific test of infectious, inflammatory, autoimmune, or malignant disease; sometimes recommended in the evaluation of anorexia nervosa
Estrogen	Mood disorders	Decreased in menopausal depression and premenstrual syndrome; variable changes in anxiety
Ferritin, serum	Cognitive/medical workup	Most sensitive test for iron deficiency
Folate (folic acid), serum	Alcohol use disorders	Usually measured with vitamin B_{12} deficiencies associated with psychosis, paranoia, fatigue, agitation, dementia, delirium
	Use of specific medications	Associated with alcoholism, use of phenytoin, oral contraceptives, estrogen
Follicle-stimulating hormone (FSH)	Depression	High normal in anorexia nervosa, higher values in postmenopausal women; low levels in patients with panhypopituitarism
Glucose, fasting blood (FBS)	Panic attacks	Very high FBS associated with delirium
	Anxiety	Very low FBS associated with delirium, agitation, panic attacks, anxiety, depression
	Delirium	
	Depression	
Glutamyl transaminase, serum	Alcohol use disorders	Increased in alcohol abuse, cirrhosis, liver disease
Gonadotropin-releasing hormone (GnRH)	Cognitive/medical workup	
	Depression	Decreased in schizophrenia; increased in anorexia; variable in depression, anxiety
	Axiety	
	Schizophrenia	
Growth hormone (GH)	Depression	Blunted GH responses to insulin-induced hypoglycemia in depressed patients; increased GH responses to dopamine agonist challenge in schizophrenic patients; increased in some patients with anorexia
	Schizophrenia	
Hematocrit (Hct); hemoglobin (Hb)	Cognitive/medical workup	Assessment of anemia (anemia may be associated with depression and psychosis)
Hepatitis A viral antigen (HAAg)	Mood disorders	Less severe, better prognosis than hepatitis B; may present with anorexia, depression
Hepatitis B surface antigen (HBsAg); hepatitis B core antigen (HBcAg)	Cognitive/medical workup	Active hepatitis B infection indicates greater infectivity and progression to chronic liver disease
	Mood disorders	May present with depression
	Cognitive/medical workup	

continues

TABLE 40–7—continued

Test	Major Psychiatric Indications	Comments
Holter monitor	Panic disorder	Evaluation of panic disorder patients with palpitations and other cardiac symptoms
Human immunodeficiency virus (HIV)	Cognitive/medical workup	CNS involvement; dementia due to HIV disease, personality disorder, mood disorder, and psychotic disorder due to a general medical condition
17-Hydroxycorticosteroid	Depression	Deviations detect hyperadrenocorticalism, which can be associated with major depressive disorder. Increased in steroid abuse
5-Hydroxyindoleacetic acid (5-HIAA)	Depression Suicide Violence	Decrease in CSF in aggressive or violent patients with suicidal or homicidal impulses. May be indicator of decreased impulse control and predictor of suicide
Iron, serum	Cognitive/medical workup	Iron-deficiency anemia
Lactate dehydrogenase (LDH)	Cognitive/medical workup	Increased in myocardial infarction, pulmonary infarction, hepatic disease, renal infarction, seizures, cerebral damage, megaloblastic (pernicious) anemia, factitious elevations secondary to rough handling of blood specimen tube
Lupus anticoagulant (LA)	Use of phenothiazines	An antiphospholipid antibody, which has been described in some patients using phenothiazines, especially chlorpromazine; often associated with elevated PTT; associated with anticardiolipin antibodies
Lupus erythematosus (LE) test	Depression Psychosis Delirium Dementia	Positive test result associated with systemic LE, which may present with various psychiatric disturbances, such as psychosis, depression, delirium, dementia; also tested for antinuclear antibody (ANA) and antiDNA antibody tests
Luteinizing hormone (LH)	Depression	Low in patients with panhypopituitarism; decrease associated with depression
Magnesium, serum	Alcohol use disorders Cognitive/medical workup	Decreased in alcoholism; low levels associated with agitation, delirium, seizures
MAO, platelet	Depression	Low in depression; has been used to monitor MAOI therapy
MCV (mean corpuscular volume) (average volume of a red blood cell)	Alcohol use disorders	Elevated in alcoholism and vitamin B12 and folate deficiency
Melatonin	Mood disorder with seasonal pattern (Seasonal affective disorder)	Produced by light and pineal gland and decreased in mood disorder with seasonal pattern
Metal (heavy) intoxication (serum or urinary)	Cognitive/medical workup	Lead—apathy, irritability, anorexia, confusion Mercury—psychosis, fatigue, apathy, decreased memory, emotional liability, "mad hatter" Manganese—manganese madness, Parkinson-like syndrome Aluminum—dementia Arsenic—fatigue, blackouts, hair loss

Test	Indication	Comment
3-Methoxy-4-hydroxyphenylglycol (MHPG)	Depression	Most useful in research; decreases in urine may indicate decreases centrally; may predict response to certain antidepressants
Myoglobin, urine	Anxiety / Phenothiazine use / Substance intoxication / Use of restraints	Increased in neuroleptic malignant syndrome; in PCP, cocaine, and lysergic acid diethylamide (LSD) intoxication; and in patients in restraints
Nicotine	Anxiety / Nicotine addiction	Anxiety, smoking
Nocturnal penile tumescence	Erectile disorder	Quantification of penile circumference changes, penile rigidity, frequency of penile tumescence / Evaluation of erectile function during sleep / Erections associated with rapid eye movement (REM) sleep / Helpful in differentiation between organic and functional causes of impotence
Parathyroid (parathormone) hormone	Anxiety	Low level causes hypocalcemia and anxiety / Dysregulation associated with wide variety of mental disorders due to a general medical condition
Partial thromboplastin time (PTT)	Treatment with antipsychotics, heparin	Monitor anticoagulant therapy; increased in presence of lupus anticoagulant and anticardiolipin antibodies
Phosphorus, serum	Cognitive/medical workup / Panic disorder	Increased in renal failure, diabetic acidosis, hypoparathyroidism, hypervitamin D; decreased in cirrhosis, hypokalemia, hyperparathyroidism, panic attacks, hyperventilation syndrome
Platelet count	Use of psychotropic medications	Decreased by certain psychotropic medications (carbamazepine, clozapine, phenothiazines)
Porphobilinogen (PBG)	Cognitive/medical workup	Increased in acute porphyria
Porphyria-synthesizing enzyme	Psychosis	Acute neuropsychiatric disorder can occur in acute porphyria attack, which may be precipitated by barbiturates, imipramine
Potassium (K), serum	Cognitive/medical workup / Eating disorders	Increased in hyperkalemic acidosis, increase in associated with anxiety in cardiac arrhythmia / Decreased in cirrhosis, metabolic alkalosis, laxative abuse, diuretic abuse; decrease is common in bulimia nervosa patients and in psychogenic vomiting, anabolic steroid abuse
Prolactin, serum	Use of antipsychotic medications / Cocaine-related disorders / Pseudoseizures	Antipsychotics, by decreasing dopamine, increase prolactin synthesis and release, especially in women / Elevated prolactin levels may be seen secondary to cocaine withdrawal / Lack of prolactin rise after seizure suggests pseudoseizure
Protein, total serum	Cognitive/medical workup / Use of psychotropic medications	Increased in multiple myeloma, myxedema, lupus / Decreased in cirrhosis, malnutrition, overhydration / Low serum protein can result in greater sensitivity to conventional doses of protein-bound medications (lithium is not protein bound)
Prothrombin time (PT)	Cognitive/medical workup	Elevated in significant liver damage (cirrhosis)
Reticulocyte count (estimate of red blood cell production in bone marrow)	Cognitive/medical workup / Use of carbamazepine	Low in megaloblastic or iron deficiency anemia and anemia of chronic diseases / Must be monitored in patient taking carbamazepine

continues

TABLE 40–7—continued

Test	Major Psychiatric Indications	Comments
Salicylate, serum	Hallucinations Suicide attempts	Toxic levels may be seen in suicide attempts; high levels may also cause salicylate-induced psychotic disorder with hallucinations
Sodium (Na), serum	Cognitive/medical workup Use of lithium	Decreased with water intoxication; SIADH Decreased in hypoadrenalism, myxedema, congestive heart failure, diarrhea, polydipsia, use of carbamazepine, anabolic steroids Low levels associated with greater sensitivity to conventional dose of lithium
Testosterone, serum	Erectile disorder Hypoactive sexual desire disorder	Increased in anabolic steroid abuse May be decreased in medical workup of impotence Decrease may be seen with hypoactive sexual desire disorder Follow-up sex offenders treated with medroxyprogesterone Decreased with medroxyprogesterone treatment
Thyroid function tests	Cognitive/medical workup Depression	Detection of hypothyroidism or hyperthyroidism Abnormalities can be associated with depression, anxiety, psychosis, dementia, delirium, lithium treatment
Urinalysis	Cognitive/medical workup Pretreatment workup of lithium Drug screening	Provides clues to cause of various cognitive disorders (assessing general appearance, pH, specific gravity, bilirubin, glucose, blood, ketones, protein, etc.): specific gravity may be affected by lithium
Urinary creatine	Cognitive/medical workup Substance abuse Lithium use	Increased in renal failure, dehydration Part of pretreatment workup for lithium; sometimes used in follow-up evaluations of patients treated with lithium
Venereal Disease Research Laboratory (VDRL)	Syphilis	Positive (high titers) in secondary syphilis (may be positive or negative in primary syphilis); RPR test also used Low titers (or negative) in tertiary syphilis
Vitamin A, serum	Depression Delirium	Hypervitaminosis A is associated with a variety of mental status changes, headache
Vitamin B₁₂, serum	Cognitive/medical workup Dementia Mood disorder Alcohol use disorders	Part of workup of megaloblastic anemia and dementia B₁₂ deficiency associated with psychosis, paranoia, fatigue, agitation, dementia, delirium Often associated with chronic alcohol abuse and dependence
White blood cell (WBC)	Use of psychotropic medications	Leukopenia and agranulocytosis associated with certain psychotropic medications, such as phenothiazines, carbamazepine, clozapine Leukocytosis associated with lithium and neuroleptic malignant syndrome

4. Contraindications
   a. Presence of upper respiratory infection or inflammation
   b. Severe hepatic or renal impairment
   c. Hypotension
   d. History of porphyria
   e. Barbiturate addiction
C. Other Laboratory Tests. Laboratory tests listed in Table 40–7 have application for clinical and research psychiatry. Standard textbooks of medicine give the laboratory values. The psychiatrist must always know the normal values of the particular laboratory performing the test, because those values vary from one laboratory to another. Two types of measurements are currently in use—the conventional and the Système International (SI) d'Unités. The latter is an international language of measurement calculated by multiplying the conventional unit by a numerical factor being adopted by many laboratories. The SI measurement system uses moles as the basic unit for the amount of a substance, kilograms for its mass, and meters for its length.

For a more detailed discussion of this topic, see Rosse RB, Deutsch LH, Deutsch SI: Medical Assessment and Laboratory Testing in Psychiatry, Sec 7.7, p 732, in CTP/VII.

41

Psychoactive Herbs

Phytomedicinals (from the Greek *phyto*, meaning plant) are herb and plant preparations that are used or have been used for the treatment of a variety of medical conditions. There are over 200 herbal drugs in use; only those with psychoactive properties are listed in Table 41–1.

Adverse effects are possible, and toxic interactions with other drugs may occur with all phytomedicinals. Adulteration is common, and there are no consistent standard preparations available for most herbs. Safety profiles and knowledge of adverse effects of most of these substances are lacking, and because of the paucity of clinical trials all of these agents should be avoided during pregnancy. Since most of these herbs are secreted in breast milk they are contraindicated during lactation.

Clinicians should always attempt to obtain a history of herbal use during the psychiatric evaluation.

It is important to be nonjudgmental in dealing with patients who use phytomedicinals. Many do so for various reasons: (1) as part of their cultural tradition, (2) because they mistrust physicians or are dissatisfied with conventional medicine, or (3) because they experience relief of symptoms with the herbal treatment. Since patients will be more cooperative with traditional psychiatric treatments if allowed to continue their herbal preparations, psychiatrists should try to keep an open mind and not attribute all effects to suggestion. If psychotropic agents are prescribed the clinician most be extraordinarily alert to the possibility of adverse effects as a result of drug-drug interactions, since many phytomedicinals have ingredients that produce actual physiological changes in the body.

For a more detailed discussion of this topic, see Kiresuk TJ, Trachtenberg A: Alternative and Complimentary Health Practices, Sec 28.98, p 2008, in CTP/VII.

TABLE 41–1
PHYTOMEDICINALS WITH PSYCHOACTIVE EFFECT

Name	Ingredients	Use	Adverse Effects[a]	Interactions	Dosage[a]	Comments
Areca, areca nut, betel nut, L. *Areca catechu*	Arecoline, guvacoline	For alteration of consciousness to reduce pain and elevate mood	Parasympathomimetic overload: increased salivation, tremors, bradycardia, spasms, gastrointestinal disturbances, ulcers of the mouth	Avoid with parasympathomimetic drugs; atropine-like compounds reduce effect	Undetermined; 8–10 g is toxic dose for humans	Used by chewing the nut; used in the past as a chewing balm for gum disease and as a vermifuge; long-term use may result in malignant tumors of the oral cavity
Belladonna, L. *Atropa belladonna*, deadly nightshade	Atropine, scopolamine, flavonoids[b]	Anxiolytic	Tachycardia, arrhythmias, xerostomia, mydriasis, difficulties with micturition and constipation	Synergistic with anticholinergic drugs; avoid with tricyclic antidepressants, amantadine, and quinidine	0.05–0.10 mg a day; maximum single dose is 0.20 mg	Has a strong smell, tastes sharp and bitter, and is poisonous
Bitter orange flower, *citrus aurantium*	Flavonoids, limonene	Sedative, anxiolytic, hypnotic	Photosensitization	Undetermined	Tincture 2–3 g per day, drug 4–6 g per day, extract 1–2 g per day	Contradictory evidence; some refer to it as a gastric stimulant
Black cohosh, L. *Cimicifuga racemosa*	Triterpenes, isoferulic acid	For premenstrual syndrome, menopausal symptoms, dysmenorrhea	Weight gain, gastrointestinal disturbances	Possible adverse interaction with male or female hormones	1–2 g per day; over 5 g can cause vomiting, headache, dizziness, cardiovascular collapse	Estrogen-like effects questionable because root may act as estrogen-receptor blocker
Black haw, cramp bark, L. *Viburnum prunifolium*	Scopoletin, flavonoids, caffeic acids, triterpenes	Sedative, antispasmodic action on uterus; for dysmenorrhea	Undetermined	Anticoagulant-enhanced effects	1–3 g per day	

continues

TABLE 41-1—*continued*

Name	Ingredients	Use	Adverse Effects[a]	Interactions	Dosage[a]	Comments
California poppy, L. *Eschscholtzia californica*	Isoquinoline alkaloids, cyanogenic glycosides	Sedative, hypnotic, anxiolytic; for depression	Lethargy	Combination of California poppy, valerian, St. John's wort, and passion flowers can result in agitation	2 g per day	Clinical or experimental documentation of effects is unavailable
Catnip, L. *Nepeta cataria*	Valeric acid	Sedative, antispasmodic; for migraine	Headache, malaise, nausea, hallucinogenic effects	Undetermined	Undetermined	Delirium produced in children
Chamomile, L. *Matricaria chamomilla*	Flavonoids	Sedative, anxiolytic	Allergic reaction	Undetermined	2–4 g per day	May be GABAergic
Corydalis, L. *Corydalis cava*	Isoquinoline alkaloids	Sedative, antidepressant; for mild depression	Hallucination, lethargy	Undetermined	Undetermined	Clonic spasms and muscular tremor with overdose
Cyclamen, L. *Cyclamen europaeum*	Triterpene	Anxiolytic; for menstrual complaints	Small doses (e.g., 300 mg) can lead to nausea, vomiting, and diarrhea	Undetermined	Undetermined	High doses can lead to respiratory collapse
Echinacea, L. *Echinacea purpurea*	Flavonoids, polysaccharides, caffeic acid derivatives, alkamides	Stimulates immune system; for lethargy, malaise, respiratory and lower urinary tract infections	Allergic reaction, fever, nausea, vomiting	Undetermined	1–3 g per day	Use in HIV and AIDS patients is controversial
Ephedra, ma-huang L. *Ephedra sinica,*	Ephedrine, pseudoephedrine	Stimulant; for lethargy, malaise, diseases of respiratory tract	Sympathomimetic overload: arrhythmias, increased blood pressure, headache, irritability, nausea, vomiting	Synergistic with sympathomimetics, serotonergic agents. Avoid with MAOIs.	1–2 g per day	Administer for short periods as tachyphylaxis and dependence can occur

Herb	Constituents	Uses	Adverse effects	Drug interactions	Dose	Comments
Ginkgo, L. Ginkgo biloba	Flavonoids, ginkgolide A, B	Symptomatic relief of delirium, dementia; improves concentration and memory deficits; possible antidote to SSRI-induced sexual dysfunction	Allergic skin reactions, gastrointestinal upset, muscle spasms, headache	Anticoagulant: use with caution because of its inhibitory effect on platelet-activating factor (PAF); increased bleeding possible	120–240 mg per day	Studies indicate improved cognition in Alzheimer's patients after 4-5 weeks of use, possibly because of increased blood flow
Ginseng. L. Panax ginseng	Triterpenes, ginsenosides	Stimulant; for fatigue, elevation of mood, immune system	Insomnia, hypertonia, and edema (called ginseng abuse syndrome)	Not to be used with sedatives, hypnotic agents, MAOIs, antidiabetic agents, or steroids	1-2 g per day	Several varieties exist: Korean (most highly valued), Chinese, Japanese, American (Panax quinquefolius)
Heather, L. Calluna vulgaris	Flavonoids, catechin, triterpenes, beta-sitosterol	Anxiolytic, hypnotic	Undetermined	Undetermined	Undetermined	Efficacy for claimed uses is not documented
Hops, L. Humulus lupulus	Humulone, lupulone, flavonoids	Sedative, anxiolytic, hypnotic; for mood disturbances, restlessness	Contraindicated in patients with estrogen-dependent tumors (breast, uterine, cervical)	Hyperthermia effects with phenothiazine antipsychotics and with CNS depressants	0.5 g per day	May decrease plasma levels of drugs metabolized by CPV450 system
Horehound, L. Ballota nigra	Diterpenes, tannins	Sedative	Arrhythmics, diarrhea, hypoglycemia, possible spontaneous abortions	May enhance serotonergic drug effects, may augment hypoglycemic effects of drugs	1-4 g per day	May cause abortion
Jambolan, L. Syzygium cumini	Oleic acid, myristic acid, palmitic and linoleic acid, tannins	Anxiolytic, antidepressant	Undetermined	Undetermined	1-2 g per day	In folk medicine, a single dose is 30 seeds (1.9 g) of powder

continues

TABLE 41-1—*continued*

Name	Ingredients	Use	Adverse Effects[a]	Interactions	Dosage[a]	Comments
Kava Kava, *L. Piperis methysticum*	Kava lactones, kava pyrone	Sedative, hypnotic antispasmodic	Lethargy, impaired cognition, dermatitis with long-term unreported usage	Synergistic with anxiolytics, alcohol; avoid with levodopa and dopaminergic agents	600–800 mg per day	May be GABAergic; contraindicated in patients with endogenous depression; may increase the danger of suicide
Lavender, *L. Lavandula angustifolia*	Hydroxycoumarin, tannins, caffeic acid	Sedative, hypnotic	Headache, nausea, confusion	Synergistic with other sedatives	3–5 g per day	May cause death in overdose
Lemon balm, sweet Mary, *L. Melissa officinalis*	Flavonoids, caffeic acid, triterpenes	Hypnotic, anxiolytic, sedative	Undetermined	Potentiates CNS depressant; adverse reaction with thyroid hormone	8–10 g per day	
Mistletoe, *L. Viscum album*	Flavonoids, triterpenes, lectins, polypeptides	Anxiolytic; for mental and physical exhaustion	Berries said to have emetic and laxative effects	Contraindicated in patients with chronic infections, e.g., tuberculosis	10 per day	Berries have caused death in children
Mugwort, *L. Artemisia vulgaris*	Sesquitemene lactones, flavonoids	Sedative, antidepressant, anxiolytic	Anaphylaxis, contact dermatitis	Potentiates anticoagulants	5–15 g per day	May stimulate uterine contractions
Nux vomica, *L. strychnos nux vomica,* poison nut	Indole alkaloids: strychnine and brucine, polysaccharides	Antidepressant; for migraine, menopausal symptoms	Convulsions, liver damage, death; severely toxic because of strychnine	Undetermined	0.02–0.05 g per day	Symptoms of poisoning can occur after ingestion of one bean; lethal dose is 1–2 g

Herb	Constituents	Actions	Adverse effects	Interactions	Dose	Comments
Oats, L. Avena sativa	Flavonoids, oligo and polysaccharides	Anxiolytic, hypnotic; for stress, insomnia, opium and tobacco withdrawal	Bowel obstruction or other bowel dysmotility syndromes, flatulence	Undetermined	3 g per day	Oats have sometimes been contaminated with aflatoxin, a fungal toxin linked with some cancers
Passion flower, L. Passiflora Incarnata	Flavonoids, cyanogenic glycosides	Anxiolytic, sedative, hypnotic	Cognitive impairment	Undetermined	4–8 g per day	Overdose causes depression
St. John's wort, L. Hypericum perforatum	Hypericin, flavonoids, xanthones	Antidepressant, sedative, anxiolytic	Headaches, photosensitivity (may be severe), constipation	Report of manic reaction when used with sertraline (Zoloft); do not combine with SSRIs or MAOIs; possible serotonin syndrome; do not use with alcohol, opioids	100–950 mg per day	Under investigation by the National Institutes of Health (NIH); may act as MAOI or SSRI; 4- to 6-week trial for mild depressive moods; if no apparent improvement, another therapy should be tried
Scarlet Pimpernel, L. Anagallis arvensis	Flavonoids, triterpenes, cucurbitacins, caffeic acids	Antidepressant	Overdose or long-term doses may lead to gastroenteritis and nephritis	Undetermined	1.8 g of powder 4 times a day	Flowers are poisonous
Skullcap, L. Scutellaria lateriflora	Flavonoid, monoterpenes	Anxiolytic, sedative, hypnotic	Cognitive impairment, hepatotoxicity	Disulfiram-like reaction may occur if used with alcohol	1–2 g per day	Little information exists to support the use of this herb in humans

continues

TABLE 41-1—*continued*

Name	Ingredients	Use	Adverse Effects[a]	Interactions	Dosage[a]	Comments
Strawberry leaf, *L. Fragaria vesca*	Flavonoids, tannins	Anxiolytic	Contraindicated with strawberry allergy	Undetermined	1 g per day	Little information exists to support the use of this herb in humans
Tarragon, *L. Artemisia dracunculus*	Flavonoids, hydroxycoumarins	Hypnotic, appetite stimulant	Undetermined	Undetermined	Undetermined	Little information exists to support the use of this herb in humans
Valerian, *L. Valeriana officinalis*	Valepotriates, valerenic acid, caffeic acid	Sedative, muscle relaxant, hypnotic	Cognitive and motor impairment, gastrointestinal upset, hepatotoxicity; long-term use: contact allergy, headache, restlessness, insomnia, mydriasis, cardiac dysfunction	Avoid concomitant use with alcohol or CNS depressants	1–2 g per day	May be chemically unstable

[a] No reliable, consistent, or valid data exist on dosages or adverse affects of most phytomedicinals.
[b] Flavonoids are common to many herbs. They are plant by-products that act as antioxidants, i.e., agents that prevent the deterioration of material such as DNA via oxidation.

42

Medication-Induced Movement Disorders

The most common medication-induced movement disorders in psychiatry are caused by drugs with dopamine receptor antagonist properties. The disorders include (1) neuroleptic malignant syndrome, (2) neuroleptic-induced tardive dyskinesia, (3) neuroleptic-induced acute dystonia, (4) neuroleptic-induced parkinsonism, (5) neuroleptic-induced acute akathisia, and (6) medication-induced postural tremor. Table 42–1 lists various drugs that may cause drug-induced disorders. The disorders are also referred to as extrapyramidal symptoms (EPS).

NEUROLEPTIC MALIGNANT SYNDROME

Neuroleptic malignant syndrome is a life-threatening complication that can occur anytime during the course of antipsychotic treatment. The motor and behavioral symptoms include muscular rigidity and dystonia, akinesia, mutism, obtundation, and agitation. The autonomic symptoms include hyperpyrexia (up to 107°F), sweating, and increased pulse and blood pressure. Laboratory findings include increased white blood cell count, creatinine phosphokinase, liver enzymes, plasma myoglobin, and myoglobinuria, occasionally associated with renal failure. The symptoms usually evolve over 24 to 72 hours, and the untreated syndrome lasts 10 to 14 days. The diagnosis is often missed in the early stages, and the withdrawal or agitation may mistakenly be considered to reflect increased psychosis. Men are affected more frequently than are women, and young patients are affected more commonly than are elderly patients. The mortality rate can reach 20 to 30 percent or even higher when depot antipsychotic medications are involved. The pathophysiology is unknown.

Treatment

The first step in treatment is the immediate discontinuation of antipsychotic drugs; medical support to cool the patient; monitoring of vital signs, electrolytes, fluid balance, and renal output; and symptomatic treatment of fevers. Antiparkinsonian medications may reduce some of the muscle rigidity. Dantrolene (Dantrium), a skeletal muscle relaxant (0.8 to 2.5 mg/kg every 6 hours, up to a total dosage of 10 mg a day), may be useful in the treatment of the disorder. Once the patient can take oral medications, the dantrolene can be given in doses of 100 to 200 mg a day. Bromocriptine (Parlodel) (20 to 30 mg a day in four divided doses) or perhaps amantadine (Symmetrel) can be added to the regimen. Treatment should usually be continued for 5 to 10 days. When antipsychotic treatment is restarted, the clinician should consider switching to a low-potency drug or to one of the new serotonin-dopamine antagonists (SDAs), which produce much less dopamine D_2 receptor

TABLE 42–1
DRUG-INDUCED MOVEMENT DISORDERS

Syndrome	Drugs Responsible	Degree	Syndrome	Drugs Responsible	Degree
Postural tremor	Sympathomimetics	++	Chorea, including tardive dyskinesia and orofacial dyskinesia	Antipsychotics	++
	Levodopa	++		Metoclopramide	++
	Amphetamines	++		Levodopa	++
	Bronchodilators	++		Direct dopamine agonists	++
	Tricyclic drugs	++		Indirect dopamine agonists and other catecholaminergic drugs[a,b]	++
	Lithium carbonate	++			
	Caffeine	++			
	Thyroid hormone	++		Anticholinergics	+
	Sodium valproate	++		Antihistaminics	+
	Antipsychotics	++		Oral contraceptives	+
	Hypoglycemic agents	++		Phenytoin (T)	+
	Adrenocorticosteroids	++		Carbamazepine (T)	+/–
	Alcohol withdrawal	++		Ethosuximide	+/–
	Amiodarone	+		Phenobarbital (T)	+/–
	Cyclosporine A	+		Lithium carbonate (T)	+/–
	MAOIs	++		Benzodiazepines	+/–
Acute dystonic reactions	Antipsychotics	++		MAOIs	+/–
	Metoclopramide	++		Tricyclic drugs	+/–
	Antimalarial agents	+		Methyldopa	+/–
	Tetrabenazine	+/–		Methadone	+/–
	Diphenhydramine	+/–		Digoxin	+/–
	Mefenamic acid	+/–		Alcohol withdrawal	+/–
	Oxatomide	+/–		Toluene (glue-sniffing)	+/–
	Tricyclic drugs	+/–	Dystonia, including tardive dystonia (excluding acute dystonic reactions)	Antipsychotics	++
Akathisia	Antipsychotics	++		Metoclopramide	++
	Metoclopramide	++		Levodopa	++
	Reserpine	++		Direct dopamine agonists[a]	+
	Tetrabenazine	++		Phenytoin (T)	+
	Levodopa and dopamine agonists	+		Carbamazepine (T)	+/–
	Ethosuximide	+/–		Trazodone	+/–
	Methysergide	+/–		Lithium	+/–
	Amoxapine	+/–			

Parkinsonism, including rabbit syndrome

Drug/Cause	
Antipsychotics	++
Metoclopramide	++
Reserpine	++
Tetrabenazine	++
Methyldopa	+
Fluoxetine	+/−
Lithium	+/−
Phenelzine	+/−
Phenytoin	+/−
Captopril	+/−
Alcohol withdrawal	+
MPTP	+
Other toxins (manganese, carbon disulfide, cyanide)	+

Myoclonus

Drug/Cause	
Cytosine arabinoside	+/−

Neuroleptic malignant syndrome

Drug/Cause	
Antipsychotics	+
Tetrabenazine with AMPT	+/−

Tics (simple and complex), including aggravation of preexisting tic disorders

Withdrawal of antiparkinsonian drugs in Parkinson's disease	+/−
Levodopa	+
Direct dopamine agonists	+
Indirect dopamine agonists	++
Antipsychotics	+
Carbamazepine	+/−

Myoclonus

Drug/Cause	
Levodopa	++
Anticonvulsants[c] (T)	++
MAOIs	++
Lithium	++
Tricyclic drugs	++
Antipsychotics	+/−
Anticonvulsants[c] (T)	++

Asterixis[d]

Levodopa	+/−
Hepatotoxins (T)	++
Respiratory depressants (T)	++

From Gershanil OS. Drug-induced movement disorders. *Curr Opin Neurol Neurosurg* 1993;6:369.
++, well documented; +, relatively well documented; common or not infrequent; uncommon; +/−, not well documented or only small number of cases in literature.
AMPT, α-methyl-paratyrosine; MAOI, monoamine oxidase inhibitor; MPTP, 1-methyl-4-phenyl-1,2,3,6-3 tetrahydropyridine; T, usually evidence of drug toxicity present (including serum drug levels).
[a] Includes apomorphine, bromocriptine, lisuride, pergolide.
[b] Includes amphetamines, methylphenidate, amantadine, pemoline, fenfluramine.
[c] Includes most categories of anticonvulsant drugs.
[d] Flapping tremor most often associated with liver damage.

blockade; however, neuroleptic malignant syndrome has also been infrequently reported to be associated with these newer treatments.

NEUROLEPTIC-INDUCED TARDIVE DYSKINESIA

Tardive dyskinesia is a delayed effect of antipsychotics; it rarely occurs until after 6 months of treatment. The disorder consists of abnormal, involuntary, irregular choreoathetoid movements of the muscles of the head, the limbs, and the trunk. The severity of the movements ranges from minimal—often missed by patients and their families—to grossly incapacitating. Perioral movements are the most common and include darting, twisting, and protruding movements of the tongue; chewing and lateral jaw movements; lip puckering; and facial grimacing. Finger movements and hand clenching are also common. Torticollis, retrocollis, trunk twisting, and pelvic thrusting are seen in severe cases. Respiratory dyskinesia has also been reported. Dyskinesia is exacerbated by stress and disappears during sleep.

About 10 to 20 percent of patients who are treated with dopamine receptor antagonists for more than a year develop tardive dyskinesia. About 15 to 20 percent of long-term hospital patients have tardive dyskinesia. Women are more likely to be affected than are men, and patients more than 50 years of age, patients with brain damage, children, and patients with mood disorders are also at high risk.

The three basic approaches to tardive dyskinesia are prevention, diagnosis (see Table 18–3 in Chapter 18), and management. Prevention is best achieved by using antipsychotic medications only when clearly indicated and in the lowest effective dosages. The new antipsychotics (e.g., risperidone [Risperdal]) are associated with less tardive dyskinesia than the old antipsychotics. Patients who are receiving an-

TABLE 42-2
ABNORMAL INVOLUNTARY MOVEMENT SCALE (AIMS) EXAMINATION PROCEDURE

Patient identification	Date
Rated by	

Either before or after completing the examination procedure, observe the patient unobtrusively at rest (e.g., in waiting room).

The chair to be used in this examination should be a hard, firm one without arms.

After observing the patient, rate him or her on a scale of 0 (none), 1 (minimal), 2 (mild), 3 (moderate), and 4 (severe) according to the severity of the symptoms.

Ask the patient whether there is anything in his or her mouth (i.e., gum, candy, etc.) and, if so, to remove it.

Ask the patient about the current condition of his or her teeth. Ask patient if he or she wears dentures. Do teeth or dentures bother patient now?

Ask patient whether he or she notices any movement in mouth, face, hands, or feet. If yes, ask patient to describe and indicate to what extent they currently bother patient or interfere with his or her activities.

0 1 2 3 4 Have patient sit in chair with hands on knees, legs slightly apart, and feet flat on floor. (Look at entire body for movements while in this position.)

0 1 2 3 4 Ask patient to sit with hands hanging unsupported. If male, between legs, if female and wearing a dress, hanging over knees. (Observe hands and other body areas.)

0 1 2 3 4 Ask patient to open mouth. (Observe tongue at rest within mouth.) Do this twice.

0 1 2 3 4 Ask patient to protrude tongue. (Observe abnormalities of tongue movement.) Do this twice.

0 1 2 3 4 Ask the patient to tap thumb, with each finger, as rapidly as possible for 10 to 15 seconds; separately with right hand, then with left hand. (Observe facial and leg movements.)

0 1 2 3 4 Flex and extend patient's left and right arms. (One at a time.)

0 1 2 3 4 ᵃ Ask patient to extend both arms outstretched in front with palms down. (Observe trunk, legs, and mouth.)

0 1 2 3 4 ᵃ Have patient walk a few paces, turn and walk back to chair. (Observe hands and gait.) Do this twice.

ᵃ Activated movements.

tipsychotics should be examined regularly for the appearance of abnormal movements, preferably by using a standardized rating scale (Table 42–2).

Treatment

Tardive dyskinesia has no single effective treatment. Discontinuing the medication, lowering the dosage of the antipsychotic, and switching to a new antipsychotic such as clozapine (Clozaril) and other SDAs are the primary treatment strategies. Vitamin E and high dosages of buspirone (BuSpar) (up to 160 mg a day) may be effective. In patients who cannot continue taking any antipsychotic medication, lithium (Eskalith), carbamazepine (Tegretol), or benzodiazepines may be effective in reducing both the movement disorder symptoms and the psychotic symptoms.

Between 5 and 40 percent of all cases of tardive dyskinesia eventually remit, and between 50 and 90 percent of all mild cases remit. However, tardive dyskinesia is less likely to remit in elderly patients than in young patients.

NEUROLEPTIC-INDUCED ACUTE DYSTONIA

About 10 percent of all patients experience dystonia as an adverse effect of typical antipsychotics, usually in the first few hours or days of treatment. Dystonic movements result from a slow, contained muscular contraction or spasm than can cause an involuntary movement. Dystonia can involve the neck (spasmodic torticollis or retrocollis), the jaw (forced opening resulting in a dislocation of the jaw or trismus), the tongue (protrusions, twisting), and the entire body (opisthotonos). Involvement of the eyes can result in an oculogyric crisis, characterized by the eyes' upward lateral movement. Other dystonias include blepharospasm and glossopharyngeal dystonia, resulting in dysarthria, dysphagia, and even trouble breathing, which can cause cyanosis. Children are particularly likely to evidence opisthotonos, scoliosis, lordosis, and writhing movement. Dystonia can be painful and frightening and often results in noncompliance with the drug treatment regimen.

Dystonia is most common in young men (less than 40 years old) but can occur at any age in either sex. Although it is most common with intramuscular (i.m.) dosages of high-potency antipsychotics, dystonia can occur with any antipsychotic. Neuroleptic-induced dystonia is least common with thioridazine (Mellaril), and it is uncommon with risperidone and other atypical antipsychotics. The mechanism of action is thought to be the dopaminergic hyperactivity in the basal ganglia that occurs when the central nervous system (CNS) levels of the antipsychotic drug begin to fall between doses. Dystonia can fluctuate spontaneously, responding to reassurance and resulting in the clinician's false impression that the movement is hysterical or completely under conscious control. The differential diagnosis of a dystonic movement should include seizures and tardive dyskinesia (Fig. 42–1).

Treatment

Prophylaxis with anticholinergics or related drugs (Table 42–3) usually prevents the development of dystonia, although the risks of prophylactic treatment weigh

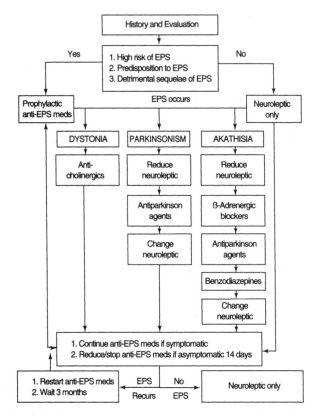

Figure 42-1. Outline of the treatment approach for major extrapyramidal symptoms.

against that benefit. Treatment with i.m. anticholinergics or intravenous (i.v.) or i.m. diphenhydramine (Benadryl) (50 mg) almost always relieves the symptoms. Diazepam (Valium) (10 mg i.v.), amobarbital (Amytal), caffeine with sodium benzoate, and hypnosis have also been reported to be effective. Although tolerance for the adverse effect usually develops, it is sometimes prudent to change the antipsychotic if the patient is particularly concerned that the reaction may recur.

NEUROLEPTIC-INDUCED PARKINSONISM

Parkinsonian adverse effects occur in about 15 percent of patients who are treated with antipsychotics, usually within 5 to 90 days of the initiation of treatment. Symptoms include muscle stiffness (lead-pipe rigidity), cogwheel rigidity, shuffling gait, stooped posture, and drooling. The pill-rolling tremor of idiopathic parkinsonism is rare, but a regular, coarse tremor similar to essential tremor may be present. A focal, perioral tremor, sometimes referred to as rabbit syndrome is another parkinsonian effect seen with antipsychotics, although perioral tremor is more likely than other tremors to occur late in the course of treatment.

TABLE 42-3
DRUG TREATMENT OF EXTRAPYRAMIDAL DISORDERS

Generic Name	Trade Name	Usual Daily Dosage	Indications
Anticholinergic			
Benztropine	Cogentin	p.o. 0.5–2 mg t.i.d.; i.m. or i.v. 1–2 mg	Acute dystonia, parkinsonism, akinesia, akathisia
Biperiden	Akineton	p.o. 2–6 mg t.i.d.; i.m. or i.v. 2 mg	
Procyclidine	Kemadrin	p.o. 2.5–5 mg b.i.d.–q.i.d.	
Trihexyphenidyl	Artane, Tremin	p.o. 2–5 mg t.i.d.	
Orphenadrine	Norflex, Disipal	p.o. 50–100 mg b.i.d.–q.i.d.; i.v. 60 mg	Rabbit syndrome
Antihistamine			
Diphenhydramine	Benadryl	p.o. 25 mg q.i.d.; i.m. or i.v. 25 mg	Acute dystonia, parkinsonism, akinesia, rabbit syndrome
Amantadine	Symmetrel	p.o. 100–200 mg b.i.d.	Parkinsonism, akinesia, rabbit syndrome
β-Adrenergic antagonist			
Propranolol	Inderal	p.o. 20–40 mg t.i.d.	Akathisia, tremor
α-Adrenergic antagonist			
Clonidine	Catapres	p.o. 0.1 mg t.i.d.	Akathisia
Benzodiazepines			
Clonazepam	Klonopin	p.o. 1 mg b.i.d.	Akathisia, acute dystonia
Lorazepam	Ativan	p.o. 1 mg t.i.d.	
Buspirone	BuSpar	p.o. 20–40 mg q.i.d.	Tardive dyskinesia
Vitamin E	—	p.o. 1,200–1,600 IU o.d.	Tardive dyskinesia

p.o., orally; i.m., intramuscular; i.v., intravenous; o.d., per day; b.i.d., twice a day; t.i.d., three times a day; q.i.d., four times a day.

Neuroleptic-induced parkinsonism affects women about twice as often as men, and the disorder can occur at all ages, although it is most common after age 40. All a dopamine receptor antagonists can cause the symptoms, especially high-potency drugs with low anticholinergic activity such as trifluoperazine (Stelazine). The pathophysiology of neuroleptic-induced parkinsonism involves the blockade of D_2 receptors in the caudate at the termination of the nigrostriatal dopamine neurons, the same neurons that degenerate in idiopathic Parkinson's disease. The differential diagnosis of the parkinsonian symptoms should include idiopathic parkinsonism, other medical causes of parkinsonism, and depression, which can also be associated with parkinsonian symptoms.

Treatment

The disorder can be treated with anticholinergic agents, amantadine, or diphenhydramine (Table 42–3). Anticholinergics should be withdrawn after 4 to 6 weeks to assess whether the patient has developed a tolerance for the parkinsonian effects; about 50 percent of patients with neuroleptic-induced parkinsonism need continued treatment. Even after the antipsychotics are withdrawn, parkinsonian symptoms may last up to 2 weeks and even up to 3 months in elderly patients. With such patients the clinician may continue giving the anticholinergic drug after stopping the antipsychotic until the parkinsonian symptoms have completely resolved.

TABLE 42-4
DRUG-INDUCED CENTRAL HYPERTHERMIC SYNDROMES[a]

Condition (and Mechanism)	Common Drug Causes	Frequent Symptoms	Possible Treatment[b]	Clinical Course
Hyperthermia (↓ heat dissipation) (↑ heat production)	Atropine, lidocaine, meperidine NSAID toxicity, pheochromocytoma, thyrotoxicosis	Hyperthermia, diaphoresis, malaise	Acetaminophen per rectum (325 mg every 4 hours), diazepam oral or per rectum (5 mg every 8 hours) for febrile seizures	Benign, febrile seizures in children
Malignant hyperthermia (↑ heat production)	NMJ blockers (succinylcholine), halothane (1:50,000)	Hyperthermia, **muscle rigidity, arrhythmias,** ischemia,[c] hypotension, **rhabdomyolysis;** disseminated intravascular coagulation	Dantrolene sodium (1–2 mg/kg/min IV infusion)[d]	Familial, 10% mortality if untreated
Tricyclic overdose (↑ heat production)	Tricyclic antidepressants, cocaine	Hyperthermia, confusion, visual hallucinations, agitation, **hyperreflexia, muscle relaxation, anticholinergic effects** (dry skin, pupil dilation), arrhythmias	**Sodium bicarbonate** (1 mEq/kg IV bolus) if arrhythmias are present, physostigmine (1–3 mg IV) with cardiac monitoring	Fatalities have occurred if untreated
Autonomic hyperreflexia (↑ heat production)	CNS stimulants (amphetamines)	Hyperthermia excitement, **hyperreflexia**	Trimethaphan (0.3–7 mg/minute IV infusion)	Reversible
Lethal catatonia (↓ heat dissipation)	Lead poisoning	Hyperthermia, intense anxiety, **destructive behavior, psychosis**	Lorazepam (1–2 mg IV every 4 hours), antipsychotics may be contraindicated	High mortality if untreated
Neuroleptic malignant syndrome (mixed: hypothalamic, ↓ heat dissipation, ↑ heat production)	Antipsychotics (neuroleptics), methyldopa, reserpine	Hyperthermia, **muscle rigidity, diaphoresis (60%), leukocytosis, delirium, rhabdomyolysis, elevated CPK,** autonomic deregulation, **extrapyramidal symptoms**	**Bromocriptine (2–10 mg every 8 hours PO or NG tube),** lisuride (0.02–0.1 mg/hour IV infusion), Sinemet (carbidopa: levodopa 25/100) PO every 8 hours), dantrolene sodium (0.3–1 mg/kg IV every 6 hours)	Rapid onset, 20% mortality if untreated

[a] Boldface indicates features that may be used to distinguish one syndrome from another. NSAID, nonsteroidal anti-inflammatory drugs; MAOI, monoamine oxidase inhibitors; NMJ, neuromuscular junction; CNS, central nervous system; DO, dopamine; CPK, creatine phosphokinase; IV, intravenously; PO, orally; NG, nasogastric.
[b] Gastric lavage and supportive measures, including cooling, are required in most cases.
[c] Oxygen consumption increases by 7% for every 1°F up in body temperature.
[d] Has been associated with idiosyncratic hepatocellular injury, as well as severe hypotension in one case.
From Theocharides TC, Harris RS, Weckstein D: Neuroleptic malignant-like syndrome due to cyclobenzaprine? (letter). *J Clin Psychopharmacol.* 1995;15:80, with permission.

NEUROLEPTIC-INDUCED ACUTE AKATHISIA

Akathisia is a subjective feeling of muscular discomfort that can cause the patient to be agitated, pace relentlessly, alternately sit and stand in rapid succession, and feel generally dysphoric. The symptoms are primarily motor and cannot be controlled by the patient's will. Akathisia can appear at any time during treatment. Once akathisia is recognized and diagnosed, the antipsychotic dosage should be reduced to the minimal effective dosage.

Treatment

Treatment can be attempted with anticholinergics or amantadine, although those drugs are not particularly effective for akathisia. Drugs that may be more effective include propranolol (Inderal) (30 to 120 mg a day), benzodiazepines, and clonidine (Catapres). In some cases of akathisia, no treatment seems to be effective.

MEDICATION-INDUCED POSTURAL TREMOR

Tremor is a rhythmical alteration in movement that is usually faster than one beat a second. Typically, tremors decrease during periods of relaxation and sleep and increase with stress or anxiety. Whereas all the above diagnoses specifically include an association with an antipsychotic, a range of psychiatric medications can produce tremor—most notably lithium, antidepressants, and valproate (Depakene).

TREATMENT

The treatment of tremor involves four general steps: (1) the lowest possible dosage of the psychiatric drug should be taken, (2) patients should minimize their caffeine consumption, (3) the psychiatric drug should be taken at bedtime to minimize the amount of daytime tremor, and (4) β-adrenergic receptor antagonists (e.g., propranolol) can be given in the treatment of drug-induced tremors.

HYPERTHERMIC SYNDROMES

Many drugs used in psychiatry and all of the medication-induced movement disorders may be associated with hyperthermia. Table 42–4 summarizes various conditions and agents associated with hyperthermia.

For a more detailed discussion of this topic, see Pi EH, Simpson GM: Medication-Induced Movement Disorders, Sec 31.4, p 2265, in CTP/VII.

43

Intoxication and Overdose

Adverse effects may occur with any drug. Although most are mild and transitory, some are severe and lethal. The prescribing psychiatrist or physician must be vigilant in determining the emergence of toxicity or signs of overdose.

A guide to the signs and symptoms and the treatment of overdose with psychotherapeutic drugs is contained in Table 43–1. The toxic dose in one person may be lethal in another person, depending on such factors as route of administration, rate of absorption, interaction with other drugs, and age and general health of the patient. It is also important to remember that a patient may have ingested more than one substance and that the clinical picture may represent polysubstance abuse. Treatment must be adjusted accordingly, and a history (from other persons) should be obtained and all drugs should be inspected. Toward that end the illustrations of the various drugs used in psychiatry at the beginning of this book can be useful.

An extreme event is an attempt by a patient to commit suicide by taking an overdose of a prescribed medication. Some are more lethal than others in overdose. Barbiturates, for example, have a higher potential for lethality than do selective serotonin reuptake inhibitors (SSRIs), and the doctor must be aware of those drugs that are more potentially lethal. It is good clinical practice to write nonrefillable prescriptions for small quantities of drugs when suicide is a consideration. In extreme cases the doctor should verify that patients are taking the medication and not hoarding the pills for a later overdose attempt. Patients may attempt suicide just as they appear to be getting better. Clinicians, therefore, should continue to be careful about prescribing large quantities of medication until the patient has almost completely recovered.

Another consideration is the possibility of an accidental overdose, particularly by children in the household. Patients should be advised to keep psychotherapeutic medications clearly labeled and in a safe place.

For a more detailed discussion of this topic, see Grebb JA: General Principles of Psychopharmacology, Sec 31.1, p 2235, in CTP/VII.

TABLE 43–1
INTOXICATION AND OVERDOSE WITH PSYCHOTHERAPEUTIC DRUGS[a]

Drug	Toxic/Lethal Dose	Signs and Symptoms	Treatment
β-Adrenergic receptor antagonists	Toxic effects with 0.8–6 g of propranolol	Hypotension, bradycardia, cardiac failure, bronchospasm, loss of consciousness, seizures	Emesis or gastric lavage; supportive care; norepinephrine or dopamine for severe hypotension; glucagon for hypotension and myocardial depression; i.v. atropine for symptomatic bradycardia, i.v. isoproterenol for persistent cases, pacemaker if refractory; diuretic or cardiac glycoside for heart failure; theophylline or β_2 agonist for bronchospasm; i.v. diazepam for seizures
Amantadine	Lethal dose of 2 g reported	Arrhythmia, tachycardia, hypertension, disorientation, lethargy, confusion, visual hallucinations, aggressive behavior, anxiety, minimally reactive and dilated pupils, ataxia, tremor, hypertonia, seizure exacerbation, coma, edema and respiratory distress, renal insufficiency, urinary retention, acid-base disturbances	Emesis or gastric lavage; supportive measures including cardiovascular monitoring, airway maintenance, and control of respiration and oxygen administration; avoid adrenergic agents as they may predispose to ventricular arrhythmias; i.v. physostigmine to treat CNS toxicity, chlorpromazine for toxic psychosis, sedation and anticonvulsants as needed; monitor urine pH, urinary output, serum electrolytes, urine acidifying agents increase rate of excretion, i.v. fluids, catheter for urinary retention
Amphetamines	Toxic effects at 30 mg, idiosyncratic toxicity as low as 2 mg, survival reported after 500 mg	Elation, irritability, hyperactivity, psychotic symptoms, depression, panic, rapid speech, confusion, anorexia, insomnia, hyperreflexia, tremor, dry mouth, hyperpyrexia, convulsions, coma, chest pain, arrhythmia, heart block, hyper/hypotension, shock, nausea, vomiting, diarrhea, abdominal cramps, tachypnea, rhabdomyolysis	Emesis or lavage, activated charcoal, cathartic (can be effective long after ingestion because of recycling through gastric mucosa); supportive care; reduce external stimuli, sedate with chlorpromazine; i.v. phentolamine for severe HTN; acidification of urine
Anticholinergics	700 mg to 7 g (doses vary depending on agent involved)	Hot, dry, flushed skin; dry mucous membranes, hyperthermia, rash, shock, tachycardia, unreactive dilated pupils, blurred vision; delirium, delusions, ataxia, hallucinations, convulsions, coma, dysphagia, nausea, vomiting, hypoactive bowel sounds, respiratory arrest, urinary retention	Emesis or lavage, activated charcoal, saline cathartics; supportive and symptomatic therapy; 1–2 mg physostigmine can reverse anticholinergic effects; cold packs, mechanical cooling devices, or sponging with tepid water for hyperthermia; continuous ECG monitoring; vasopressors and fluid therapy for shock, i.v. propranolol for supraventricular tachyarrhythmias, avoid dopamine receptor antagonists; local miotics for mydriasis; diazepam for agitation

continued

TABLE 43–1—*continued*

Drug	Toxic/Lethal Dose	Signs and Symptoms	Treatment
Antihistamines	2.8 g diphenhydramine, 1.75–17.5 g hydroxyzine	Disorientation, drowsiness, excitation, depression, hallucinations, anxiety, delirium, hyperthermia, tachycardia, hypotension, arrhythmias, seizures	Emesis or lavage; support cardiorespiratory function; i.v. fluids and vasopressors for hypotension; caffeine and sodium benzoate to counteract CNS depressant effects; physostigmine for anticholinergic effects; diazepam for seizures; sponge baths with tepid water (not alcohol) or cold packs for hyperthermia
Barbiturates	10 times the daily dose or 1 g of most barbiturates causes severe toxicity 2–10 g fatal	Delirium, confusion, excitement, headache, CNS and respiratory depression (somnolence to coma), Cheyne-Stokes respiration, areflexia, shock, miosis, oliguria, tachycardia, hypotension, hypothermia	Emesis or lavage, activated charcoal, saline cathartics; supportive treatment, including maintaining airway and respiration and treating shock as needed; maintain vital signs and fluid balance; alkalinizing the urine increases excretion; forced diuresis if renal function is normal; hemodialysis in severe cases
Benzodiazepines	Toxic dose: diazepam 2 g, chlordiazepoxide 6 g	CNS depression ranging from drowsiness to coma, slurred speech, ataxia, confusion, hyporeflexia, hypotension, hypotonia	Emesis or lavage, saline cathartic and activated charcoal; supportive care, monitor vital signs, maintain airway; i.v. fluids and norepinephrine for hypotension; the benzodiazepine antagonist flumazenil can be used with caution and only in hospitalized patients
Bromocriptine	Survival after 225 mg; 1 death of unknown dosage	Severe hypotension, nausea, vomiting, psychosis	Lavage and aspiration; i.v. fluids for hypotension
Bupropion	Survival after 0.85–4.2 g; deaths reported in massive overdoses	Seizures, loss of consciousness, hallucinations, tachycardia	Lavage and activated charcoal, emesis not recommended; supportive care, maintain airway and respiration, EEG, ECG, and vital signs monitoring for 48 hours, provide fluids; i.v. benzodiazepines for seizures
Buspirone	Toxicity at 375 mg; fatal dose unknown	Dizziness, drowsiness, nausea, vomiting, miosis, gastric distress	Emesis or lavage; symptomatic and supportive care, monitor vital signs
Calcium channel inhibitors	10.8 g diltiazem and 9 g of nifedipine has been survived; 9.6 g verapamil—fatal	Confusion, headache, nausea, vomiting, seizures, flushing, constipation, hyperglycemia, metabolic acidosis, hypotension, bradycardia, AV block, cardiac failure, arrhythmias, noncardiogenic pulmonary edema with verapamil	Emesis or lavage, activated charcoal; supportive care, monitor for cardiovascular and respiratory function, observation for at least 48 hours; i.v. calcium chloride 10–20 mg/kg in 10% solution with normal saline over 30 min and repeated as needed: atropine or isoproterenol for bradycardia or AV block, a pacemaker may be needed; inotropes and diuretics for cardiac failure, CPR for asystole; fluid and vasopressors for hypotension

Drug	Overdose data	Signs and symptoms	Treatment
Carbamazepine	30 g in adults and 10 g in children have been survived; lethal doses of 3.2 g in adults and 1.6 g in children reported	Drowsiness, coma, seizures, dizziness, ataxia, agitation, tremor, athetoid movements, opisthotonos, ballism, abnormal reflexes, adiadochokinesis, nystagmus, mydriasis, nausea, vomiting, flushing, cyanosis, urinary retention, hypo/hypertension, arrhythmias, tachycardia, shock, respiratory depression	Emesis or lavage, activated charcoal and laxatives; supportive care, respiratory support; monitor vital signs, ECG, kidney function, and pupillary reflexes; forced diuresis, dialysis in severe poisoning with renal failure; i.v. fluids and vasopressors for hypotension; diazepam for seizures
Chloral hydrate	30 g has been survived; lethal dose of 10 g reported	Coma, confusion, drowsiness, miosis, respiratory depression, hypotension, hypothermia, vomiting, gastric necrosis and perforation, esophageal stricture, hepatic and renal injury	Lavage: supportive care, maintain airway, cardiorespiratory function, and body temperature; hemodialysis or peritoneal dialysis may be of use; saline enema if drug was administered rectally
Clonidine	100 mg has been survived, 0.1 mg toxic in children; no deaths with clonidine alone, 2 deaths from mixed overdoses	Hypertension (followed by hypotension), bradycardia, arrhythmia, cardiac conduction defects, respiratory depression, apnea, hyporeflexia or areflexia, seizures, miosis, weakness, irritability, sedation, coma, hypothermia	Lavage, activated charcoal, and a saline cathartic, emesis not recommended; supportive treatment, maintain airway and respiration; i.v. furosemide, β-adrenergic receptor antagonists, or diazoxide for hypertension; i.v. fluids, vasopressors, and Trendelenburg's position for hypotension; i.v. atropine for symptomatic bradycardia; naloxone for respiratory depression, hypotension, and coma; i.v. benzodiazepines for seizures
Clozapine	>4 g has been survived; lethal dose >2.5 g	Delirium, drowsiness, coma, respiratory depression, tachycardia, arrhythmias, hypotension, hypersalivation, seizures	Activated charcoal with sorbitol (may be as or more effective than lavage or emesis); supportive and symptomatic treatment, maintain airway and respiration; cardiac and vital signs monitoring; epinephrine, quinidine, and procainamide are to be avoided; patient should be observed for several days for delayed effects
Dantrolene	No overdose data available	Muscular weakness, lethargy, coma, crystalluria, diarrhea	Lavage; supportive care, maintain airway and respiration, careful observation of patient; ECG monitoring; large quantities of i.v. fluids to avert crystalluria
Disulfiram	≥6 deaths with 0.5–1 g disulfiram with BAL of 1 mg/mL; 30 g ingestion produces serious toxicity	Headache, peripheral or optic neuropathy, psychotic behavior, mucous membrane injury, rash, respiratory depression, cardiovascular collapse, arrhythmias, myocardial infarction, acute CHF, unconsciousness, convulsions, death	Lavage; supportive care; restore blood pressure and treat shock; monitor potassium levels; maintain airway and respiration; i.v. antihistamines, vitamin C, and ephedrine sulfate may be of benefit
Dopamine receptor antagonists	Chlorpromazine: 26 g adult fatality, 0.35 g child fatality; thiothixene: 2.5–4 g fatal; phenothiazines: 1.05–10.5 g fatal	CNS depression from somnolence to coma, extrapyramidal symptoms, agitation, restlessness, convulsions, fever, dry mouth, ileus, hypotension, tachycardia, arrhythmias, ECG changes (prolonged QT interval and wide QRS complexes with risperdal)	Lavage, saline cathartic, activated charcoal: emesis is not recommended; symptomatic and supportive care, monitor vital signs and ECG; maintain airway and respiration; i.v. fluids and norepinephrine or phenylephrine for hypotension, avoid dopamine and epinephrine; antiparkinsonism drugs, anticholinergics, and diphenhydramine (Benadryl) may be useful for extrapyramidal symptoms; stimulants such as amphetamines or caffeine with sodium benzoate if desired,

continues

TABLE 43-1—continued

Drug	Toxic/Lethal Dose	Signs and Symptoms	Treatment
			avoid picrotoxin and pentylenetetrazol; antiarrhythmics such as neostigmine, pyridostigmine, and propranolol, disopyramide, procainamide, and quinidine should be avoided; diazepam for convulsions
Ethchlorvynol	50–100 g has been survived; 6 g lethal	Hypotension, hypothermia, severe respiratory depression, apnea, prolonged coma (can last days to weeks), areflexia, mydriasis, bradycardia, nystagmus, pancytopenia	Lavage: supportive treatment; maintain airway and respiration, maintain cardiorespiratory function and body temperature; monitor blood gases and vital signs; hemoperfusion using Amberlite column technique hastens drug elimination; hemodialysis, peritoneal dialysis, or forced diuresis may be useful in increasing urinary output
Fluoxetine	3 g has been survived; lethal dose unknown, 2 deaths in combination with other drugs	Nausea, vomiting, CNS excitation, restlessness, agitation, hypomania, tachycardia, hypertension, seizures	Lavage and activated charcoal, emesis not recommended; supportive and symptomatic care; maintain airway and respiration; monitor ECG and vital signs; i.v. diazepam for ongoing seizures
Fluvoxamine	10 g has been survived; 2 deaths of unknown dosages solely due to fluvoxamine	Drowsiness, vomiting, diarrhea, dizziness, coma, tachycardia, bradycardia, hypotension, ECG abnormalities, liver function abnormalities, convulsions	Lavage and activated charcoal; supportive care; maintain airway and respiration; monitor ECG and vital signs
Glutethimide	5 g severe intoxication, but survived; 10–20 g fatal	Hypotension, prolonged coma, shock, respiratory depression, hypothermia, fever, inadequate ventilation, apnea, cyanosis, fixed and dilated pupils, ileus, bladder atony, dry mouth, hyporeflexia, areflexia, intermittent spasticity or flaccidity	Lavage using 1 to 1 mixture of castor oil and water may be more effective than aqueous lavage, leave 50 mL castor oil in stomach as a cathartic, activated charcoal; maintain airway and cardiorespiratory function; hemodialysis with activated charcoal or soybean dialysate; hemoperfusion with Amberlite XAD-2 resin; charcoal hemoperfusion; continue drug removal for at least 2 hours after the patient regains consciousness; maintain urinary output but avoid overhydration
Levodopa	≥8 a day causes toxicity	Palpitations, arrhythmias, spasm or closing of eyes, psychosis	Lavage; supportive and symptomatic treatment; maintain airway; ECG monitoring; i.v. fluids; treat arrhythmias as necessary
Lithium	Lethal dose produces serum levels >3.5 mEq/L 12 hours after ingestion	Diarrhea, nausea, vomiting, drowsiness, tremor, muscle weakness, giddiness, ataxia, vertical nystagmus, tinnitus, diabetes insipidus, multiorgan toxicity	Emesis or lavage: infuse 0.9% sodium chloride i.v. if toxicity is due to sodium depletion; hemodialysis for 8–12 hours if fluid and electrolyte imbalance does not respond to supportive measures; repeated courses of dialysis are needed if level > 3 mEq/L or if level is 2–3 mEq/L and patient is deteriorating, or if level has not decreased 20% in 6 hours; goal is level < 1

meq/L 6 hours after dialysis is completed; ured, mannitol, and aminophylline increase lithium excretion

Meprobamate	40 g has been survived; 12 g lethal	Stupor, drowsiness, lethargy, ataxia, coma, respiratory depression, hypotension, shock	Emesis or lavage and activated charcoal; supportive care; maintain airway, respiration, and blood pressure; pressor agents if necessary; CNS stimulants; elimination may be enhanced by forced diuresis, hemodialysis, peritoneal dialysis, or osmotic diuresis; monitor urine output
Methadone	40–60 mg lethal in nontolerant persons	CNS depression (stupor to coma), pinpoint pupils, cold and clammy skin, bradycardia, hypotension, shock, respiratory depression, cardiac arrest, cyanosis, apnea, skeletal muscle flaccidity, Cheyne-Stokes respiration	Lavage; supportive care; i.v. fluids and vasopressors; maintain airway and respiration; i.v. naloxone to treat clinically significant respiratory or cardiovascular depression, monitor continuously for recurrence of respiratory depression, treat repeatedly with naloxone until patient's status is stable (initial adult dose of naloxone is 0.4–2 mg IV every 2–3 minutes)
Methylphenidate	2 g	Delirium, confusion, agitation, hallucinations, hyperpyrexia, mydriasis, tremors, muscle twitching, seizures, coma, hyperreflexia, euphoria, headache, palpitations, tachycardia, arrhythmias, hypertension, vomiting, sweating, flushing, dry mucous membranes	Lavage, activated charcoal, and cathartics; in severe toxicity use a carefully titrated dose of short-acting barbiturate before lavage; supportive care; maintain respiratory and circulatory function; isolation to reduce external stimuli; protection against self-harm; external cooling procedures for hyperpyrexia
Mirtazapine	No deaths reported solely due to mirtazapine	Disorientation, drowsiness, impaired memory, tachycardia	Emesis or lavage and activated charcoal; supportive care; monitor cardiac and vital signs, maintain airway and respiration
Monoamine oxidase inhibitors (MAOIs)	600 mg severe toxicity; single doses of 1.75–7 g fatal	Dizziness, drowsiness, irritability, insomnia, headache, confusion, hyperactivity, agitation, anxiety, hallucinations, trismus, opisthotonus, rigidity, convulsions, coma, hypertensive crisis (mainly seen in conjunction with tyramine), tachycardia, hypotension, arrhythmia, diaphoresis, chest pain, shock, hypertension, respiratory depression, faintness, hyperpyrexia	Emesis or lavage and activated charcoal; symptomatic and supportive care; maintain airway and respiration; monitor vital signs; maintain fluid and electrolyte balance; treat hypotension and shock with i.v. fluids and vasopressors (adrenergics may produce a markedly increased pressor response, therefore administer carefully); i.v. diazepam for convulsions; phenothiazine derivatives and CNS stimulants should be avoided; manage hyperpyrexia intensively with external cooling; hypertensive crisis: discontinue MAOIs and treat with 5 mg i.v. phentolamine by slow injection; toxic effects may be delayed therefore observe patient for at least 1 week; never use meperidine (Demerol)
Naltrexone	≥1000 mg/kg toxic	Salivation, depression, convulsions, tremors, reduced activity	Supportive care and symptomatic treatment
Nefazodone	1–11.2 g toxicity; death reported in combination with alcohol	Nausea, vomiting, somnolence	Lavage (emesis is not recommended); supportive care; maintain airway and respiration; monitor ECG and vital signs

continues

TABLE 43-1—continued

Drug	Toxic/Lethal Dose	Signs and Symptoms	Treatment
Olanzapine	300 mg has been survived	Drowsiness, slurred speech, shock	Lavage, activated charcoal, and laxatives (emesis not recommended); maintain airway and respiration; continuous cardiovascular and ECG monitoring; i.v. fluids and vasopressors for hypotension and shock; avoid beta agonists; avoid epinephrine and dopamine in the presence of α-adrenergic blockade
Paroxetine	2 g has been survived	Nausea, vomiting, sedation, dizziness, sweating, facial flush	Lavage and activated charcoal (emesis not recommended); maintain airway and respiration; monitor ECG and vital signs
Pemoline	2 g	Agitation, euphoria, delirium, hallucinations, tremors, hyperreflexia, convulsions, coma, headache, mydriasis, flushing, hyperpyrexia, vomiting, hypertension, tachycardia; hepatic effects not due to overdose	Lavage, activated charcoal, and cathartic; symptomatic treatment; chlorpromazine to decrease CNS stimulation and sympathomimetic effects; protect against self-injury and external stimuli that would aggravate overstimulation
Risperidone	20–300 mg has been survived	Drowsiness, sedation, tachycardia, hypotension, extrapyramidal symptoms, hyponatremia, hypokalemia, prolonged QT interval, widened QRS complex conversions	Establish and maintain airway; gastric lavage; activated charcoal; continuous cardiovascular monitoring; disopyramide, procainamide, and quinidine should be avoided in the presence of arrhythmias; fluid management of hypotension; avoid epinephrine and dopamine in the presence of α-adrenergic receptor blockade; anticholinergics for extrapyramidal symptoms
Sertraline	0.5–6 g toxicity; no deaths with sertraline alone, 4 deaths in combination with other drugs and alcohol	Somnolence, nausea, vomiting, tachycardia, ECG changes, anxiety, mydriasis	Lavage, charcoal, and cathartics; supportive care; maintain airway and respiration; monitor vital signs and cardiac function; hydration
Tacrine	2 g toxic	Cholinergic crisis: nausea, vomiting, salivation, perspiration, bradycardia, hypotension, collapse, convulsions, increasing muscle weakness (death if respiratory muscles involved)	Supportive care; tertiary anticholinergics such as i.v. atropine titrated to effect. Initial dose 1–2 mg in adults, 0.05 mg/kg in children, subsequent dosing every 10–30 minutes
Thyroid hormones	0.3 g/kg desiccated thyroid—severe toxicity	Thyrotoxicosis: nervousness, sweating, palpitations, abdominal cramps, diarrhea, tachycardia, hypertension, headache, arrhythmias, tremors, cardiac failure, angina, insomnia, increased appetite, weight loss, heat intolerance, fever, menstrual irregularities	Emesis or lavage, charcoal and cholestyramine to interfere with thyroxine absorption; supportive care; control fluid loss, fever, hypoglycemia; maintain airway and respiration; β-adrenergic receptor antagonists such as propranolol (1–3 mg i.v. over 10 minutes) can be used to counteract increased sympathetic activity

Drug	Toxicity/dose	Symptoms	Treatment
Trazodone	7.5–9.2 g has been survived	Lethargy, vomiting, drowsiness, headache, orthostasis, dizziness, dyspnea, tinnitus, myalgias, tachycardia, incontinence, shivering, coma	Emesis or lavage; supportive care; forced diuresis may enhance elimination; treat hypotension and sedation as appropriate
Tricyclics and tetracyclics	0.7–1.4 g: toxicity; 2.1–2.8 g: fatal; amitriptyline: 10 g has been survived, 0.5 g lowest known fatality; imipramine: 0.5 g fatal (30 mg/kg average lethal dose)	Initial CNS stimulation, confusion, agitation, hallucinations, hyperpyrexia, nystagmus, hyperreflexia, parkinsonian symptoms, mydriasis, seizures, CNS stimulation followed by depression, hypothermia, respiratory depression, hypotension, coma, arrhythmias, QRS prolongation (degree indicates severity of the overdose), impaired cardiac contractility, vomiting, polyradiculoneuropathy, stupor, drowsiness	Lavage and activated charcoal, emesis is not recommended; symptomatic and supportive care; monitor ECG and vital signs; maintain airway and respiration; minimum of 6 hours observation with cardiac monitoring; i.v. diazepam for seizures; i.v. sodium bicarbonate to maintain pH of 7.45–7.55 to help treat arrhythmias, hyperventilation and/or antiarrhythmics such as lidocaine may be needed, type 1A and 1C antiarrhythmics contraindicated; physostigmine not recommended except for life-threatening treatment-refractory anticholinergic toxicity and then only in consultation with poison control center
Valproic acid	36 g has been survived, patients with blood levels of 2120 µg/mL have survived; fatalities of unknown dose reported	Somnolence, coma, heart block	Value of emesis or lavage varies with time since the drug has rapid absorption; supportive measures; maintain adequate urinary output; naloxone may reverse CNS depressant effects of overdose but may also reverse anticonvulsant effects and should be used with caution
Venlafaxine	6.75 g has been survived; fatalities reported in combination with other drugs and alcohol	Somnolence, convulsions, prolonged QT interval, mild sinus tachycardia	Lavage and activated charcoal, emesis not recommended; supportive and symptomatic care; maintain airway and respiration; monitor vital signs and cardiac rhythm

*The clinician should always consult *Physicians Desk Reference* (PDR) or contact the manufacturer of the drug for the latest information on toxicity and lethality.

Index

Page numbers followed by an *f* denote figures; those followed by a *t* denote tables.

A

Absorption of drugs, 2
  in elderly, 24*t*
Abuse of drugs
  potential, DEA schedule on, 7
  urine screen for, 279, 279*t*
Acebutolol, 35–41
  dosage guidelines on, 37*t*, 40
  molecular structure of, 36*f*
Acetaminophen
  with barbiturates in combination products, 59*t*
  in hyperthermia, drug-induced, 302*t*
Acetazolamide, interaction with lithium, 144*t*
Acetophenazine, 113–134
  dosage and potency of, 114*t*
  preparations of, 131*t*
Adalat. *See* Nifedipine
Adapin. *See* Doxepin
Adderall. *See* Amphetamines, with
    dextroamphetamine
Adipex-P. *See* Phentermine
Adipost. *See* Phendimetrazine
α_2-Adrenergic receptor agonists, 29–34
  adverse effects of, 32–34
  in children, 31, 33*t*
  dosage guidelines on, 33*t*, 34
  indications for, 29–32
  molecular structure of, 30*f*
β-Adrenergic receptor antagonists, 35–41
  adverse effects of, 39, 40*t*
  dosage guidelines on, 37*t*, 40–41
  indications for, 35–39, 36*t*
  interaction with other drugs, 39–40, 57*t*, 128*t*
  molecular structure of, 36*f*
  in movement disorders, 301*t*
    in lithium-induced tremor, 38, 139
  toxic levels of, 305*t*
Adverse effects of drugs, 8*t*, 8–13, 9*t*
  in children, 23*t*
  in drug-drug interactions, 13–14
  in elderly, 24
  history-taking on, 15
  hyperthermic syndromes in, 302*t*, 303
  movement disorders in, 295–303. *See also*
    Movement disorders, drug-induced
  in overdose. *See* Overdose of drugs
  treatment of, 9–12
  withdrawal symptoms in, 13. *See also*
    Withdrawal symptoms
Aggressive behavior
  α_2-adrenergic receptor agonists in, 31
  β-adrenergic receptor antagonists in, 38
  buspirone in, 80, 81
  carbamazepine in, 88, 89

dopamine receptor antagonists in, 117
lithium in, 135, 137
serotonin-dopamine antagonists in, 208
valproate in, 254
Agitation, 10
  carbamazepine in, 88, 89
  dopamine receptor antagonists in, 117
  from selective serotonin reuptake inhibitors, 10,
    189
  serotonin-dopamine antagonists in, 207
  trazodone in, 238
  valproate in, 252, 254
Agoraphobia and panic disorder, tricyclic and
    tetracyclic antidepressants in, 243
Agranulocytosis
  from serotonin-dopamine antagonists, 211, 217,
    218
  treatment of, 274*t*
Akathisia, 10, 296*t*, 303
  β-adrenergic receptor antagonists in, 38
  anticholinergic drugs in, 46, 48, 303
  antihistamines in, 50
  benzodiazepines in, 69
  from dopamine receptor antagonists, 123
  from serotonin-dopamine antagonists, 212, 213
  symptoms in, 303
Akinesia, dopamine receptor agonists and
    precursors in, 108, 110
Akineton. *See* Biperiden
Alcohol dependence and withdrawal
  α_2-adrenergic receptor agonists in, 29
  β-adrenergic receptor antagonists in, 38
  benzodiazepines in, 69
  carbamazepine in, 89
  disulfiram in, 105–107
  gabapentin in, 180
  naltrexone in, 158, 161, 163
  valproate in, 254
Alcohol interaction with antipsychotic drugs, 128*t*
Allegra. *See* Fexofenadine
Allergic reactions
  to dopamine receptor antagonists, 121
  to selective serotonin reuptake inhibitors,
    197–198
  to tricyclic and tetracyclic antidepressants, 247
Alprazolam, 63–74
  in children, 21*t*
  dosage and half-life of, 67*t*
  in elderly, 25*t*
  molecular structure of, 64*f*
Alurate. *See* Aprobarbital
Alzheimer's disease
  cholinesterase inhibitors in, 98, 99–100, 101
  dopamine receptor antagonists in, 117
Amantadine, 42–44